Artificial Intelligence in Public Health

Min Wu

Artificial Intelligence in Public Health

Springer

Min Wu
Zilber College of Public Health
University of Wisconsin-Milwaukee
Milwaukee, WI, USA

ISBN 978-3-032-15871-0 ISBN 978-3-032-15872-7 (eBook)
https://doi.org/10.1007/978-3-032-15872-7

This Springer imprint is published by the registered company Springer Nature Switzerland AG
The registered company address is: Gewerbestrasse 11, 6330 Cham, Switzerland

Preface

Artificial intelligence (AI) is a hot new "tool" and is a fast-moving field. AI researchers from all over the world release new models every month. There is a massive need for education on AI in all fields, including the growing role of AI in public health. There is an increasing demand for AI literacy, particularly in public health. This AI book will add value, given the focus on public health.

This book has the potential to make an original contribution to the field of public health informatics, particularly in how it addresses the intersection of AI and public health from both a pedagogical and practical perspective. Its emphasis on design principles, design models, evaluation frameworks, and case studies (combined with its AI approach to public health practices) sets it apart from existing literature. Given the fast pace of advancements in AI, significant elements of the book, such as its focus on design and evaluation models and pedagogy (e.g., ready-to-use "meta-AI homework" and grading rubric), will likely give it more lasting relevance.

To design AI in public health, I started with a concept-based approach that AI mirrors human cognitive processes. This approach inspired non-technological readers (e.g., public health students) to conceptually design AI applications in public health (e.g., break down complexity or spot innovation gaps). Following the technology-based AI approaches, AI's "non-human (or superman) strengths" were introduced, and alternatives were provided for further design and implementation of AI applications in public health. "Encoding justice" is the only design principle in this textbook. As a professor of health informatics for over twenty years, I've seen that core concepts remain valuable even as technology rapidly evolves. I've developed conceptual frameworks such as EquiRisk, PMCO-AI, PAPO, and ATPM to show how AI can strengthen public health practice.

The idea of AI in public health is timely. This book is needed as few AI books are dedicated to public health. This book is written for students and faculty at all levels, public health practitioners, and policymakers. As AI continues to grow more powerful, courses related to AI in public health have the potential to become a core component of the curriculum in undergraduate and graduate public health degree programs. This textbook would be used for advanced courses (e.g., AI applications in public health) or entry-level courses (e.g., Introduction to AI literacy for public health). In this textbook, "meta-AI homework" is defined and prepared for students to practices.

After reading this textbook, you will understand different AI definitions and learn to move beyond seeing AI as just a new "tool" to treat it as a "thinking partner". My hope is that some of you will be inspired to design or evaluate AI applications in public health in the future.

Finally, I thank my family for their love and support: my wife, Qun Tang, and my twin boys, Edwin and Melvin Wu.

Milwaukee, WI, USA Min Wu

Competing Interests The author has no competing interests to declare that are relevant to the content of this manuscript.

Contents

Part VI Future

About the Author

Min Wu has held a Ph.D. in medical informatics from the University of North Carolina at Chapel Hill since 2003. Now an associate professor in the Zilber College of Public Health at the University of Wisconsin, Milwaukee, his research focuses on identifying unmet public health needs and implementing technological solutions. His writing has appeared in the *Journal of Medical Informatics*, the *Journal of Medical Systems*, and *Academic Radiology*. Dr. Wu is a past recipient of the Best Article Award for his work in the *Journal of Digital Imaging*. Dr. Wu has taught health informatics graduate courses for over 20 years and gained a deep and broad understanding of biomedical informatics. Recently, Dr. Wu published review articles on "Big data application on biomedical research and Health care" and "Wearable technology application in Health care" and closely tracks AI's impact on public health issues to prevent disease, promote health and prolong life.

About the Author

List of Figures

List of Tables

Part I
Introduction

Chapter 1
Introduction

1.1 What is AI?

What is artificial intelligence (AI)? Below are technical, role-based, concept-based, and ethical-based definitions of AI.

Technical-based AI Definition

A technical-based AI definition helps you understand how AI works. Suppose you are a developer, engineer, or researcher focusing on building and improving AI applications. In that case, you should know the specific technologies you need to master or innovate upon. For example, suppose you plan to be a robot engineer who fixes robots as a job in the future. In that case, you should know the technical-based AI definition. You will be clarified about what AI can and cannot do based on current technological capabilities and limitations.

Some literature about AI definitions from technology perspectives (Liu et al., 2021) (Davenport et al., 2019) will provide background information for you to understand what AI is. Let me define AI from a technology perspective as below:

> **Technical-based AI definition:** "AI is a field of computer science and uses technologies like neural networks, machine learning, deep learning, transformer models, natural language processing (NLP), computer vision, reinforcement learning, and robotics to replicate or augment human cognitive functions."

The technical-based AI definition identifies key technologies of AI applications, so it'll be helpful for you to track and assess new technological advancements and breakthroughs in AI. For example, you will understand new developments in transformer models (e.g., Generative Pre-trained Transformer (GPT)) directly influence AI capabilities. If you want to become a developer of AI applications, now you know what you need to get started learning in Chapter 2.

M. Wu, *Artificial Intelligence in Public Health*,
https://doi.org/10.1007/978-3-032-15872-7_1

Role-based AI Definition

The role-based AI definition will be used to communicate with general AI application users and the public. It helps you understand how AI affects the world and results it produces.

Some literature about AI definitions from role perspectives (Mishra et al., 2023) (Huang et al., 2021) will provide background information for you to understand what AI is. Let me define AI from a role perspective as below:

> **Role-based AI definition:** "AI is a field of computer science that designs systems to amplify human problem-solving, created by builders and guided by bridges, to perform reasoning, prediction, or action at scale."

In short, technologists are builders, and domain experts are bridges. From the builder's perspective, AI is a system of algorithms and data structures that can perform tasks requiring pattern recognition, learning from experience, and decision-making. From the bridge's perspective, AI is *a thinking partner* that helps humans analyze complexity, test options, and accelerate insight. AI still needs human values, context, and interpretation.

Public health informatics students and more public health experts will become the bridges (human-AI integrators). They should understand the public health problem deeply, know how to work with AI tools, and translate human needs into machine capabilities.

Concept-based AI Definition

Based on Merriam-Webster dictionary, "Intelligence" is "*the act of* ***understanding,***" and "Artificial" is "*made, produced, or done by humans especially to seem like something natural*" (Merriam-Webster, 2025).

Some literature about AI definitions from conceptual perspectives (Stead, 2018) (Maddox et al., 2019) will provide background information for you to understand what AI is. Let me define AI from a conceptual perspective as below:

> **Concept-based AI definition:** "AI is a field of computer science that develops systems capable of simulating or mimicking human cognitive functions to understand the world."

Human cognitive function (HCF) abstraction is a powerful way to explore AI applications, especially for complex tasks. Chapter 3 will further discuss their features in concept-based design models. It breaks down the complex and spots innovation gaps. Focusing on insight and creativity, this approach inspires non-technical readers to conceptualize AI applications. The limitations of this definition are obvious. This is a human-centered approach. You should know technology-based AI definitions, which show AI's "non-human (or superman) strengths" (e.g., massively parallel processing), and AI does not only mimic human cognitive functions. AI's non-human functions are most powerful and potentially most dangerous.

Ethical-based AI definition

AI safety (AI operates beyond human understanding) and alignment (how do you align a system that thinks differently?) are central to those AI's non-human strengths. Chapter 3 will further discuss their features in technology-based design models (mainly non-human functions). An ethics-based AI definition is needed for us to address those issues. Let me define AI from an ethical perspective as below:

> **Ethical-based AI definition:** "AI is a field of computer science that develops systems to achieve human-intended goals while aligning with moral values, legal standards, societal expectations, and ensuring safety through the prevention of unintended behaviors, misuse, or harm."

AI Hallucination

The AI hallucination is an elephant in the room. This is a new type of cognitive overload for us: making judges contend with AI-generated hallucinations daily. Living in the AI era, we have no choice but to face it. Let me define it first.

> **AI hallucination:** AI generates false or fabricated information.

For example, your prompt for a generative AI (e.g., chatbots) is "*Give me peer-reviewed studies about meta-AI homework in 2025. Citation in RIS (Research Information Systems) format.*" AI quickly provides some citations. When you try to retrieve full articles based on AI references, you find that AI invents (fabricates) author names, journal titles, and URLs (Uniform Resource Locators). They are all fake information.

Why? What Happened?

Firstly, "meta-AI homework" is a recent topic that has limited training data. The "meta-AI homework" topic emerged after the AI's knowledge cutoff or has sparse coverage. Secondly, AI doesn't have direct access to the literature archive database. Requests for citations are beyond AI's reach. AI does not know the answers, but the AI model insists on answering them, filling the gaps by inventing fake or irrelevant information.

For another example, your prompt for a generative AI (e.g., chatbots) is "*Analyze the correlation between national green tea consumption and bicycle accident rates. Show your work and conclude if green tea causes bicycle accidents.*" AI quickly provides its answers, which are not "I don't know."

Why? What Happened?

Besides data issues, there are issues with evaluation metrics for AI models. AI prioritizes helpfulness (fulfilling users' prompts) over the truth. A SAT (Scholastic

Aptitude Test) score is essential for high school students admitted to college. MMLU (Massive Multitask Language Understanding) score is significant for AI models. MMLU is a standardized test for AI models, and there is no penalty for incorrect answers. The early SAT tests do not penalize students for guessing incorrectly. Now, the SAT test has been reformed and deducts 0.25 points for a wrong answer. The current MMLU score setting is an incentive for AI models' guessing, so we do not get honest answers: "I don't know," instead of a low probability guess (incorrect answers).

1.2 Why do we use AI in Public Health?

We have some AI definitions in the previous section. Let's find out what public health is. My understanding of public health is "*to prevent diseases, live longer, and live better through organized efforts of societies.*"

Big Data in Public Health

The key factors that reduce AI hallucinations are having high-quality data (e.g., structured data in databases or spreadsheets), frequent updates, standardized terminology, and verifiable sources (e.g., peer-reviewed papers). The good news for AI in public health is that public health does have high-quality datasets (e.g., meaningful use of EHRs (Electronic Health Records), WHO (World Health Organization), and CDC (Center of Disease Control and Prevention)), peer-reviewed studies, and real-time surveillance. Compared with other fields, such as politics (opinion-based), AI ethics (too new), and ancient history (too old), AI in public health has great potential to succeed with fewer AI hallucinations.

More than eight billion people live on the earth (United Nations Population, 2025). Public health targets the entire population and has big data for population-level health issues. As a part of data-driven (evidence-based) approaches in public health, traditionally, biostatistics in public health handles big data. Biostatistics uses predictive modeling, statistical analysis, and epidemiological modeling to predict disease spread, assess health risks in populations, and evaluate the effectiveness of public health interventions. Public health workers also focus on behavioral modeling to understand community health habits and risks (e.g., modeling smoking rates and exercise levels). AI naturally upgraded those statistical analyses of a community's health and can provide more efficient and reliable ways to diagnose community health. AI relies on data to train models, make predictions, and solve problems. AI could help to identify health trends, track diseases, and design interventions.

Public health data are aggregated from various disciplines, such as demographic information, epidemiology data, health surveys, environmental factors (air quality, access to healthcare), and social factors (e.g., income, education, housing conditions). Another promising field is bioinformatics, which can be integrated with public health informatics. Suppose we have human genome sequences for all eight billion people on earth. In that case, our humans can live longer based on new genetic knowledge (such as genetic marks or profiles) through organized society efforts. We will discuss big data in public health in Chapters 5 and 6 in detail.

Complex Problems in Public Health

Public health applies everywhere, including industrial and occupational health, substance misuse, sanitation, environmental factors (climate changes), etc. Public health aims at population health management and health outcomes at a societal level. Public health informatics aims to identify unmet needs in public health and implement IT/AI as a part of their solutions. Public health is interdisciplinary and integrates epidemiology, social sciences, policymaking, and medicine. We need many organized efforts to solve public health problems, such as policy, education, and community-level interventions. AI aims to solve complex problems across industries. For example, AI can help build consensus among all partners and integrate workflow. AI can optimize frameworks (who to target, when to screen/treat, etc.). Public health issues, such as obesity and healthy eating, are deeply intertwined with sociological and behavioral factors.

Uncertainty in Public Health

Public health information inherently carries a lot of uncertainty (Hancock et al., 2019)(Han et al., 2011). Public health relies on statistical modeling, surveys, and clinical trials, all with limitations and biases. Many health outcomes are multi-causal, making it difficult to establish absolute truths. There are complex causal relationships in public health. Usually, we use probability to describe uncertainty. Public health relies heavily on probability, statistics, and predictive models, which are inherently uncertain. For example (confounding variables), lifestyle, genetics, environment, and healthcare access affect outcomes, making it difficult to control all variables. Public health is not just scientific; it is also political and ethical, leading to uncertainty in policy decisions. Due to evolving science, data limitations, and ethical considerations, uncertainty is fundamental to public health. Current new AI models are data-driven and statistics-based. Uncertainty is also a fundamental characteristic of data-driven AI models (Sáez et al., 2024) because these models rely on probabilities and approximations rather than absolute certainty. User acceptance of AI applications in public health could be better than in other fields, based on the tolerance of uncertainty in public health. The urgency of health issues may also reduce hesitancy toward AI solutions (Benda et al., 2024). AI tools can help public health practitioners quantify and predict uncertainty, handle incomplete or noisy public health data, and reduce decision-making biases.

Ethical Considerations of Public Health

Public health involves service for all citizens instead of patients, including most people at the bottom of the economic pyramid. Public service areas, such as transportation, often have a low-profit margin for private companies' participation, so the government should play a vital role in those areas, such as public health. Baby boomers in the US are retiring and need more public health services (long-term care) to live longer. Public health grapples with issues like equity, resource allocation, and informed consent. Public health analyzes patterns of health inequities and recommends policies or actions to address health disparities.

Regulatory Oversight into Public Health

AI applications in public health may be guided by guidelines from public health organizations (e.g., WHO, CDC) or government health agencies. However, compared to medical AI applications, public health AI applications have less direct regulations (Edelstein et al., 2024). It provides more freedom for you to design and develop a new AI application in public health, such as AI applications involved in health surveillance, policy-making, and social interventions. Your AI application in public health may be subject to broader health regulations and policies. Still, it generally falls outside the more stringent medical device regulations. Suppose you design an AI application in medicine. In that case, it will be subject to strict regulatory oversight and approval processes from organizations, such as FDA (Food and Drug Administration).

1.3 The Organization of the Book Content

This book's content spans a wide range of essential topics in six parts, from an overview of AI fundamentals and AI application modeling to data acquisition, algorithm development, user acceptance, workforce, and future challenges. The various AI definitions are provided in Chapter 1. There is a brief introduction of key AI components in Chapter 2. Design models for AI applications in public health are proposed in Chapter 3. The emphasis on evaluating AI applications in public health is an essential aspect of the book in Chapter 4. Few resources in this area provide in-depth discussions on how to systematically assess the effectiveness and impact of AI tools in real-world public health settings. AI heavily depends on data. Data issues and domain data in public health are summarized in Chapters 5 and 6 from an AI pipeline perspective. A wide range of AI applications in public health are explored, including many case scenarios in Chapters 7 and 8. Use acceptance for AI is discussed in Chapter 9. The relationships between AI and the public health workforce are presented in Chapter 10. Finally, this book identifies a list of challenges and opportunities of AI in public health in the future in Chapter 11.

The textbook has didactic elements that enhance learning, such as discussion questions and case studies. A large project will require you to develop a sequence of questions for AI tools during the thinking process. The meta-AI homework project sample, development framework, and grading rubric have been designed for teachers (see Appendix). They will provide hands-on exercises or opportunities for students to engage directly with AI. These projects aim to develop subject matter understanding and AI literacy by guiding students to reflect on how they use AI, why they use it, and what they learn from it. This innovative approach combines AI education, metacognitive learning, and public health. It shifts homework from outcome-based to process-oriented.

1.4 Discussion Questions

Question 1.1. How do different ways of defining AI (technical-based, role-based, concept-based, ethical-based) shape how we understand its applications in public health?

Question 1.2. How would you explain "AI" to a public health professional with no technical background? Why is it essential for future public health professionals to develop a clear and practical concept of AI before applying it?

Question 1.3. What does "AI hallucination" mean, and why is it imperative to address it in public health applications?

Question 1.4. What unique advantages does AI offer over traditional methods in addressing public health challenges (e.g., disease outbreaks, heatwaves)? Can you think of potential risks or limitations?

References

Benda, N. C., Desai, P., Reza, Z., Zheng, A., Kumar, S., Harkins, S., & Turchioe, M. R. (2024). *Patient Perspectives on AI for Mental Health Care*: Cross-Sectional Survey Study (Preprint). https://doi.org/10.2196/preprints.58462

Davenport, T. H., & Kalakota, R. (2019). The Potential for Artificial Intelligence in Healthcare. *Future Healthcare Journal, 6*(2), 94–98. https://doi.org/10.7861/futurehosp.6-2-94

Edelstein, M., & Haroz, E. E. (2024). Mapping Artificial Intelligence Governance for Public Health Applications. *Sais Review of International Affairs, 44*(2), 57–74. https://doi.org/10.1353/sais.2024.a950957

Han, P. K. J., Klein, W. M. P., & Arora, N. K. (2011). Varieties of Uncertainty in Health Care: A Conceptual Taxonomy. *Medical Decision Making, 31*(6), 828–838. https://doi.org/10.1177/0272989x11393976

Hancock, J., & Mattick, K. (2019). Tolerance of Ambiguity and Psychological Well-being in Medical Training: A Systematic Review. *Medical Education, 54*(2), 125–137. https://doi.org/10.1111/medu.14031

Huang, J., Saleh, S., & Liu, Y. (2021). A Review on Artificial Intelligence in Education. *Academic Journal of Interdisciplinary Studies, 10*(3), 206. https://doi.org/10.36941/ajis-2021-0077

Liu, N., Shapira, P., & Yue, X. (2021). Tracking Developments in Artificial Intelligence Research: Constructing and Applying a New Search Strategy. *Scientometrics, 126*(4), 3153–3192. https://doi.org/10.1007/s11192-021-03868-4

Maddox, T. M., Rumsfeld, J. S., & Payne, P. (2019). Questions for Artificial Intelligence in Health Care. *Jama, 321*(1), 31. https://doi.org/10.1001/jama.2018.18932

Merriam-Webster. (2025). Merriam-Webster Dictionary. https://www.merriam-webster.com/

Mishra, V., Ugemuge, S., & Tiwade, Y. (2023). Artificial Intelligence Changing the Future of Healthcare Diagnostics. *Journal of Cellular Biotechnology, 9*(2), 161–168. https://doi.org/10.3233/jcb-230118

Sáez, C., Ferri, P., & García-Gómez, J. M. (2024). Resilient Artificial Intelligence in Health: Synthesis and Research Agenda Toward Next-Generation Trustworthy Clinical Decision Support. *Journal of Medical Internet Research, 26*, e50295. https://doi.org/10.2196/50295

Stead, W. W. (2018). Clinical Implications and Challenges of Artificial Intelligence and Deep Learning. *Jama, 320*(11), 1107–1108. https://doi.org/10.1001/jama.2018.11029

United Nations Population. (2025). *World Population Prospects: 2024 Revision (Medium-Fertility Variant).* https://www.worldometers.info/world-population/

Chapter 2
AI Components

2.1 AI: Ecosystem

Artificial intelligence (AI) is considered an ecosystem that has many components in a multilayer structure (see Fig. 2.1). With society's massive demand for AI tools, huge investments have flowed into AI development.

At the bottom, you need a lot of electricity from energy companies to support your AI computing centers or data centers. In the future, we want to have more new energy sources. If your city is located near the ocean, you have the potential to develop "offshore wind power plants." If your town is close to deserts with a lot of sunshine, you can go for solar power plants. Suppose you live close to mountains, where those mountains collect and store large amounts of precipitation, providing a significant water source for surrounding areas. In that case, you can go for hydroelectric power plants. You may go for an underground energy source on earth (geothermal energy) or mini nuclear power plants if you have none. "Energy-rich" or "energy-constrained" regions will become new essential terms in the AI ecosystem. Hopefully, more societies recognize electricity and AI as shared lifelines, not just private assets.

The middle layer of AI ecosystems is hardware companies for computing power, which will design and develop computing and storage semiconductor chips for computer systems. Advanced computing infrastructures for AI are developed. AI growth depends on sufficient GPU (Graphics Processing Unit)/TPU (Tensor

---

Suppose you do not have a math or information technology (IT) background and are unfamiliar with AI, so some content in this chapter may be too complex for you. There is a risk of overwhelming you or oversimplifying AI key components. The balance between simplifying technical concepts and retaining sufficient depth could be challenging. AI is a fast-moving field, and AI researchers world-wide release new models every month. Given the fast pace of advancements in AI models, significant elements of Chapter 2 will likely have less lasting relevance when you read this book. The basic ideas behind those models will be focused on instead of the details of the AI model architecture.

M. Wu, *Artificial Intelligence in Public Health*,
https://doi.org/10.1007/978-3-032-15872-7_2

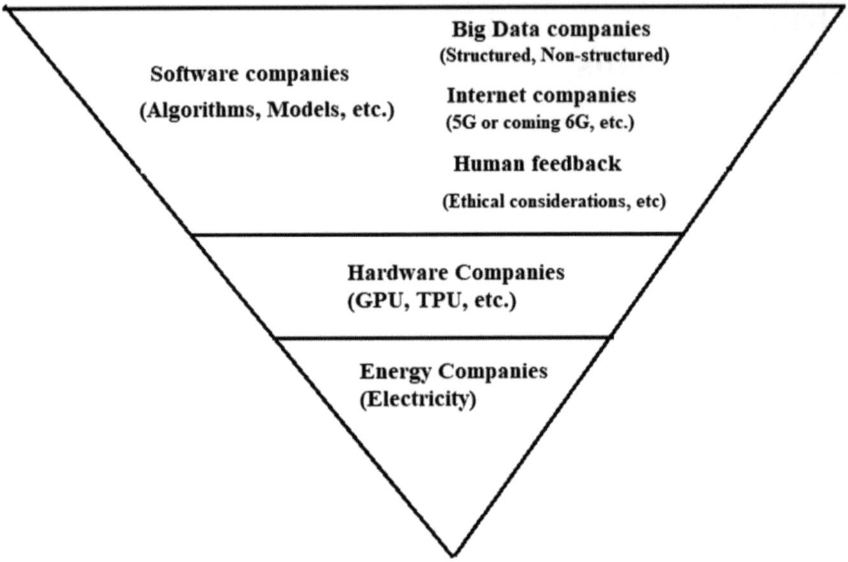

Fig. 2.1 Multilayers of AI ecosystem

Processing Unit) capacity for both research and commercial deployment. Bottlenecks in supply or pricing can slow innovation.

The top layer is software companies that provide general and specialized AI applications for the public. Software companies compete intensively on all sides, including model architecture, optimization, and fine-tuning techniques. AI needs high-quality, diverse training data from big data companies. Other key forces for AI development are human feedback and ethical consideration. Open-source AI is critical for the healthy growth of the AI ecosystem. It accelerates both general-purpose AI applications (such as chatbots, coding assistants, and analysis tools) and specialized, vertical AI software in the public health sector.

The inverted pyramid hints at the fragility of our AI ecosystem: the base may not be large enough to sustainably support the rapidly expanding top layers in the future. A healthy AI ecosystem requires investment in foundational layers (energy and hardware) and responsible scaling at the top. Based on Fig. 2.1, we should expand the base to invest in renewable energy, energy-efficient AI chips, and next-gen infrastructure.

An AI application will have three key components: data, algorithm/model, and computing power. For AI applications in public health, data can be open-source text, device/sensor signals, genomic data, or administrative data (See Chapters 5 and 6). Algorithms/models can be traditional biostatistics models, machine learning, or large language models (See Chapters 7 and 8). Evaluations for AI applications in public health are vital to control misinformation risk. Evaluation in public health is hard, and evaluation is a gap for public health AI model development (See Chap. 4). Computing power can be lightweight for statistical surveillance. National-scale projects (or genomic projects) need robust computing power.

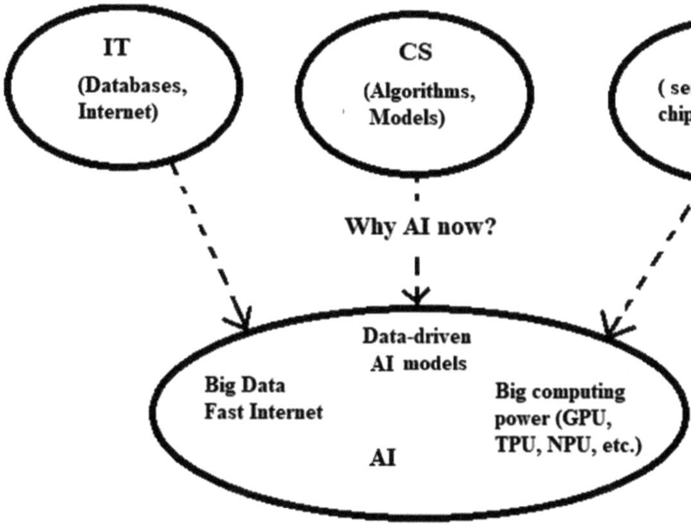

Fig. 2.2 Why AI now?

One of the future trends (See Chap. 11) is community-based AI applications in public health. Based on the key features of AI applications, community-level trust makes data availability much better than in fragmented national systems. AI can help with data standardization in public health. Bias, incompleteness, or incorrectness are easier to spot and correct by AI at the community level than at the national scale. Computing power can be lightweight at the community scale. The challenge is to develop high-level AI frameworks/models that address communities' urgent needs daily in public health.

This chapter will introduce key algorithms and models used in AI applications one by one. Big data is generated and processed in the top layer, which will be explained in Chapters 5 and 6.

2.2 Why AI Now?

AI is not novel. Many AI ideas are old at the software level and continue to grow or be revised. At the hardware level, changes in quantity lead to changes in quality. Why AI now? What are the turning points for AI development? The short answer is "fast computing, big data with fast internet, and the breakout of AI algorithms."

The long answer will discuss the progress in information sciences (IT), computer sciences (CS), and electronic engineering (EE), shown in Fig. 2.2. In the past half-century, computers were invented, providing excellent digital memory (such as databases) for humans with 100% accuracy in copying/pasting a file.

Let's introduce you to a fantastic rule, Moore's Law. In the past 50 years, half a century, there have been well-organized community efforts among scientists/ engineers worldwide, following many 5-year roadmaps from semiconductor associations. One of the remarkable achievements of humans is the complement of Moore's law: "The number of transistors in an integrated circuit (IC) doubles roughly every two years." (Liu et al., 2017) At the same time, in the public health domain, our human effort, through organized community efforts following WHO (World Health Organization) roadmaps on clean water and sanitation, successfully reduced the spread of waterborne diseases like cholera and typhoid. A crucial prerequisite of "artificial intelligence" is to access "big data" related to human behaviors. 5G or the coming 6G internet will be a key component of the AI ecosystem. n the 2010s, data-driven AI models allow humans to handle complex human cognitive functions, such as human language processing. Our human life is full of uncertainty and is a complex world. Uncertainty is a fundamental characteristic of data-driven AI models because these models rely on probabilities and approximations rather than absolute certainty.

As an informatics student, you know that "intelligence" is "understanding." Natural language processing (NLP) by computer was only feasible in IBM computing centers many years ago. When your phones have more computing power than the most potent IBM supercomputers 20 years ago, suddenly, you feel your phone is much more "understanding" you. Artificial Intelligence (AI) times are coming. Based on our concept-based AI definition, this "man-made understanding" is to simulate human cognition. We will discuss the breakout of AI algorithms in the following sections, such as Transformer in 2017.

2.3 Rule-Based Systems (RBS) and Expert Systems (ES)

To mimic human cognition (make decisions or perform reasoning), early and more traditional approaches to AI are rule-based systems. These rules are created manually by domain experts and programmers to capture knowledge and logic. The rule-based systems use explicitly defined "if-then" rules. For example, hypertension is that your blood pressure is too high (140/90 mmHg or higher) (Chobanian et al., 2003). The rule is "*IF blood pressure > 140/90mmHg, THEN hypertension.*"

An expert system is a rule-based system that mimics human expertise in a specific domain. Expert systems are built on rule-based logic but incorporate more sophisticated reasoning methods and domain-specific knowledge. Usually, an expert system has a knowledge base containing facts and a collection of "if-then" rules derived from domain experts (see Fig. 2.3). For example, MYCIN (Medical Diagnosis for Infectious Diseases) (Geng et al., 2014) was one of the first expert systems. Patient data (symptoms) will trigger inference engines to the medical knowledge base and provide recommendations for diagnosing diseases.

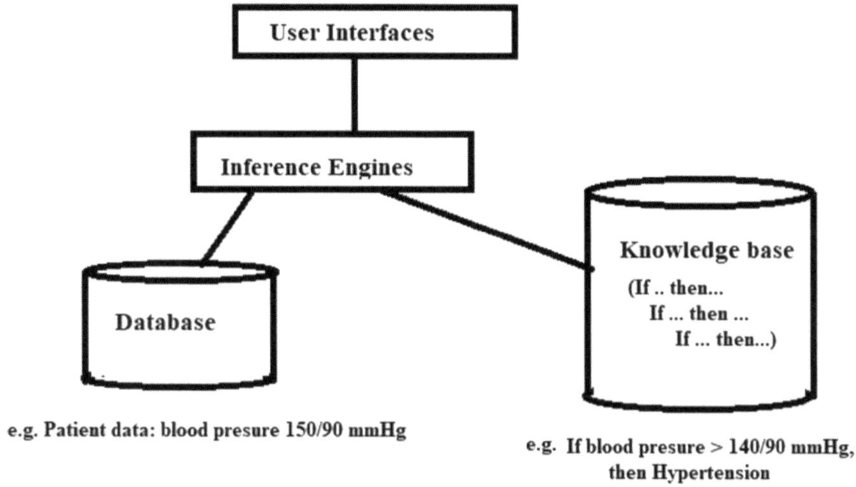

Fig. 2.3 Expert Systems

If there are clear, well-defined rules exist, such as clinical guidelines (based on best practices), and regulatory compliance is strict, such as FDA approval, the rule-based systems are still used in many applications, such as computer decision support systems (CDSS) in electronic medical records systems (EMR). Another clear advantage of RBS is transparency. These RBSs provide clear explanations for their decisions based on the predefined rules, making them easier to understand and trust. Hence, the user acceptance of RBS is high. When we integrate CDSS into CPOE (computer physician order entry) in EMR, we find many benefits of those rule-based systems, such as consistency and reliability (use the same set of rules and reduce human errors) and ease of implementation (well-defined pick-up lists or guidelines, etc.)

Modern approaches to AI are moving to machine learning (ML) and data-driven AI models. What's wrong with rule-based systems? What are the limitations of rule-based systems in AI? Rule-based systems really depend on expert knowledge. The effectiveness of rule-based systems depends heavily on the expertise that goes into defining the rules. Incomplete or outdated knowledge can lead to suboptimal decisions. The rule-based system has limited adaptability. Rule-based systems are only as good as the rules they are built on. Unlike machine learning systems, they cannot learn or adapt automatically to new patterns or knowledge. Many situations are complex and must handle vague or incomplete information. There are no clear rules that exist. If there are some rules in your cases, unfortunately, those rules are too many (thousands) and too complex to manage. It's tough to maintain those rules. Any changes require manual updating of rules, so running a rule-based system on a large-scale level in real time is impractical. In the following section, let's study the main AI models in machine learning.

2.4 Data-Driven AI Models

2.4.1 Machine Learning (ML)

In my first computer programming class at UNC-Chapel Hill 25 years ago, my CS professor trained us a skill to "abstract" the world. We practiced in the classroom and abstracted a TV and a car. Based on the abstract rules for various scenarios, we start explicitly programming it. The traditional approaches of computer tools depend on rules abstracted by humans.

Modern techniques are data-driven approaches instead of "rule-based" approaches. In many case scenarios, it's hard for humans to abstract clear rules, but we have a lot of data about those complex cases. Instead of specifying rules, we feed machine learning models with examples (data). For example, the input-output pairs (data) can be images and their annotations (labels). The machine learning models are trained using many examples. In the training stage, the model finds relationships and patterns in data by adjusting its internal parameters. The "new rules" are generated by machine learning. Next, the model applies the "new generalized rules" to new, unseen data. The model can be trained over time and continuously improve if there is more data. Machine learning models can handle complex and dynamic environments better than manual coding. Our times are information overload, and we have big data in every part of our lives, including the public health domain.

A successful story of machine learning is spam detection in our email system. There are no clear, well-defined rules for "good" or "bad" emails, but we have thousands of emails in our inbox folders. The computer model "learns" "the rules" from data about "spam" or "not spam." The most beautiful part of this story is that when there is new spam in the email over time, this machine learning model will automatically adapt and improve without needing new rules written manually.

ML models learn from data without explicit programming. ML models generalize from past experiences and adjust their behavior accordingly, making them highly flexible and efficient in complex tasks. Another example of machine learning is the customer recommendation system, which learns user preferences to suggest products.

2.4.2 Neural Networks (NNs)

Neural Networks (NNs) are math models first constructed in the 1950s (Rosenblatt, 1958). A neural network is the fundamental AI model and will be introduced to you as a valuable cognitive resource. Neural networks consist of layers, which are given information in *the input* and *output* layers. There is a *black box* in the middle. For example, patient symptoms and historical data can be input for medical reasoning. Pathological testing information confirming whether patients have diseases or not will be the output data. The network aims to learn some associations between input and output layers. We consider this AI model because it mimics the human cognitive processes of understanding the world based on the concept-based AI definition. For example, one of the human cognitive processes is physicians' medical reasoning through patient symptoms to final medical diagnoses. This model can be learned by modifying the connection weights between parameters. The network is learning from examples (data) to determine the weights by trial and error.

A typical NN project has two stages: training and testing. The training stage is where the NN learns from the data. It involves feeding input data to the model, adjusting the model's parameters (weights and biases), and minimizing the error using optimization techniques. NN requires careful tuning of parameters to achieve optimal learning performance. In the past, this learning process was often manual, time-consuming, and required expertise. The good news is that a new strategy is to use automated machine learning. Complex NN with millions or billions of parameters require substantial memory resources.

As the basis of AI models, NN has the same limitations as AI. You will understand what AI can and cannot do. NN struggles with tasks outside the distribution of the training data. In the testing stage, NN will fail to extrapolate effectively to new situations not represented in training. You will understand that AI suits repeated tasks but not new situations. For example, an autonomous vehicle trained on urban roads may struggle when encountering rural or extreme weather conditions.

The fundamental limitation of NN is computing power. In the previous section, we discussed *why AI now*. After half a century of Moor's law achievement in computing resources, we are better positioned to apply AI models like NN.

Neural networks are susceptible to variations or noise in input data. Small changes in input can cause significant changes in predictions. "Garbage in, garbage out" means that if you feed your model garbage, you will get garbage. The key limitation of NNs is the requirement for substantial data quantity (big data) and quality (labeled data). The structured data (annotated or labeled data) require expert domain knowledge. The electronic medical records (EMR) will be discussed in Chap. 5.

For the medical examples, another limitation of NNs is that it's difficult to interpret how NN arrives at specific decisions in those "black boxes" to physicians. The lack of transparency of NN hinders its adoption in medical fields. There is more discussion in Chap. 9, which discusses user acceptance of AI.

2.4.3 Deep Learning (DL)

Deep learning (DL) is a machine learning subset involving multilayered neural networks. We know that neural networks need a lot of computing power to implement. When we have apparent achievements of Moor's Law and reach a significant level of computing power, the interest in neural networks is growing. Traditional (shadow) neural networks with no hidden layers often overfit (low training error, high test error) to training data and fail to generalize well.

At the same time as computing power (hardware) progressed, AI models (software) made some breakthroughs in the 2000s. Dr. Geoffrey Hinton in Canada and his team made multi-layered neural networks feasible by using a technique called greedy layer-wise pretraining (Hinton et al., 2006). Basically, hidden layers are introduced in traditional (shadow) neural networks. The deep learning revolution began, and it reduced the need for large, labeled datasets. It can handle non-linear relationships within the data. Hidden layers allow the model to extract meaningful features from raw input data. In deep networks, each hidden layer can learn different levels of abstraction from the input.

More revisions of deep learning models were developed in image recognition (computer vision). A significant breakthrough occurred when Alex Krizhevsky, Ilya Sutskever, and Geoffrey Hinton introduced AlexNet in computer vision in 2012 (Krizhevsky et al., 2012). There are many innovations introduced by AlexNet, such as the ReLU activation function to help speed up training, dropout regularization to prevent overfitting, leveraged GPUs, and overlapping pooling to improve feature retention. It popularized deep learning in computer vision by showing that deep networks can outperform traditional methods.

2.4.4 Transformers (T)

Google proposed the Transformer model in 2017 in the paper titled "*Attention Is All You Need,*" authored by Vaswani et al. (Vaswani et al., 2017). It consists of two main components: encoder and decoder. The goal of the encoder is to understand relationships between words and their meanings within the context. The input raw text is tokenized. Embedding is to map tokens to numerical vectors for processing. Self-attention layers analyze relationships between words. The goal of the decoder is to convert processed data back to human-readable text.

A famous transformer model is the "Generative Pre-trained Transformer" (GPT), developed by OpenAI company. The breakthrough model is GPT-3, launched in 2020. It is well known for generating human-like text and revolutionizing natural language processing (NLP). The training dataset includes books, Wikipedia, and web pages. GPT-3 became a "true AI tool," mimicking human cognition to understand the world. It seems that GPT-3 can understand human language and can write, code, and even think of ways to solve problems. The GPT-4 was launched in 2023, and it enhanced multimodal capabilities. ***ChatGPT*** is an interactive chatbot application built on GPT models (such as GPT-4) optimized for conversational interactions with users.

The transformer can work on many tasks, such as machine translation, text summarization, text generation, question answering, sentiment analysis, text classification, code completion, and image captioning.

2.4.5 *Mixture of Experts (MoE)*

The Mixture of Experts (MoE) concept is to divide complex tasks among specialized sub-models (experts) (Shazeer et al., 2017). Unlike traditional neural networks that use all parameters during inference, MoE models activate only a subset of experts, significantly reducing computational requirements. Experts can run in parallel across multiple processing units. ***DeepSeek-V3*** (DeepSeek, 2024) is a MoE language model with 671 billion parameters, with 37 billion activated for each token. This design aims to enhance inference speed and efficiency.

2.4.6 *FP8 (8-Bit Floating Point)*

FP8 is a lower-precision numerical format used in AI models to optimize computation and memory efficiency while maintaining accuracy. Adopting FP8 precision in AI models is an emerging trend to enhance computational efficiency without compromising accuracy.

2.4.7 *Reinforcement Learning (RL)*

The main idea of an RL model is to enable an agent to learn how to make optimal decisions by interacting with an environment, receiving rewards or penalties, and adjusting its actions to maximize long-term rewards (Sutton et al., 2018). The RL model revolves around "trial and error" learning. First, the AI agent observes the current state of the environment, then takes an action based on its current policy (a strategy for choosing actions), and then receives feedback as a reward or penalty. Lastly, it updates its policy to improve future decision-making based on past experiences. Over time, the agent aims to maximize cumulative rewards by learning the best sequence of actions.

DeepSeek-R1 (Deep Seek, 2024) is an open-source AI model developed by *Deep Seek*. This model also employs reinforcement learning techniques to enhance its reasoning capabilities. This model allows AI applications to be designed for mathematics, coding, and reasoning tasks.

2.4.8 *Large Language Models (LLMs)*

LLMs (such as GPT or Gemini) can handle many data types, including text, code, images, audio, and multimodal data. Large language models in AI are designed to understand and generate human language, so LLM mainly focuses on human-generated or human-related data. For example, the limits of our human vision will decide the major image formats (resolutions) on the Internet, such as 1920x1080 pixel dimension, an image resolution often used for web images. We may accept a lower-precision numerical format (such as FP8 or FP16 (16-bit Floating Point)) to handle those human data. One of the benefits of using FP8 in LLMs is that we need less computing power with increased speed, reduced memory, etc. When we handle scientific computing with non-human data (such as environmental or biological data), we often use other AI models with high-precision numerical formats, such as FP16 or FP32 (32-bit Floating Point).

2.4.9 Natural Language Processing (NLP)

In the early years of NLP research, rule-based systems and symbolic AI were used. Symbolic approaches faced challenges due to language complexity, leading to the decline of interest. We call it AI winter, and it's hard to simulate human cognition to understand the world. In the 1980s, NLP shifted towards statistical models like the hidden Markov model (HMM). In the 1990s, data-driven approaches became mainstream. In 2017, Google introduced the transformer model for NLP. In the 2020s, large-scale language models such as GPT-3 and GPT-4 recently demonstrated impressive generative capabilities, making NLP more accessible and practical across industries.

The most common NLP applications are text processing and analysis, machine translation, speech recognition, and voice assistants, chatbots and conversational AI, information retrieval and search engines, text generation and auto-completion, document classification and spam filtering, optical character recognition, question answering systems, sentiment and emotion detection in social media, text-to-speech (TTS: converts written text into spoken words), fraud detection and compliance monitoring, personalized recommendations, extracting critical information from medical records and assisting with diagnoses, clinical decision support, and legal document processing, etc. If you want to use those AI roles in public health, you can go to Chap. 3 and learn how to design AI applications in public health.

The performance of NLP models is typically evaluated using a variety of quantitative metrics and qualitative assessments that measure their accuracy, efficiency, and robustness. The key performance indicators (PIs) for NLP models are grouped into accuracy-based metrics, language understanding metrics, computational efficiency metrics, robustness and generalization metrics, user-centric metrics, data-related metrics, ethical and fairness metrics, and business and impact-oriented metrics (Jurafsky et al., 2023). Selecting the right performance indicators group ensures that the NLP model is optimized for accuracy, efficiency, and real-world effectiveness. You can find more information about how to evaluate AI applications in public health in Chap. 4.

2.4.10 Computer Vision (CV)

Like NLP, computer vision (CV) is an important AI task that allows machines to interpret and understand visual data (images or videos) from the world. Pattern recognition was a rule-based model in the 1970s. In the 1980s, statistical methods like principal component analysis (PCA) were introduced to reduce image dimensionality for facial recognition (Sirovich et al., 1987). In the 2000s, image classification and object detection advancements were made through statistical models such as Hidden Markov Models (HMMs) and Bayesian networks. In the 2010s, large datasets like ***ImageNet,*** developed by Fei-Fei Li and her team (Deng et al., 2009), were a benchmark for training computer vision models. ***AlexNet***, a deep learning model developed by Alex Krizhevsky and his team (Krizhevsky et al., 2012), demonstrated the power of deep learning in image recognition. Recently, AI trends have been holistic, multimodal AI models, combining vision with language and audio.

Images or videos are used everywhere, so computer vision (CV) AI models can be used everywhere, such as healthcare and medical imaging, autonomous vehicles and transportation, security and surveillance, retail and e-commerce, agriculture and farming, manufacturing and industrial automation, entertainment and media, robotics and automation, defense and military applications, finance and banking, sports analytics, education and e-learning, smart cities and urban planning, and environmental monitoring. The most common CV applications are facial recognition systems and autonomous vehicles (using cameras to navigate and understand their environment).

2.4.11 Combined "Rule-Based" and "Data-Driven" Models

Public health is to solve population problems through organized efforts of societies, and there are no simple solutions for complex problems. Combining "rule-based" and "data-driven" models is a practical approach to address public health issues. For example, this textbook proposes some combined conceptual frameworks, such as the "Equity-aware risk stratification" (EquiRisk) model (See Session 7.5) and the "Policy-aware personalized opportunities" (PAPO) model (See Session 8.7). Equity and policies in public health are rules, and risk stratifications or personalized opportunities are typical applications of data-driven AI models. Many real public health issues are best addressed with hybrid models because of the complexity of health problems. Public health often deals with messy, multi-factor matters (e.g., social, biological, behavioral, and policy-driven). Purely data-driven models may miss context, while rules alone can't capture evolving patterns.

2.5 Robotics, AI Agent and Networks of AI Agents

Robotics.[1]

In the 1980s and 1990s, researchers began to combine AI with robotics, leading to robots. AI integrated into robots allows machines to perceive, act, and make decisions in the physical world. Nowadays, modern robotics research has several areas, such as humanoid robots (closely resemble human appearance and behavior), robotic process automation (RPA) (automating business processes), collaborative robots (Cobots) (working alongside humans in shared spaces), and autonomous vehicles and drones (self-driving cars and autonomous drones).

Robot training needs huge physical environmental "spatial data," like Internet website "text data" for LLMs training. For example, a standardized new house or apartment may have more 3D virtual demonstration "spatial data" (about the physical world) available for robot training.

AI Agent

> Due to the advancement of AI technologies, "*AI Agent*" has become a hot keyword and has gained more prominence in recent years. What is an AI Agent? As informatics students, you must establish a clear concept. In 2020, Stuart Russell defined *AI Agents* in his textbook (*Artificial Intelligence: A Modern Approach) as***AI Agent:** "An entity that perceives its environment through sensors and acts upon that environment through actuators, aiming to achieve specific goals or maximize performance based on an objective function." (Stuart Russell, 2020) The three key features of an AI agent are perception, decision-making, and action toward achieving goals autonomously.

Suppose a robot operates purely based on pre-programmed instructions without decision-making abilities, learning, or adaptive behavior. In that case, it is not considered an AI agent based on the definition. For example, a basic robotic arm performs repetitive tasks in a factory without responding to environmental changes.

Suppose a robot has an AI-based control system capable of reasoning, learning, and decision-making. In that case, it qualifies as an AI agent. For example, autonomous drones have cameras that allow them to perceive the environment. It has actuators (motors) that enable it to interact with the physical world, and it has an AI-based control system to make rational decisions based on its perception and goals.

Besides robotics (AI agents), AI agents are used in many domains, such as virtual assistants (e.g., Apple Siri), chatbots and customer service agents, recommendation systems (e.g., Netflix's AI agent), online search engines (e.g., Google search

[1] AI-powered robots and smart home technologies are advancing rapidly. When I become old, I wish to stay home rather than move to a nursing home. Hopefully, robots can provide care and companionship at home at that time.

agent), financial trading agents (e.g., high-frequency trading), autonomous vehicles, email filters and spam detection, video games and game AI, healthcare and diagnostic AI (e.g., IBM's Watson Health), fraud detection and security, autonomous software agents in business operations, intelligent tutors and educational AI, personal finance management, voice-activated smart devices, and natural language processing applications.

Every day, new AI agents are launched worldwide. It's information overload for all of us. A book, *Artificial Intelligence: A Modern Approach*, written by Stuart Russell and Peter Norvig, was first published in 1995. In that book (Stuart Russell, 2020), AI agents were grouped into five types. They are simple reflex agents (make decisions based on current perceptions alone), model-based reflex agents (use internal models to keep track of the world and make decisions based on both current perceptions and memory of past states), goal-based agents (choose actions based on their goals and consider the future consequences of their actions to achieve those goals.), utility-based agents (aim to select actions that maximize overall utility), and learning agents (learn from experience and improve their decision-making over time). The classifications of AI agents will help us understand and use them in the future. We will likely see more AI agents for public health-related tasks in the future.

Networks of AI Agents

A traditional network model needs two basic components: node names/IDs (e.g., IP address) and communication rules/network protocols (e.g., TCP/IP) among nodes. To create a network of AI agents, we must define standards for AI agents' unique IDs and create communication standards among AI agents. Stakeholders are AI developers, governments, ethicists, legal experts, and end-users (e.g., the healthcare sector). AI agents learn and adapt, making standardization harder. For AI agents, it may not be a traditional network model (peer-to-peer relationships). However, it could be a hierarchical model (parent-to-children relationships). Many ideas (protocols) will be proposed by stakeholders about how to communicate among AI agents and what relationships are among them. Those specific frameworks/protocols will compete, and the market will widely adopt one or two protocols for networks of AI agents in the future (like TCP/IP for the Internet).

2.6 Computing Power

In the 2010s, AI researchers began using large Graphics Processing Units (GPU) clusters to train AI models. GPUs allow training on datasets with millions of images. Cloud computing platforms offered scalable infrastructure for AI, enabling researchers and organizations to leverage vast computing power without owning hardware. Companies are developing specialized hardware like Tensor Processing Units (TPUs) and GPUs. One of the bottlenecks for AI development is high computational cost. Those deep learning models require significant computational resources to train. Besides data centers for computing power, there are edge computing approaches. AI can run on edge devices (e.g., smartphones, drones, IoT devices) to reduce the need for constant communication with cloud servers. NPUs (Neural Processing Units) are specialized hardware accelerators in AI computing. NPUs are optimized for low power consumption and high efficiency in AI tasks (such as transformer models). They are used in edge AI devices, autonomous vehicles, and embedded AI systems. DeepSeek models may attract more attention to NPUs. Quantum computing is still in its early stages. Still, companies like IBM, Google, and D-Wave are investing heavily in developing quantum computers that could potentially revolutionize AI by solving complex problems much faster than classical computers. Energy consumption in AI data centers is a significant concern. Energy-efficient AI model design, like the Mixture of Experts (MoE) model, will be critical for the future of AI.

In addition, you need to know units for measurement of computing power in AI. One of the units is FLOPS, which stands for Floating Point Operations Per Second. TFLOPS is trillions of FLOPS. MLOps is Machine Learning Operations. In practice, MLOps ensure that AI systems have access to the computing power they need (e.g., GPUs, cloud clusters, or edge devices) while automating tasks such as data processing, model retraining, and performance monitoring.

2.7 Internet and Internet of Things (IoT)

The Internet and AI are deeply intertwined. The Internet is a data source for AI. For example, NLP models, such as GPT, use huge text corpora from the Internet to learn language patterns and generate responses. The Internet is a platform for AI deployment. In cloud computing, the cloud has become the primary platform for hosting and deploying AI models.

The Internet of Things (IoT) is a network of connected devices. With IoT devices connected to the Internet, AI systems can process real-time data to make decisions. For instance, AI can monitor healthcare devices in real time via the Internet. In the future, smart homes, wearable devices, autonomous vehicles, and smart cities will all rely on AI to analyze data from connected devices, optimize systems, and provide real-time feedback to users. The Internet serves as the communication channel between these devices and AI systems. IoT can be widely used in AI applications in public health. You can explore "City-oriented IoT" for public health systemic factors (See Chap. 7) and "Personal-oriented IoT" for public health personal responsibilities (See Chap. 8).

Internet speed is a critical enabler of AI performance. Whether for autonomous systems, cloud-based AI models, or real-time AI-powered applications, high-speed internet is essential for AI solutions' scalability, responsiveness, and accuracy. 6G internet technology is expected to have a strong connection to satellite communications. As technologies like 5G and 6G continue to evolve, the role of speed and low latency will become even more central to the advancement of AI.

2.8 General Development Processes of AI Models

Currently, most AI models are data-driven models instead of rule-based models. It's useful for you to understand the general development process of an AI model so you can communicate effectively with developers who come from engineering backgrounds. Basically, there are two steps in the development of an AI model, training and testing (Schmidhuber, 2015). Overfit means that there are low training errors, but it has high test errors.

The training process generally includes data preparation (e.g. splitting the dataset, normalizing or standardizing the data, data augmentation, etc.), forward propagation (input data passes through the network layers and predictions are generated), loss calculation (e.g., mean squared error for regression, cross-entropy for classification, etc.), backward propagation (gradients of the loss function and optimization algorithms), evaluation on validation set (evaluated on the validation set), and hyper-parameter tuning (parameters are fine-tuned for optimal performance). The training aims to minimize the error (loss) and make the model generalize well to new data.

The testing process mainly includes data preparation (using a separate test dataset for unbiased evaluation), model inference (running the trained model on the test data to generate predictions), performance evaluation (e.g., accuracy, precision, recall, and F1-score, mean absolute error, root mean squared error, etc.), and error analysis (examining misclassifications or high-error cases to gain insights). Testing aims to verify the model's ability to perform well on real-world or unseen data without overfitting.

2.9 AI Ethical Guidelines and Governance Frameworks

AI will grow faster beyond many people's expectations. One of the reasons is simple; machines are digital and have different memory mechanisms. Basically, AI knowledge can be copied and shared among machines immediately, while humans are biological bodies, and we have organic growth, such as human education. We cannot stop AI growth because of competition among corporations and countries. The only thing we can do is to regulate AI's development.

The fundamental idea of the regulations in AI is our human safety. Maybe we can borrow some ideas from the regulations of nuclear weapons. Humans need comprehensive global regulations on AI development in the long run. We can focus on that AI tools will do good instead of harming in the short term. For example, we want AI to provide facts and knowledge (truth). It may not be the "whole truth," but the "partial truth." You do not want to have fake/biased/error information from AI tools, such as phony information of corporation advertisements. AI models should measure errors/biases and correct them.

Begin with the end in mind. Ethical guidelines and governance frameworks of AI are emerging. The resulting effect of the regulations in AI is to make human life safer.

We need to figure out how many regulation components are needed for AI development to protect humans in the future. It should include human rights, fairness and non-discrimination, transparency and explainability, accountability and responsibility, privacy and data protection, safety and security, a human-centric approach, sustainability and environmental impact, inclusivity and accessibility, ethical use of AI in warfare and autonomous weapons, governance and regulation, and comprehensive global regulations (Selbst et al., 2019) (National Institute of, 2023).

AI industries faced increasing pressure to ensure AI models are fair, transparent, and auditable. AI development needs new project management methodologies like Model Lifecycle Management (MLM) (Kreuzberger et al., 2023). MLM is the process of managing the entire lifecycle of a machine learning (ML) or AI model from its initial development to deployment, monitoring, and eventual retirement or updating. One of the key components should be "*compliance and ethical AI*."

Given the global nature of public health challenges, Chap. 3 has more discussions on regulatory frameworks like the EU's AI Act and the FDA's (Food and Drug Administration) guidance on AI applications in healthcare. Recently, the Department of HHS created an assistant secretary for technology policy. To design AI applications in public health, you need to better understand the legal and ethical landscapes of AI applications in public health.

2.10 Discussion Questions

Question 2.1. How does viewing AI as an ecosystem (energy, hardware, and software layers) help us understand both its potential and its vulnerabilities? How can public health professionals effectively engage with the AI ecosystem without requiring technical expertise, and what knowledge is most essential for them to possess?

Question 2.2. Why is the availability of energy and computing infrastructure a critical factor in the sustainability of AI applications?

Question 2.3. The middle layer (hardware) and top layer (software) depend on each other. How do advancements in semiconductor chips (e.g., faster GPUs) enable new AI applications? Conversely, how might software demand drive innovation in hardware design?

Question 2.4. The chapter mentions introducing key AI algorithms/models. Before reading, what algorithms do you expect to be most relevant for public health? How might they address challenges like disease prediction or resource allocation?

Question 2.5. How do different AI models and algorithms—such as neural networks, machine learning, deep learning, transformers, and reinforcement learning—differ in their applications to public health?

Question 2.6. What are the strengths and weaknesses of natural language processing (NLP) when applied to analyzing health data or communicating public health information?

Question 2.7. How might AI agents be designed to act responsibly in sensitive domains like public health?

Question 2.8. Why are ethical guidelines and governance frameworks necessary to balance innovation with accountability in the AI ecosystem?

References

Chobanian, A. V., Bakris, G. L., Black, H. R., Cushman, W. C., Green, L. A., Izzo, J. L., & Roccella, E. J. (2003). Seventh report of the joint National Committee on prevention, detection, evaluation, and treatment of high blood pressure. *Hypertension, 42*(6), 1206–1252. https://doi.org/10.1161/01.hyp.0000107251.49515.c2

Deep Seek. (2025). Deep Seek-R1: Advancing Retrieval-Augmented Generation with Large Language Models. https://deepseek.com

Deng, J., Dong, W., Socher, R., Li, L.-J., Li, K., & Fei-Fei, L. (2009, 2009//). *Image Net: A Large-Scale Hierarchical Image Database.* Paper presented at the IEEE Conference on Computer Vision and Pattern Recognition (CVPR), 248–255. https://doi.org/10.1109/CVPR.2009.5206848

Geng, S., & Zhang, Q. (2014). Clinical Diagnosis Expert System Based on Dynamic Uncertain Causality Graph. 233–237. https://doi.org/10.1109/itaic.2014.7065041

Hinton, G. E., Osindero, S., & Teh, Y.-W. (2006). A fast learning algorithm for deep belief nets. *Neural Computation, 18*(7), 1527–1554. https://doi.org/10.1162/neco.2006.18.7.1527

Jurafsky, D., & Martin, J. H. (2023). *Speech and Language Processing*: Pearson. https://web.stanford.edu/~jurafsky/slp3/

Kreuzberger, D., Kühl, N., & Hirschl, S. (2023). Machine learning operations (MLOps): Overview, definition, and architecture. *IEEE Access, 11*, 31866–31879. https://doi.org/10.1109/ACCESS.2023.3262138

Krizhevsky, A., Sutskever, I., & Hinton, G. E. (2012, 2012). *Image Net Classification with Deep Convolutional Neural Networks.* Paper presented at the Advances in Neural Information Processing Systems 25 (NIPS 2012). https://papers.nips.cc/paper/2012/hash/c399862d3b9d6b76c8436e924a68c45b-Abstract.html

Liu, T. J. K. (2017). Extending the Era of Moore's Law. 1. https://doi.org/10.1117/12.2286671

National Institute of, S., & Technology. (2023). AI Risk Management Framework (AI RMF 1.0). https://www.nist.gov/itl/ai-risk-management-framework

Rosenblatt, F. (1958). The perceptron: A probabilistic model for information storage and Organization in the Brain. *Psychological Review, 65*(6), 386–408. https://doi.org/10.1037/h0042519

Schmidhuber, J. (2015). Deep learning in neural networks: An overview. *Neural Networks, 61*, 85–117. https://doi.org/10.1016/j.neunet.2014.09.003

Selbst, A. D., Boyd, D., Friedler, S. A., Venkatasubramanian, S., & Vertesi, J. (2019). *Fairness and Abstraction in Sociotechnical Systems.* Paper presented at the Proceedings of the Conference on Fairness, Accountability, and Transparency. 59–68. https://doi.org/10.1145/3287560.3287598

Shazeer, N., Mirhoseini, A., Maziarz, K., Davis, A., Le, Q. V., Hinton, G. E., & Dean, J. (2017). *Outrageously Large Neural Networks: The Sparsely-Gated Mixture-of-Experts Layer.* Paper presented at the International Conference on Learning Representations (ICLR). https://arxiv.org/abs/1701.06538

Sirovich, L., & Kirby, M. (1987). Low-dimensional procedure for the characterization of human faces. *Journal of the Optical Society of America A, 4*(3), 519–524. https://doi.org/10.1364/JOSAA.4.000519

Stuart Russell, P. N. (2020). *Artificial Intelligence: A Modern Approach* (4th ed.): Pearson. https://aima.cs.berkeley.edu/

Sutton, R. S., & Barto, A. G. (1998). Reinforcement learning: An introduction. *IEEE Transactions on Neural Networks, 9*(5), 1054–1054. https://doi.org/10.1109/tnn.1998.712192

Vaswani, A., Shazeer, N., Parmar, N., Uszkoreit, J., Jones, L., Gomez, A. N., & Polosukhin, I. (2017). Attention is all you need. *Advances in Neural Information Processing Systems, 30*, 5998–6008. https://arxiv.org/abs/1706.03762

Part II
Modeling of AI Applications for Public Health

Chapter 3
Design Models for AI in Public Health

A Big Picture for Solving Public Health Problems with AI

Let me provide a big picture for solving public health problems with artificial intelligence (AI). The end results for applications in public health are clear and straightforward: prevent diseases, live longer, and live better. Visions of public health applications will have specific health ideas about what the public wants. For example, specific public health issues include vaccines, antibiotic resistance, air pollution, clean water, diabetes, mental health, substance abuse, etc. We need a lot of effort to determine the current realities (starting points) of public health issues in your community, city, state, and country. The big picture for solving public health problems has two steps in Fig. 3.1: (1) understanding the current realities and (2) choosing appropriate approaches (acting) for the end results.

In this big picture, applications' visions and end results are clear, and circles are drawn in solid lines in Fig. 3.1. We know what we want in the end. Unfortunately, we cannot accurately describe current realities. There are distortions of current public health reality. For example, how many people will ask for help with mental health issues? How many of them can get affordable mental health care? Fig. 3.1 shows the starting zone circles in the dotted lines for "unknown" areas.

In Fig. 3.1, you will get a big picture of AI's impact on public health. AI can help us better understand current public health realities in the first step, empower current approaches or provide new AI-driven solutions, and help us choose wisely in the second step. You will find that AI-driven new approaches are shown in the dotted lines in Fig. 3.1 because AI agents for public health are still under design and development. Hopefully, you will be involved in this process to solve public health problems with AI.

It's an exciting era of innovation, such as AI. You are lucky to have witnessed and benefited from AI in your lifetime. AI is transforming everything, including public health. This chapter discusses design models for AI in public health.

M. Wu, *Artificial Intelligence in Public Health*,
https://doi.org/10.1007/978-3-032-15872-7_3

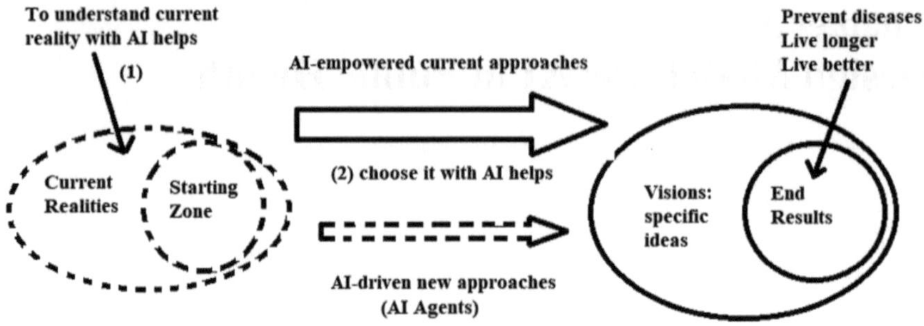

Fig. 3.1 A big picture for solving public health problems with AI

3.1 Design Principle

For our public health informatics students who will design AI applications in the future, a simple design principle is proposed as follows:

Design principle: "Encoding Justice (EJ)." "Justice" includes health equity, procedural fairness, distributive justice, anti-oppression, and more.

Justice should not be treated as something to fix after deployment or via external regulation. The AI ethics should not be a regulatory add-on. "Encoding justice" should be your design principle. It's your design choices (e.g., data, labeling, model objectives) to pre-wire the AI system for equity or harm prevention.

AI cannot solve structural justice issues on its own. Historical biases in data, systemic inequalities, and entrenched institutional policies are deeply embedded and complex. However, AI can help reduce harm, depending on how it is designed and implemented. For example, incorporating equity auditing directly into the architecture of an AI system is one way to promote fairness and accountability.

One of the goals of this textbook is to introduce this design principle to the next generation of designers of AI applications in public health, "***encoding justice at the design level***." This design principle will serve as an "adoption accelerator" for your AI applications. In public health, our communities, professionals, and regulators will adopt your AI application more quickly when trust is built into the design model.

3.2 Software Development Process Model for Designing AI Applications

Begin with the end in mind. The designer should clearly list the goals of AI applications for public health in their mission statements and objective statements. Let's review the public health definition: "prevent diseases, live longer and live better through organized society's efforts." The people's health should be the primary goal for designers. There are other aims to develop AI applications in public health, such as financial, legal, research, administrative goals, etc. The first goal for designing AI applications for public health could be "To take care of population health." The goal for designing an EMR (Electronic Medical Record) system is to "take care of the patient." In developing AI applications in public health, equity is foundational to population health. You should center equity in AI design and deployment. When AI designers forget the principles (Encoding Justices), AI has unintended consequences in public health, such as exacerbating health inequities.

3.2.1 Waterfall Process Model

Our public health informatics students need to know a simple process model to design AI applications that are easy to understand and follow. One of the earliest and most structured software development methodologies is the waterfall model (Boehm, 1976). It includes requirement analysis, system design, implementation, testing, deployment, and maintenance. Designing an AI application is a structured process that requires careful planning, data preparation, algorithm selection, model development, and testing. As informatics students, you can contribute a lot to the whole AI application development team and play a key role in aligning the AI solution with user needs and the public health problem you're trying to solve.

3.2.2 Project Process Management Methodology

AI projects are complex and require a systematic project management methodology. This methodology manages key factors during development, such as quality, time, and cost. Designers or developers of AI applications need to know some project management methodologies, such as waterfall, Agile, Scrum, and Crisp-dm. Table 3.1 lists some AI project management (PM) methodologies. Using a project management methodology is like following a recipe when cooking a complex dish. You only need to select one method that fits your taste and stick to it.

Table 3.1 Some AI project management methodologies

Methodology	Descriptions (key features)	Best For
Waterfall	A linear, sequential approach where each structured phase of the project is completed before moving to the next (see Fig. 3.2)	Projects with well-defined requirements and minimal expected changes such as infrastructure upgrades or legacy system migrations
Agile/scrum	Agile is an iterative and incremental approach. Its advantages include flexibility, faster delivery, and improved stakeholder engagement Scrum is an Agile framework that organizes work into fixed-length iterations and uses roles. Its advantages include high transparency, regular feedback loops, and adaptability	Projects with evolving requirements, such as AI-driven applications Projects such as AI model training require flexibility, frequent feedback, and iterative development
Hybrid (Agile-waterfall mix)	Uses Waterfall for upfront planning and Agile for execution and iteration	Projects need both structured planning and agility
CRISP-DM	CRISP-DM is a specialized methodology for data mining and AI/ML projects. It includes phases like business understanding, data preparation, modeling, evaluation, and deployment. It is structured yet flexible and tailored for data science workflows	AI and data science projects such as predictive modeling or data-driven solutions

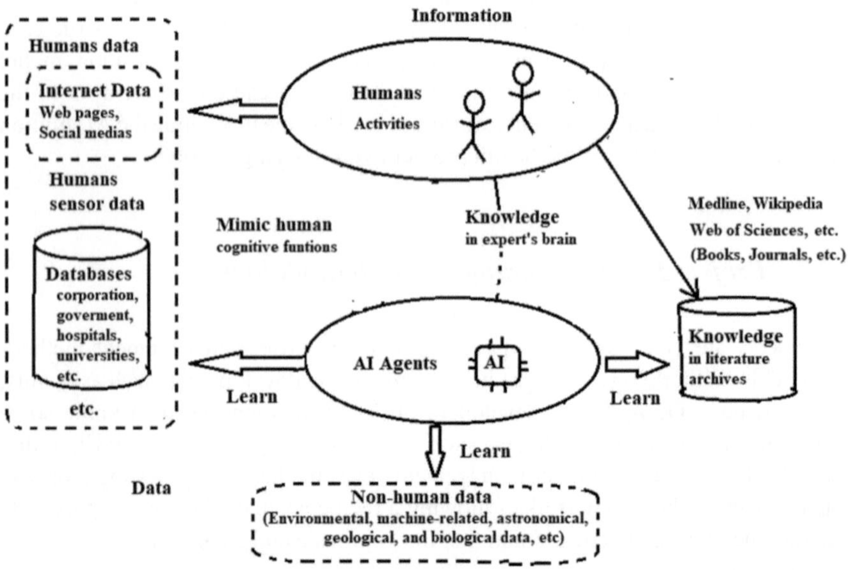

Fig. 3.2 Concept-based definition of AI

3.3 Understand Current Public Health Reality with AI

3.3.1 What is Health? Health Outcomes

"*Health is a state of complete physical, mental, and social well-being, not merely the absence of disease or infirmity*" defined by the World Health Organization (WHO) in 1948 (World Health Organization, 1948). Well-being is how you feel about yourself and your life. Public health focuses on the overall health outcomes of a group of people. It aims to improve people's well-being through organized efforts of societies.

How do we measure health outcomes? Many descriptive public health data focus on disease. For example, the typical rates used in health outcome measurement are mortality rate (death rate), incidence rate, or prevalence rate (about infectious or chronic diseases). When data indicate a lack of or a relatively low level of disease, they consider the level of health to be high. In many situations, health is not measured directly. It's different from the WHO's definition (not merely the absence of disease).

In the AI era, our health data (not only disease data) may be directly collected by sensors (wearable devices), smartphones, telehealth technologies, and AI tools. To better understand the reality of current public health, new health outcome indicators about people's health could be measured directly in the future. For example, Health-Related Quality of Life (HRQoL) is an indicator that measures physical, mental, and social well-being (World Health Organization, 1995). It's back to the original meaning of health, defined by WHO half a century ago. When public health focuses on more citizens instead of patients, we can design more AI applications on the primary prevention (prevent a new disease) than the secondary prevention (handle existing disease) in public health.

One of the end results in Fig. 3.1 is to live longer. Life expectancy at birth is an indicator, which is the average number of years a newborn is expected to live. The current reality about US life expectancy is only 78.4 years in 2023, while life expectancy in Europe (EU) was estimated at 81.5 years in 2023. Nobody likes being the bearer of bad news, but delivering tough news in public health is necessary. AI tools could help us explore and improve the affordability and accessibility of the US healthcare system in the long run.

3.3.2 Systemic Factors and Personal Responsibilities

Empowered by AI, designers of AI applications in public health should fully understand current public health realities first. Many health issues should be explored from both individual choices and systemic factors. Table 3.2 lists systemic factors and personal responsibilities in the top 10 public health problems worldwide. For example, obesity is the top health issue in many US cities. Firstly, personal preferences include poor diet and unhealthy eating habits (e.g., drinking too many sodas with sugar). But there are some food desert areas, and people have limited choices. AI tools can help us understand all systemic factors and identify those food deserts. AI could help us emphasize systemic issues and personal responsibility for those public health problems equally. Public health informatics aims to identify unmet public health needs and implement IT/AI as their solutions. The designers of AI applications for public health could find unmet public health needs/gaps in Table 3.2, either a systemic factor problem or an individual choice issue. You could design AI applications as their solutions.

In Chap. 7, AI applications for public health systemic factors will be discussed. Chapter 8 will discuss AI applications for public health personal responsibilities.

One of the public health realities is the lack of funding. AI could explore this complex question, "*Is public health spending wasteful?*" There is intense short-term funding when public health emergencies (e.g., infectious disease outbreaks) exist. Those long-term health issues such as mental health and chronic disease prevention are underfunded. "*Can preventative care save money by reducing long-term healthcare costs?*" We hope AI can help us discover the facts about this question.

3.3.3 Realized Needs

A realized need in AI refers to an existing demand where AI has been successfully applied to address a challenge. These needs emerge from real-world AI problems, often validated by successful implementations. For example, like an autopilot keeping a plane on course, AI automates repetitive tasks, allowing humans to focus on more significant decisions. When computers get smart, we realize that some tedious, time-consuming, repetitive tasks like data entry will be replaced by AI automation. Just like an oracle predicts the future, AI analyzes massive amounts of weather data to forecast storms, heat waves, and climate patterns more accurately than ever before. Our lives depend on weather forecasts. Instead of guessing the future, AI analyzes patterns to predict what's coming, like a crystal ball that works with real data. Another example of transportation is self-driving cars. More humans believe self-driving cars can simplify life, and AI is required to help autonomous vehicles navigate roads. Table 3.3 directly shows some examples of realized needs for AI in public health.

3.3.4 Unrealized Needs

Public health informatics aims to identify unmet public health needs and implement AI as a solution. You should review the design models in this chapter. They summarize many systemic factors and personal responsibilities for top public health issues. Hopefully, you can open minds and explore those unmet or unrealized needs for AI applications in public health.

Table 3.2 Systemic factors and personal responsibilities

Public health problems	Examples of systemic factors	Examples of personal responsibilities
Part I		
Cardiovascular Diseases (CVDs)	Healthcare system and access to care (e.g., Health disparities) Socioeconomic and educational factors (e.g., Income inequality) Food System and diet-related issues (e.g., Food deserts; processed food availability) Environmental and urban planning factors (e.g., Air pollution; lack of walkable cities) Government policies and public health initiatives (e.g., Tobacco and alcohol regulations)	Diet & nutrition choices Physical activity and exercise Avoiding tobacco and limiting alcohol Managing stress & mental health
Infectious diseases and pandemics	Healthcare system and access to care (e.g., Overloaded healthcare systems) Globalization and travel (e.g., Supply chain issues) Climate change and environmental factors (e.g., Rising temperatures and habitat destruction) Government policies and public health infrastructure (e.g., Vaccine policies) Misinformation and public trust issues (e.g., Distrust in governments and scientists)	Vaccination and immunization Hygiene and sanitation Wearing protective gear and social distancing Safe food and water practices Responsible travel and exposure prevention Combating misinformation and promoting public health awareness
Mental health disorders (Slade et al., 2015)	Healthcare system and access to mental health care (e.g., Shortage of mental health professionals; High cost of care) Socioeconomic and workplace factors (e.g., Poverty and financial stress; Unemployment and underemployment) Education and awareness issues (e.g., mental health stigma; Misconceptions about mental illness) Social and community factors (e.g., Family and childhood experiences; Social isolation) Environmental and digital factors (e.g., Urban stressors; Social media impact) Government policies and public health initiatives (e.g., Weak mental health policies; Inadequate workplace protections)	Seeking HELP AND TREATMENT (e.g., Reach out for professional help) Practicing self-care and stress management (e.g., Engage in relaxation techniques) Maintaining a healthy lifestyle (e.g., Exercise regularly) Strengthening social connections (e.g., Join support groups) Being mindful of triggers and emotional well-being (e.g., Identify stressors)

(continued)

Table 3.2 (continued)

Public health problems	Examples of systemic factors	Examples of personal responsibilities
Part II		
Cancer	Healthcare system and access to cancer care (e.g., Limited access to early detection and screening; Expensive treatments) Environmental and occupational exposure (e.g., Air and water pollution; Workplace carcinogens) Government policies and public health infrastructure (e.g., Lack of strong anti-tobacco regulations) Socioeconomic and lifestyle factors (e.g., Poverty and financial stress; Urbanization and sedentary lifestyles)	Cancer screening and early detection (e.g., Get regular screenings) Healthy lifestyle choices (e.g., Avoid tobacco and smoking) Reducing Environmental and occupational risks (e.g., Minimize exposure to harmful chemicals) Vaccination and preventive care (e.g., Get the HPV vaccine) Advocacy and awareness (e.g., Spread awareness)
Obesity (Swinburn et al., 2019)	Food environment and accessibility (e.g., Food deserts; Unhealthy food availability) Socioeconomic and educational factors (e.g., Low-income communities at higher risk) Built environment and physical activity (e.g., Car-dependent infrastructure) Healthcare system and policy gaps (e.g., Limited insurance coverage for obesity treatment) Psychological and cultural factors (e.g., Emotional eating and stress; Cultural norms around food)	Healthy eating habits (e.g., Choose nutrient-dense foods) Regular physical activity Building healthy lifestyle habits (e.g., Get enough sleep) Seeking medical and professional support Raising awareness and advocacy
Diabetes (Powers et al., 2020)	Healthcare system and access to diabetes care (e.g., Limited access to preventive healthcare) Food environment and nutrition accessibility (e.g., High availability of processed and sugary foods) Socioeconomic and educational barriers (e.g., Lower-income populations at higher risk) Built environment and physical activity (e.g., Lack of safe spaces for exercise) Policy and government regulations (e.g., Inadequate public health policies)	Healthy eating habits (e.g., Monitor carbohydrate intake) Regular physical activity Monitoring and preventive healthcare (e.g., Check blood sugar levels regularly) Managing Stress and Sleep Medication and treatment compliance (e.g., Follow doctor's recommendations) Raising awareness and advocacy

(continued)

Table 3.2 (continued)

Public health problems	Examples of systemic factors	Examples of personal responsibilities
Part III		
Dementia (Livingston et al., 2020)	Healthcare system and access to dementia care (e.g., Limited access to early diagnosis) Socioeconomic and educational factors (e.g., Lower education levels linked to higher risk) Aging population and life expectancy (e.g., Aging is the biggest risk factor) Lifestyle and built environment (e.g., Lack of community programs) Government policies and public health initiatives (e.g., Limited public awareness campaigns)	Brain health and cognitive engagement (e.g., Stay mentally active) Healthy lifestyle choices (e.g., Exercise regularly) Monitoring and preventive healthcare (e.g., Get regular checkups) Reducing risk factors (e.g., Avoid smoking & excessive alcohol; Prioritize sleep) Caregiver preparedness and advocacy (e.g., Plan ahead)
Environmental health and climate change (Romanello et al., 2023)	Industrial pollution and greenhouse gas emissions (e.g., Fossil fuel dependence) Urbanization and infrastructure challenges (e.g., Insufficient waste management; Air pollution) Water and food security risks (e.g., Contaminated water sources) Public health and climate-driven disease burden (e.g., Vector-borne diseases expanding) Government policies and corporate responsibility (e.g., Weak environmental regulations)	Reducing carbon footprint Waste reduction and recycling Water and air quality protection (e.g., Use water efficiently) Advocacy and community engagement (e.g., Support environmental policies) Disaster preparedness and health protection (e.g., Stay informed on climate risks)
Antimicrobial Resistance (AMR)	Overuse and misuse of antibiotics in healthcare (e.g., Excessive antibiotic prescriptions) Antibiotic use in agriculture and livestock (e.g., Widespread antibiotic use in farming) Inadequate infection prevention and control (IPC) in Healthcare (e.g., Poor hospital hygiene) Globalization and spread of resistant pathogens (e.g., International travel and trade) Weak regulations and pharmaceutical industry Practices (e.g., Weak antibiotic regulations)	Responsible antibiotic use (e.g., Only take antibiotics when prescribed) Infection prevention and hygiene practices (e.g., Wash hands regularly) Reducing antibiotic exposure through food and environment (e.g., Choose antibiotic-free meat and dairy) Advocating for stronger policies and education (e.g., Raise awareness)

(continued)

Table 3.2 (continued)

Public health problems	Examples of systemic factors	Examples of personal responsibilities
Substance abuse and addiction (Alcohol, Tobacco, and Drugs)	Socioeconomic inequality and unemployment (e.g., Poverty and lack of opportunities; Neighborhood conditions) Healthcare system barriers (e.g., Limited access to mental health care) Prescription drug misuse and overprescribing (e.g., Easy access to opioids and painkillers) Cultural and social influences (e.g., Peer pressure and social norms) Weak law enforcement and drug policies (e.g., Inconsistent drug policies; Lack of prevention programs)	Making healthy lifestyle choices (e.g., Avoid recreational drug use) Seeking help early (e.g., Recognize early warning signs) Advocating for prevention and awareness (e.g., Educate others) Reducing social and peer pressure (e.g., Surround yourself with positive influences) Supporting harm reduction and recovery (e.g., Use harm reduction strategies)

Table 3.3 Examples of realized needs for AI applications in public health

Domains	Examples of realized needs for AI in public health
Disease detection and diagnosis	AI-powered medical imaging analysis AI symptom checkers AI-powered pathogen identification: use rapid genetic sequencing
Outbreak prediction and surveillance	AI-powered epidemiological modeling AI-powered wastewater surveillance AI-powered early warning systems:
Drug discovery	AI-driven drug discovery AI-powered clinical trial optimization: identify suitable patients
Personalized medicine	AI-powered genomics and precision medicine: AI personalizes treatments based on patient genetic profiles
Telehealth services	AI chatbots and virtual health assistants AI in remote patient monitoring: Wearables and AI analyze heart rate, glucose levels, and sleep patterns to alert doctors of health risks AI-powered telemedicine
Health systems optimization and resource allocation	AI-powered scheduling Smart ambulance dispatching AI in supply chain management
Public health policy and decision support	Policy impact simulation AI for health economics Misinformation detection
Mental health and well-being	AI mental health chatbots AI suicide prevention tools AI for stress and burnout detection

Education in AI is critical; you can understand what AI can and cannot do. Improving public health staff's AI literacy can help them identify their unrealized needs for public health using new innovative AI functions or AI agents launched every month worldwide.

Instead of directly showing unrealized AI needs in public health, we provide some approaches to identify them. Table 3.4 lists some approaches with examples.

When we face "unknown" areas in public health, your own speculations (guesses) may be distortions of reality. AI is a powerful cognitive resource and helps find facts and solutions. As a designer of AI applications in public health, you must be precise about current public health reality and objectively observe public health issues. That will be the starting point for designing practical AI applications in public health.

Table 3.4 Some approaches identifying unrealized needs in public health

Approaches	Descriptions	Examples of unrealized AI needs
Data-oriented approach	Data gaps and inefficiencies; analyze data for hidden patterns and gaps	Explore manual processes in public health that could be automated Identify the situations where there is a lack of accurate, timely health data Explore recurring health system inefficiencies Identify health conditions that are neglected and underreported
Health disparities approach	Explore health disparities	Explore what populations lack access to quality healthcare Reduce healthcare costs for underserved communities Map healthcare access gaps Explore neglected diseases in certain areas
Negative events approach	Study near-miss events and system failures: errors reveal hidden problems that AI can solve	Explore trends in medical errors, misdiagnoses, or preventable hospital readmissions Examine cases where harm was avoided by chance Optimize crisis response for pandemics, natural disasters, and disease outbreaks
Community-oriented approach	Explore community and behavioral insights: unrealized needs often come from frontline community public health workers who experience daily challenges	Explore health behaviors contribute to preventable diseases Explore how AI personalize interventions to change behavior, such as malnutrition tracking Conduct interviews and focus groups with community workers for unrealized AI needs Conduct observation studies on public health workers
Global perspective approach	Explore emerging global public health challenges	Identify poorly addressed health threats (climate change, antimicrobial resistance) Explore how AI help mitigate the impact of future pandemics

(continued)

Table 3.4 (continued)

Approaches	Descriptions	Examples of unrealized AI needs
Future-threats approach	Explore emerging health threats	Predict how climate change will impact infectious disease spread, heat-related illnesses, and waterborne diseases Monitor antibiotic resistance trends Track psychological and behavioral health trends, such as social isolation
Interdisciplinary approach (Kivits et al., 2019)	Create cross-sector collaboration to explore unrealized AI needs	Integrate healthcare with urban planning, education, or agriculture to improve health outcomes AI models that detect financial fraud can be repurposed for medical insurance fraud AI that optimizes delivery routes in e-commerce could improve medical supply chain efficiency

3.4 Empower Current Public Health Approaches with AI

"Empowered by AI" means that AI is a supporting tool, and human oversight is essential. AI enhances existing processes but is not the core technology driving the system. AI provides insights, automation, and decision support but doesn't operate independently.

Data collection, entry, and processing are significant challenges in public health. Currently, vast amounts of public health data come from surveys, hospital health records, clinics, labs, research studies, etc. Data sources are inconsistent and lack standardized formats across different health systems. Public health involves large populations with more duplicate records and missing data. Manual data entry increases errors and delays because overburdened human staff leads to fatigue and mistakes. Privacy concerns and strict HIPAA (Health Insurance Portability and Accountability Act) regulations in the U.S. may delay data collection and make them more inefficient. Public health data is critical and impacts policy decision-making and resource allocation. One of the key roles of AI is automation, which automates repetitive or time-consuming tasks. AI applications can empower current public health approaches to standardize the processes, reduce the need for human intervention, and free up human resources for more complex activities. Part III of this book will discuss big data in public health with AI in detail.

Data processing and analysis in public health are always facing Big Data challenges. Public health data on populations has millions of records and needs fast processing. Before data-driven AI models were available, old software (biostatistics software) struggled to analyze big data in public health. Empowered by AI, current data analysis and decision support tools for public health (such as biostatistics tools, etc.) could analyze large datasets to uncover insights, patterns, and trends that inform decision-making processes. For example, AI analyzes big data to predict air pollution risks during and after California fires. AI-powered early warning systems can analyze global health data to predict disease outbreaks. AI-empower tools can optimize vaccine distribution, allocating vaccines efficiently based on demand and priority groups. AI can help optimize current processes, improving efficiency and resource allocation in public health. Empowered by AI, we can monitor social media for public health. For example, AI could detect disease outbreaks early based on social media discussions.

3.4.1 Primary Prevention

Primary prevention in public health is to prevent new cases of diseases. It includes both health promotion and specific preventive measures. Health promotion involves health education and providing conditions that influence health, such as adequate food, housing, clothing, etc. Specific preventive measures include clean water, immunization, and protection from occupational hazards or accidents.

Health Outcome Indicators

To better understand the reality of current public health in your community, new health outcome indicators about people's health could be measured directly in the future, such as Health-Related Quality of Life (HRQoL), which is an indicator that measures physical, mental, and social well-being (Ware & Sherbourne, 1992). It focuses on primary prevention (preventing a new disease) rather than secondary prevention (handling existing disease) in public health. The health outcome indicators can be assessed as a starting point, and you can evaluate whether AI applications in public health enhance those indicators. AI can enhance the measurement, analysis, and application of HRQoL indicators by automating data collection, analyzing trends, and providing personalized insights.

Immunization

Let's look at the case of AI applications for immunization. Immunization is one of the most important public health interventions that save millions of lives annually. Vaccines help prevent infectious diseases, protect communities, and reduce healthcare costs. AI can automate data entry and verification in immunization registries, reducing errors and improving tracking. AI can predict vaccine demand, ensure timely supply, and reduce waste. It helps identify potential vaccine candidates faster and optimize clinical trial designs.

Older Adults

As populations live longer, societies must address the challenges and opportunities of aging to ensure healthy, independent, and dignified lives for older adults. In AI-powered nursing homes or communities, health care for older adults can be personalized. AI tailors services or experiences to individual users based on their preferences, behaviors, or needs.

Personally, I prefer to stay at home when I am old. Hopefully, AI-powered robots and telehealth systems will be intelligent enough to allow me to age in place rather than move to a nursing home. AI technologies will enhance independence, safety, health monitoring, and companionship, reducing reliance on full-time caregivers (Yousefi et al., 2023).

3.4.2 Secondary Prevention

Current public health approaches focus on diseases related to secondary prevention (with existing diseases). They involve screening, early disease detection, and early treatment, often allowing for the reversal or delay of the progression from preclinical to clinical disease. AI can empower those routine diagnostics. For example, AI models can analyze medical images (e.g., X-rays, CT scans, MRIs) for early detection of diseases like cancer, heart disease, or tuberculosis, automating the initial diagnostic process. AI can provide health screening automation. For example, routine screening tests for conditions like diabetes, hypertension, or cholesterol levels can be automated using AI.

Cardiovascular Diseases (CVDs)

Let's look at the case of AI applications on heart health. AI could automate data collection, entry, and process in heart health. Heart health is a significant public health issue worldwide. Cardiovascular diseases (CVDs) include heart disease, stroke, high blood pressure, and heart failure. AI can monitor heart rate, blood pressure, oxygen levels, and ECG (Electrocardiogram) remotely using wearables or home devices and flag anomalies for telemedicine practitioners to act upon (Bashkirtsev et al., 2023). Smartphone Apps with AI integration can collect daily data on physical activity, stress levels, diet, and sleep patterns. This data can be used by healthcare providers to offer personalized lifestyle recommendations to prevent heart diseases.

Dementia

Let's look at the case of AI applications for dementia. AI tools can empower current public health strategies in screening and early detection of dementia. Dementia is a significant public health issue. Over 55 million people worldwide live with dementia, and the aging population means cases will double every 20 years. It's a public health issue. Lack of early diagnosis leads to increased emergency room visits and hospitalizations. Current screening tools for dementia include clinical questionnaires, such as the Mini-Mental State Examination (MMSE) (Folstein et al., 1975). In our AI era, AI can empower those screen tools. Virtual reality (VR) video games could be screening tools for early recognition of dementia (Zygouris & Tsolaki, 2015). Those VR and AI tools could generate a 3D (Three-Dimensional) virtual reality environment where users perform screening tasks. Those simulated daily living environments can be kitchens or shopping malls. When dementia goes undiagnosed, families often struggle to understand changes in their loved ones' behavior. This can lead to stress, frustration, and confusion before diagnosis. AI can help them to detect dementia early.

Cancer

Cancer is a big public health concern. It is one of the leading causes of death and significantly impacts healthcare systems, economies, and communities (Sung et al., 2021). Finding a cure for cancer is complex. There is significant hope in ***bioinformatics*** for advancing cancer treatment and potentially finding cures (Tr, 2015). In integrating bioinformatics with public health, we need to face big data of human genome and genetic knowledge (genetic marks, genetic profiles, etc.), and we need AI tools to help us with this. AI is not optional but is required in bioinformatics and public health informatics.

3.5 Develop New AI-Driven Public Health Approaches

"AI-driven" means that artificial intelligence plays a central role in analyzing data and influencing decisions, which may be fully or partially automated. AI is at the core of the process, making decisions without or with minimal human input. AI actively learns, adapts, and executes decisions based on data and patterns. In Chap. 2, we define AI agents, which are AI-driven systems. "Embedded AI" also means that AI is a core function within a big system, allowing it to function autonomously.

AI Agents for Health Education

Personal responsibility is crucial for addressing public health issues, so individuals contribute significantly to health outcomes. In the past, it was impossible to increase health literacy and reduce the health knowledge gap between laypeople and healthcare providers. The AI era is happening due to advancements in big data, hardware (like Moore's Law), and algorithms (like Transformers). With the breakout of AI in natural language processing, AI can facilitate communication between humans and machines using natural language, enabling tasks like language translation, chatbots, and voice assistants. AI agents, like virtual assistants, can answer health questions for us. AI health agents can educate citizens about the risk factors of diseases. AI agents can automate routine public health communication, such as reminding people about vaccinations, preventive health screenings, or outbreak alerts. Chatbots or AI-powered virtual assistants can provide 24/7 information about health conditions, answer common questions, and direct people to appropriate resources without human intervention. For example, AI agents can provide mental health education, one of the top public health issues worldwide.

When your friends or neighbors have family members who are healthcare professionals, you may envy them. They can conveniently ask their son or daughter health questions at any time. Suppose a family's average level of health education is raised, and we can expect the level of health of this family to be promoted. Health AI Agents could be your "family members" with medical knowledge in the future. I think this will be the most promising and exciting area for AI to significantly impact public health. In Chap. 8, we will discuss improving health literacy with AI in detail.

AI Agents for Immunization

The AI agent keeps your immunization registries records. When AI agent perceives/identifies public health concerns, such as virus breakouts. AI agents can detect misinformation online, and provide accurate, science-based information for you. This individualized AI virtual assistant can assess individual and community-level risk factors, helping tailor vaccination campaigns to specific demographics. It can provide personalized vaccine recommendations to you and set up reminders for implementation.

AI Agents for Occupational Hazards

Public health informatics aims to identify unmet public health needs and implement IT or AI as their solutions. Suppose an occupation has severe occupational hazards; it will go against our public health goals: live longer and better. Letting AI agents replace dangerous tasks in those jobs is a preventive measure for public health. Let's look at the top ten occupations with severe occupational hazards (U.S. Bureau of Labor Statistics, 2024) in Table 3.5, which are unmet public health needs.

3.6 Ethical Considerations and Regulations

Let's discuss the ethical issues related to AI applications for public health. Why is this topic so important? First, we must prevent AI from harming humans in the long run. Legal and ethical standards for AI are required, and all AI developers must comply with them. The short-term goal to protect humans is to avoid AI-driven misdiagnosis, discrimination, or misinformation. The second reason is that it's a human right to health services. We must defend human rights to ensure fair, unbiased, and equitable AI applications for public health. Another important reason is that we need to build public trust for AI applications for public health. We need to increase transparency and accountability and make AI more acceptable. A solid business model can help AI applications for public health survive from AI bubbles. Ethical issues are essential for multi-criteria public health decision-making. Hopefully, ethical AI will enhance reliability in public health decisions.

Table 3.5 The top ten occupations with severe occupational hazards

Occupation	Examples of occupational hazards	Needs
Healthcare workers	Exposure to infectious diseases (e.g., COVID-19, tuberculosis, HIV (Human Immunodeficiency Virus)) Needle-stick injuries Burnout/Stress	Protect the well-being of doctors, nurses, paramedics, etc.
Construction workers	Exposure to dust (e.g., silica, asbestos) Falls from heights Heavy machinery accidents Hearing loss from loud noises	Protect the well-being of construction workers
Miners	Exposure to toxic gases, dust (e.g., coal dust, silica) Cave-ins Explosions Hearing damage	Protect the well-being of miners
Firefighters	Smoke inhalation Toxic chemical exposure Extreme heat Psychological trauma Burns	Protect the well-being of firefighters
Agricultural workers	Pesticide exposure Zoonotic diseases Sun exposure (skin cancer risk) Heavy machinery accidents	Protect the well-being of farmers and pesticide handlers, etc.
Industrial and factory workers	Exposure to hazardous chemicals (e.g., benzene, lead, asbestos) Repetitive strain injuries Toxic fumes	Protect the well-being of factory workers
Offshore Oil workers	Harsh weather conditions Drowning risk Exposure to oil spills Dangerous machinery	Protect the well-being of oil workers
Transportation workers	Long working hours Sleep deprivation High stress Exposure to diesel fumes Accidents	Protect the well-being of truck drivers, pilots, train operators, etc.

(continued)

Table 3.5 (continued)

Occupation	Examples of occupational hazards	Needs
Waste and sanitation workers	Exposure to infectious waste Hazardous chemicals Biohazards Rodents	Protect the well-being of garbage collectors, sewage workers
Law enforcement and military personnel	Exposure to violence High stress PTSD (Post-Traumatic Stress Disorder) Toxic substances (e.g., tear gas, explosives)	Protect the well-being of policemen and soldiers

3.6.1 Big Picture of Ethical Issues for AI in Public Health

Preventing AI Harm Humans

Uncertainty is inherent in data-driven AI models, and this uncertainty arises from data quality, model assumptions, and real-world variability. The goal of protecting humans is to avoid AI-driven misdiagnosis, discrimination, or misinformation. War causes harm to humans on a massive scale, and we should carefully think about the ethical use of AI in warfare.

Human Rights to Health

The right to health is a fundamental human right, including access to public health services, essential healthcare, and disease prevention measures without discrimination. Public health is deeply concerned with addressing health inequities; we should explore how AI could either help reduce disparities or potentially worsen them. More emphasis should be put on how AI applications can be designed to promote equitable health outcomes. AI must ensure equal access to healthcare services and avoid exacerbating health inequalities.

Ethical AI Access

Open-source AI tools and free AI models and frameworks can help make AI more accessible. We should prioritize open-source AI solutions for low-income countries. For example, public health officials in low-income countries should have access to AI-powered disease prediction models for infectious disease detection in their regions.

AI education is essential. Only a privileged few can develop and control AI without AI education, leading to technological and economic gaps. Only educated users can detect AI applications' biases, misinformation, and risks. *The unmet need for our public health informatics is to promote AI literacy for all.* We hope to help all citizens make informed decisions about AI in healthcare and public health services.

Hopefully, this book can contribute a little to public health informatics students, all students in public health schools, and public health practitioners. We hope to see more AI education in high schools and colleges with more AI education curricula. AI training should be available for all citizens, teaching AI basics to the public.

AI can automatically code and replace part of programmers' tasks. AI-Integrated Development Environments (IDEs) can help improve access to AI by lowering technical barriers and enabling more people, including non-experts, to develop AI applications. Decentralized AI initiatives can help prevent AI monopolization and encourage public involvement. Hopefully, our public health informatics students can lead some community-based AI development in the future.

Privacy and Data Protection

AI must protect sensitive medical and personal data to prevent misuse. Modern AI models are data-driven, not rule-based, so AI relies heavily on large datasets, often containing sensitive personal information. AI should not exploit personal data for profit or manipulation without user consent. Without privacy protection, people may fear and reject AI technologies. Privacy and AI often involve a trade-off, and humans face the challenge of balancing AI with ethical responsibility. For example, AI-powered facial recognition and tracking systems can violate privacy rights. AI must comply with GDPR (General Data Protection Regulation) (Europe) (Voigt & von dem Bussche, 2017), HIPAA (US), and other privacy regulations.

3.6.2 *Ethical Issues in the AI Application Level*

Fairness and Non-discrimination (Mehrabi et al., 2021)

AI must not reinforce biases against certain populations based on gender, race, age, disability, or socioeconomic status. AI models should be trained in diverse populations to avoid bias in healthcare recommendations. For example, AI-powered telemedicine services in remote areas provide healthcare access to low-income populations. AI systems must undergo ethical review before deployment. For example, WHO's AI Ethics Framework sets global AI ethical standards for healthcare.

Transparency and Explainability (Barredo Arrieta et al., 2020)

Are the AI's decision-making processes explainable to users? Unlike rule-based systems, data-driven AI models learn patterns from large datasets in a way often not directly interpretable by humans. Unfortunately, transparency and explainability are significant weaknesses of many data-driven AI models, especially complex ones like deep learning and large language models. Hopefully, user education and communication could provide understandable insights into how AI models work. It's a challenge to simplify explanations of AI for end users. Another way is to engage domain experts, policymakers, and affected communities in the AI development process. We will try to improve transparent and explainable AI (XAI) in decision-making. For example,

AI-powered cancer treatment ensures patients understand why AI recommends a specific therapy.

Accountability and Responsibility

Is there a mechanism to address errors or harm caused by the AI application? Who is responsible when AI makes a mistake in a medical decision? It is a legal question in a lawsuit. We need related laws (such as consumer protection, anti-discrimination, etc.) available then. EU AI Act and WHO AI Ethics Guidelines ensure clear accountability for AI errors in public health decisions. In court, we can align AI with legal liability principles and clearly define who is legally responsible for AI-driven harm (developer, company, or end-user). To address accountability and responsibility, we should provide human oversight and intervention. A human-in-the-loop (HITL) system was designed to ensure AI systems augment rather than replace human decision-making. For example, we use human verification in high-risk AI applications. Humans' continuous monitoring and feedback loop mechanisms are required to monitor AI behavior post-deployment and update models to correct unintended consequences.

Informed Consent

Do users understand how their data is being used? AI must respect patients' autonomy by ensuring they understand AI-based decisions. AI systems should provide clear, human-readable explanations. Patients must have the right to opt out of AI-driven decisions.

3.6.3 Regulations for AI in Public Health

The AI models keep changing with innovative technologies, and governments (such as the FDA (Food and Drug Administration) and HHS (U.S. Department of Health and Human Services)) must implement AI ethics guidelines for public health applications. AI is a fast-growing field, so we expect AI governance and regulations to be dynamically updated. The key ideas behind some legal and ethical standards are discussed in this section. The updated details of regulations will be available from their official websites.

3.6.3.1 Legal Standards and Regulations

HIPAA (Health Insurance Portability and Accountability Act) (Annas, 2003)

HIPAA is a U.S. federal law enacted in 1996. While HIPAA has not been officially updated to address AI, this law protects patient data privacy and security. AI applications handling electronic health records (EHRs) must comply with HIPAA's Privacy and Security Rules.

GDPR (General Data Protection Regulation) (Vimercati et al., 2019)

GDPR is a European Union (EU) law enacted in 2016. GDPR regulates how personal data is collected, processed, and stored. GDPR requires that AI decisions affecting individuals must be explainable, requires explicit patient consent for AI to process health data, and should guarantee data minimization (only the minimum amount of personal data necessary) and security for AI-driven health analytics.

FDA (U.S. Food and Drug Administration) AI Regulations (Benjamens et al., 2020; Warraich et al., 2025)

FDA AI Regulations are not a single law, but a set of guidelines and regulatory frameworks developed by the FDA. They oversee AI and machine learning use in medical devices, drugs, and biological products. For example, the FDA released the first proposed regulatory framework for AI/ML in medical devices in 2019. FDA released the Good Machine Learning Practice (GMLP) guiding principles in 2021. FDA is not a formal law, but FDA-enforced regulations apply under existing laws like the FDCA (Federal Food, Drug, and Cosmetic Act). AI-based medical devices must go through FDA approval if they affect treatment or diagnosis. AI-driven medical products must comply with FDA guidelines.

WHO Guidance on AI in Public Health (Katirai, 2023)

WHO AI guidelines are not legally binding like national laws. However, many countries use WHO recommendations to develop AI healthcare policies. WHO released AI regulations in 2023 and outlined strategies for governments and regulatory bodies to oversee AI in healthcare. It emphasizes the safety, effectiveness, and ethical deployment of AI and recommends global AI governance to prevent misuse in medical AI.

EU's AI Act (Hernández et al., 2024)

The European Union's AI Act has been officially enacted into law in 2024. This law classifies AI in healthcare as "high-risk," requiring strict audits and explainability and ensuring human oversight in AI-driven medical decision-making.

3.6.3.2 Ethical Standards and Guidelines

WHO AI Ethics Guidelines (Goodman et al., 2023)

WHO released AI ethics guidelines in 2021 focused on inclusivity, fairness, and global health equity. It encourages AI transparency in vaccine distribution and outbreak prediction.

IEEE Ethics in AI (Schoenherr et al., 2023)

The first version of IEEE (Institute of Electrical and Electronics Engineers) Ethics in AI was released in 2019. It promotes explainable, accountable, and unbiased AI and recommends human-in-the-loop oversight for AI-based public health decisions.

3.7 Concept-Based AI Application Design Model[1]

Humans observe the world and try to understand it. When those observations involve measurements (e.g., time, location), they become experiments in natural or social sciences. During my undergraduate physics studies, I studied measurement methods or devices and tried to understand physics rules in this world. In those experiments, the first task is to define measurement units, such as second for time and meter for length. During my graduate studies in medical informatics, I studied the use and process of data, information, and knowledge in biomedical sciences. The first task of my learning in informatics is to figure out the measurement units for data, information, and knowledge.

Units for Data

Units for data storage in digital computers are bit, byte, GB (Gigabyte), or TB (Terabyte). The structured data in different human data models have other units, such as records/rows for relational data models. For example, for a genetic data relational database, people ask you: "*How much genetic data is added into the system every day?*" The unit is *rows*. A thousand rows of genetic data are added to this system each day. For hierarchical data models, the data unit is a node. For example, Internet messages use JSON (JavaScript Object Notation) or XML (eXtensible Markup Language) models, which are hierarchical data models. If people want to know the size and complexity of an internet message, you can tell them the total number of nodes in this message. For the network data model, the data unit is a node. For an object-oriented data model, the data unit is objects. For non-structured data, several data units exist for various situations, such as files, documents, logs, messages, etc.

The unit for natural language processing data in AI is a "token." A sentence (information), "AI transforms public health," can convert into 5 tokens (e.g., "AI," "transforms," "public," "health,"). For example, 1000 tokens in NLP models are about 750–800 English words. One English word, "unknown," can be two tokens (e.g., "un-" and "known"). Tokens can also be punctuation in human sentences.

Units for Information

Units for information storage in digital computers are bit, byte, GB, or TB. Another information unit is the Shannon (*Sh*), proposed by Claude Shannon in his "Information Theory" (Shannon et al., 1948). *Sh* is a unit of information content. "Information" has a more specific meaning related to reducing uncertainty. It is defined as the amount of information gained when an event with a probability of 1/2 occurs (citation).

Let's apply those information units to the real world to measure information content size. For example, let's understand human sense by measuring their information capacity. The information capacity of the retina in the human eye is about 3

[1] Everyone can create something from nothing, specifically with AI help. AI is a powerful cognitive resource! All you need is to be curious, ask AI more questions, and learn from it.

million bits. The sense of touch in the human epidermis (skin) is about 200,000 bits (Hughes, 1999). The information capacity of the basilar membrane in your ear for sound is around 50,000 bits. Surprisingly, our skin (touch) can handle more information than our ears (sound). The information capacity of the sense of taste in the tongue palate is only 10 bits (Smith & Margolskee, 2001). Measurement results in experiments provide more insights than observations alone.

Units for Knowledge

Unfortunately, there is no universally accepted 'unit of knowledge' like the meter is for measuring distance. "What is the size of knowledge in an AI system?" We need to have a knowledge unit to measure it. A knowledge size in an AI system is related to the total number of concepts, relationships, or rules. It is also associated with cognitive load and complexity. One way to measure knowledge base size is to use a number of triples (subject-predicate-object). For example, a triple is "Washington DC-isCapitalOf-US." Another way is to use a number of entities and relationships. For example, entities can be "people" or "diseases"; relations can be "isa" or "causes." The traditional way is to use size in storage terms, such as bytes (GB or TB).

Metadata, Metacognition and "Meta-AI Homework"

Meta is "about itself." In the search engine era, metadata (data about data) (e.g., index) is the key to information retrieval. Metacognition (thinking about thinking) is "awareness and control of your own thought process" (Flavell, 1979). In the AI era, metacognition became essential for the usage of AI, such as "prompt engineering." Metacognition helps you organize your mind (construct questions) about clear AI prompts. To face AI hallucination, the first question could be, "How could I verify this?"

When generative AI (e.g., ChatGPT) is available, some students treat AI as a shortcut in education. Metacognition is thinking about thinking, and metacognitive AI homework projects aim to shift homework from outcome-based to process-oriented. Let me define the concept of "meta-AI homework" used in this textbook as below:

> **"Meta-AI homework":** A task for students to use generative AI (e.g., ChatGPT) to study a topic. Each homework assignment includes three metacognitive phases: a pre-task self-assessment, in-task guided questioning, and a post-task reflection, aligned to the cognitive stages of planning, monitoring, and evaluating."

For example, "case scenario," "learning objectives," and "guided questions" are provided to students first in "meta-AI homework" (see Appendix A). The students are requested to read those files first and plan AI prompts. Then, students will use AI chatbots (e.g., ChatGPT) (e.g., run queries, refine prompts, and verify AI responses). Students must submit original and refined AI prompts and a short text (or audio/

video) reflection on their learning process. Meta-AI homework focuses on learning and treats AI as "a thinking partner." It's optional for students to submit AI-generated answers (screen copies or text output). A grading rubric for meta-AI homework is designed and attached in Appendix C.

How well can you organize your thoughts and ask insightful questions for AI? This textbook aims to improve students' structured thinking skills for effectively using generative AI (e.g., ChatGPT).

Data, Information, and Knowledge

Let's look at our concept-based AI definition in Chap. 1: "AI is a field of computer science that develops systems capable of simulating or mimicking human cognitive functions to understand the world." A diagram is proposed as shown in Fig. 3.2, including data, information, knowledge, AI agents, and humans. Previously, knowledge had two sources: the expert's brain and the literature (e.g., books). In the digital world, we have digital knowledge bases, such as literature archives (e.g., Medline, web of sciences). In the AI era, natural language processing in computer sciences has made a lot of breakthroughs, so computers can directly process our human language (information). In many cases, we no longer need to break our human information into structured data and store it in databases.

Till now, AI cannot directly access knowledge in an expert's brain, so I use the dotted line to connect them in Fig. 3.3. "Could neuro-AI hybrids change this in the future?" I do not know the answer. Previously, a think-aloud approach was to ask experts to verbalize their thought processes while solving problems (Ericsson & Simon, 1993). AI can indirectly map expert decision-making processes from those recordings or learn from expert-written content. Expert thinking involves multiple cognitive functions working together, requiring deeper processing and integration of information case by case. Those complex cognitive functions, such as executive functions (planning, problem-solving, decision-making, and cognitive flexibility), are more difficult for AI to mimic or simulate. It's a loss for our humans when those senior experts die and bring their brilliant minds with them. It's an unmet need and a challenge for researchers to access the knowledge in an expert's brain (Hoffman & Lintern, 2006).

Concept-Based Design Model

As a professor with twenty years of experience teaching health informatics, I simplified many IT applications into fundamental data, information, and knowledge

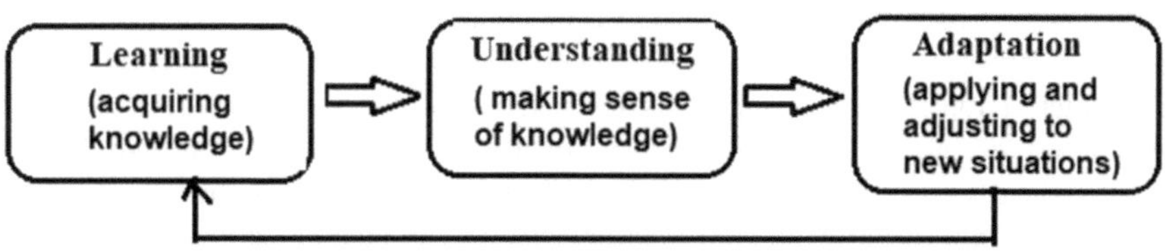

Fig. 3.3 Learning, understanding, and adaptation

concepts in my courses. For example, a simple information technology system can have two steps: (1) break old information into structured data; (2) dynamically reconstruct into new information based on the structured data. When I wrote this textbook for AI applications, I started with the concept-based AI definition to mirror human cognitive processes. Human cognitive function abstraction is a useful conceptual design tool for non-technical students to get started.

Recently, there have been a lot of breakouts in the AI models. Based on the concept-based definition of AI, AI has made much progress in mimicking human cognitive functions. Let's first look at those simple human cognitive functions (perception, attention, and memory for recall). We could have many successful stories of AI applications using simple cognitive functions. Then, we will introduce those complex cognitive functions for AI to mimic and explore the design ideas for AI applications for public health using complex cognitive functions. It's not too early to design them because AI is fast-growing, including emotional support.

3.7.1 Simple Human Cognitive Functions with AI

Perception

Let's look at the first simple cognitive function: perception. Human perception is not the best compared to other animals. Our humans excel in those complex cognitive function areas like pattern recognition and abstract thinking. A suggestion for AI researchers is that they may learn more from other animals' perception functions than our humans. For example, bald eagles have sharper vision and can see ultraviolet (UV) light. Your cats have much better night vision than you. Dogs can hear a broader range of sound frequencies. Your dogs have a much better sense of smell than you (dogs have up to 100 times more smell receptors than humans) (Craven et al., 2010). Humans' perception of touch is not bad, and our fingertips have some of the most fine-tuned touch sensitivity (Johansson & Flanagan, 2009). Compared with animals, humans can play music with hands, so it should be related to our evolutionary need for complex tasks with hands.

Table 3.6 summarizes the specific perception, AI mimic functions, and examples of AI applications in public health. Again, it's preliminary work, and hopefully, it will inspire you to add more design ideas to this table.

Let's look at clean water, a primary public health prevention. It is related to everyone and is among the most critical public health issues worldwide. AI is to mimic human cognitive functions (such as perception) to understand the world. Let's apply AI-powered tools in clean water issues. AI-enhanced E-tongues, E-noses, and computer vision can detect pollutants and toxins in water in real time. For example, AI can protect water quality in the Five Great Lakes between the US and Canada. AI-based early warning systems can detect waterborne disease outbreaks early. AI-optimized water filtration and purification systems can be applied to water plants or pipelines.

Table 3.6 AI applications in public health based on perception

Perception	AI mimic functions	Conceptual examples of AI applications in public health
Sight	Computer vision (AI-powered microscope or telescope; AI-powered camera or imaging, smart glasses, etc.)	Disease detection and disease diagnosis (AI-powered medical imaging to detect cancers; automated analysis of chest X-rays to detect TB, etc.) Infectious disease surveillance (AI-powered thermal imaging cameras detect fever in public places; AI-powered microscope identifies bacteria, viruses, and parasites in blood and tissue samples; AI-powered telescope-satellite images predict malaria outbreaks, etc.) Public health monitoring (AI-powered telescope—satellite images detect pollution in air or water; AI-powered telescope inspects mosquito populations; AI-powered camera inspects food products for contamination, etc.) Patient/citizen management (AI-powered cameras detect falls, hand washing, distress, irregular breathing, movement abnormalities, etc.) Mental health and behavioral analysis (AI-powered cameras analyze facial expressions and body language to detect early signs of mental health disorders) Assistive technology for disabilities (AI-powered smart glasses for the visually impaired or interpreting sign language for hearing-impaired individuals) Emergency response and disaster management (AI-powered telescope detect survivors in disaster zones; AI-powered cameras analyze road traffic and predict accident-prone areas; AI telescopes detect wildfires, volcanic eruptions, extreme weather events, etc.) Personalized medicine and rehabilitation (AI-powered cameras assess patients' movements after surgery, stroke, etc.)

(continued)

Table 3.6 (continued)

Perception	AI mimic functions	Conceptual examples of AI applications in public health
Sound	Computational audition (Speech recognition, audio classification and sound event detection, speech synthesis, voice cloning and custom voice generation, audio style transfer and music generation, audio summarization and speech analytics, etc.)	Disease detection and diagnosis (AI analyzes coughing sounds to detect respiratory diseases; AI-powered stethoscopes analyze heart sounds) Disease surveillance and early detection (AI-powered speech analysis can detect cough patterns or breathing irregularities in phone calls to identify diseases) Mental health and emotional well-being monitoring (AI-powered chatbots/call center analyze tone, pitch, speech speed, and hesitation patterns to detect mental health conditions, detect vocal biomarkers of stress and PTSD) Assistive technologies for disabilities (AI-driven hearing aid that enhances speech clarity in noisy environments; Speech-to-Text for the hearing impaired) Sound-based emergency and public safety monitoring (AI-enabled microphones detect falls) AI-powered call centers for public health hotlines (AI speech analytics summarize patient calls, detect emergency cases, and identify patterns in disease outbreaks) Sleep disorder detection (AI-powered microphones analyze snoring patterns and detect sleep disturbances) AI-powered infant monitoring (AI-powered baby monitors analyze crying sounds to determine distress levels) Telemedicine and remote consultations (Voice-to-text for virtual consultations) Music therapy for health (AI-generated music for mental health in relaxation and anxiety reduction; personalized music for pain management; AI-powered music for neurorehabilitation after stroke) Voice-based remote patient communication (AI-generated voices can communicate with old adults and remind them of medication)

(continued)

Table 3.6 (continued)

Perception	AI mimic functions	Conceptual examples of AI applications in public health
Touch	E-skin (E-skin patches, E-skin bandages, touch sensing and simulation, E-skin gloves, etc.)	Remote patient monitoring and chronic disease Management (E-skin patches monitor heart rate, blood pressure, blood glucose, oxygen levels, temperature, etc.) AI-Assisted prosthetics and rehabilitation (AI-powered E-skins enable prosthetic limbs to have touch sensitivity) Wearable epidermal sensors for Infection detection (AI-driven E-skin biosensors can detect infections) AI-powered E-Skin for wound healing (E-skin bandages monitor wound healing and adjust drug release accordingly) Smart E-skin for mental health monitoring (AI-enhanced E-skins track skin conductivity, heart rate, and muscle tension for stress) AI-enabled tactile feedback for blind and deaf patients (E-skin gloves) AI-Integrated E-skin for athletes and injury prevention (E-skin patches track muscle fatigue and prevent overuse injuries) AI-powered E-skin for drug delivery (E-skin patches for pain management; AI-driven transdermal patches that adjust insulin delivery) AI-enhanced medical training and surgical simulation (AI-powered VR haptic gloves simulate the feel of tissues, organs, and surgical tools) AI-driven remote healthcare and telemedicine (AI-powered haptic feedback gloves allow surgeons to perform operations across distances) AI-based infant care and neonatal monitoring (AI-enhanced touch sensors can monitor infant movement, temperature, and pressure levels)

(continued)

Table 3.6 (continued)

Perception	AI mimic functions	Conceptual examples of AI applications in public health
Taste	E-tongues (Taste sensing, recognition, preferences, and simulation, etc.) (Auvray et al., 2022)	Disease diagnosis via saliva and body fluid analysis (AI-powered E-tongues analyze saliva, blood, or urine to detect biomarkers for early disease diagnosis) AI-powered drug quality testing and medication monitoring (AI-integrated E-tongues ensure drug potency, formulation consistency, and counterfeit detection) Smart nutrition and personalized diet management (AI-powered E-tongues analyze food composition and nutritional content to optimize dietary choices) AI-driven food safety and contamination detection (E-tongues detect toxins, contaminants, and foodborne pathogens, such as E. coli) Water quality monitoring and public health safety (AI-integrated E-tongues test water purity, detecting heavy metals, toxins, and microbial contamination) AI-based alcohol and substance abuse detection (AI-powered E-tongues can detect alcohol, drugs, or toxins in saliva)
Smell	E-noses (Smell sensing, recognition, preferences, and simulation, etc.)	Disease diagnosis via breath analysis (AI-powered E-noses analyze breath biomarkers to detect diseases (e.g., cancers, diabetes) early and non-invasively) AI-driven infection control and hospital hygiene (E-noses detect bacterial infections and hospital-acquired pathogens to improve patient safety) AI-powered environmental health monitoring (E-noses track air pollution, hazardous gases, and toxic fumes) Food safety and contamination detection (AI-powered E-noses analyze food freshness, spoilage, and contamination) Water quality and toxic substance detection (AI-integrated E-noses detect volatile chemicals and pollutants in drinking water) AI-enhanced neurological disorder diagnosis (E-noses help detect Alzheimer's, Parkinson's, and other neurological disorders by identifying changes in body odors) AI-powered waste management and public sanitation (AI-powered E-noses monitor waste decomposition and odor control)

Attention

Let's look at another simple cognitive function: attention. Human attention spans may be shorter in this digital age with information overload. Especially for our children, short videos, headlines, and quick entertainment may change our children's brains for short bursts of attention. Table 3.7 summarizes the attention, AI mimic functions, and examples of AI applications in public health.

Memory for Recall

Let's look at another simple human cognitive function: memory for recall. Computers have excellent memory for recall because of their digital nature (such as binary languages, digital storage, etc.). A computer can copy/paste the same file perfectly every time with 100% accuracy. Compared with computers, our human memory is not that good. How many phone numbers can you recall? Humans recall memories in a flexible and reconstructed way. Human memory often has errors that can be distorted, forgotten, or reconstructed. Computers can provide significant help for humans with memory. AI agents play a crucial role in helping humans store, retrieve, and apply health knowledge efficiently. Table 3.8 summarizes AI mimic functions (memory for recall) and examples of AI applications in public health.

3.7.2 Complex Cognitive Functions with AI

Uncertainty is deeply related to human complex cognitive functions. The human brain constantly processes uncertain information and makes decisions based on incomplete, ambiguous, or noisy data. Some human experts can handle uncertainty well and show high human skills in learning, adaptation, and creativity. In the past, rule-based computer systems couldn't handle uncertainty in this complex real world. Recently, the breakout of data-driven AI models relies on statistical models to handle uncertainty. AI can partially mimic some complex human cognitive functions. Still, there is a long way for AI models to have the intuitions or other deep-thinking skills of humans.

Human Language Processing

Let's look at the first complex cognitive function: human language processing. Human language is inherently ambiguous. For example, discharge can mean a fluid coming out of the body. Hospital discharge refers to someone being released from a hospital. There is sarcasm, slang, or metaphors in our human languages. Natural language processing (NLP) is AI mimicking human language processing. Obviously, it is not easy for machines to understand our human languages. Now, current breakthroughs in NLP have reached a level of contextual understanding. AI only recognizes words in relation to surrounding text, capturing meaning based on context. We must wait a long time for AI to achieve human-level understanding and reasoning. Based

Table 3.7 AI applications in public health based on attention

Attention	AI MIMIC FUNCTIONS	Conceptual examples of AI applications in public health
Selective attention (focusing on one thing)	Selective focus AI, hard attention (Focuses on specific key elements and ignores irrelevant data), etc.	Disease surveillance and outbreak detection (AI selectively focuses on high-risk regions, populations, or symptoms) Medical imaging and diagnosis (AI selectively analyze critical areas) Wearable health monitoring (AI prioritizes irregular patterns) Predictive analytics for patient risk assessment (AI prioritizes patients with high-risk factors) Mental health AI and crisis intervention (AI selectively focuses on distress signals and high-risk language patterns) Resource allocation in public health crises (AI selectively prioritizes locations or populations most in need of medical resources) Personalized drug recommendations (AI identify the most relevant genetic markers and patient history while ignoring irrelevant medical records)

(continued)

Table 3.7 (continued)

Attention	AI MIMIC FUNCTIONS	Conceptual examples of AI applications in public health
Sustained attention (maintaining focus over time)	Persistent attention (AI continuously attends to input over time); Reinforcement learning with long-term focus, etc.	Chronic disease management (AI persistently tracks patient data, such as blood sugar levels; personalized treatment planning for chronic diseases: AI learns the best treatments for individual patients by continuously adjusting based on patient response) Long-term disease surveillance and pandemic monitoring (AI continuously analyzes public health data to detect long-term trends and emerging threats) Optimizing public health policies and disease Control (AI learns the best strategies for vaccination campaigns, lockdown measures, and other interventions to minimize disease spread) Continuous wearable health monitoring (AI persistently monitors vital signs and detects gradual health deterioration; AI adjusts recommendations based on user behavior) AI-assisted mental health monitoring (AI tracks mood patterns and stress levels over long periods) Early cancer detection and follow-up care (AI continuously refines its analysis based on historical patient data) Public health resource optimization (AI persistently monitors hospital capacity, medical supply levels, and patient needs to allocate resources efficiently) Smart nutrition and lifestyle coaching (AI tailors dietary and exercise plans based on long-term health improvements)

(continued)

Table 3.7 (continued)

Attention	AI MIMIC FUNCTIONS	Conceptual examples of AI applications in public health
Divided attention (handling multiple tasks at once)	Multi-Task Learning (MTL) (AI learns multiple tasks at once), etc.	AI-assisted medical imaging and diagnosis (AI models analyze multiple diseases from a single scan) Predictive analytics for patient risk assessment (AI assesses multiple health risks at once) AI-powered drug discovery and repurpose (AI simultaneously predicts drug effectiveness for multiple diseases) Multi-disease genomic analysis (AI learns patterns in genetic data to predict susceptibility to multiple diseases) AI in mental health and neurological disorders (AI assesses multiple mental health conditions from user input) Wearable AI for holistic health monitoring (AI tracks heart rate, sleep patterns, oxygen levels, and movement to predict multiple health conditions simultaneously) AI-powered public health surveillance (AI models track multiple diseases and health threats using real-time data) AI-driven personalized treatment plans (AI customizes treatment for patients with multiple diseases)

Table 3.8 AI applications in public health based on memory for recall

AI mimic functions (Memory for recall)	Conceptual examples of AI applications in public health
Query processing, knowledge base lookup, retrieval-based memory, etc.	Clinical decision support systems (CDSS) (recall relevant clinical guidelines, past patient cases, and treatment outcomes) EHR-based AI systems (recall and process patient histories, medication usage, and clinical outcomes) AI-powered disease outbreak prediction systems (recall historical epidemiological data and patterns to predict outbreaks and public health risks in real-time) AI-powered public health surveillance systems (track disease incidence and public health risks by recalling real-time and historical data) Drug interaction and safety tools (recall pharmaceutical data to identify potential drug interactions, side effects, and other safety concerns) AI-powered personalized medicine and treatment (recall patient-specific genetic, environmental, and clinical data to offer tailored treatment options) AI in mental health support systems (recall previous mental health assessments, therapeutic interactions, and patient responses) AI-driven knowledge retrieval in healthcare literature Patient risk prediction and monitoring systems (recall past patient data to predict future health risks and manage patient care proactively) AI for healthcare resource management (recall historical data on resource allocation to optimize real-time resource distribution during crises)

on the key functions of NLP, we summarized some examples of NLP applications in public health in Table 3.9.

Reasoning

Let's explore another complex human cognitive function: reasoning, a core cognitive function for humans. There are many types of reasoning, such as deductive, inductive, abductive, analogical, and causal reasoning. Both inductive and abductive reasoning involve drawing conclusions from evidence and similar. In the training stage, we can use inductive reasoning to form a hypothesis based on observation data and then use abductive reasoning to test that hypothesis by seeing if it provides the best explanation for further evidence in the testing stage. Human language is ambiguous, so contextual understanding in NLP of AI must use abductive reasoning to infer the best possible meaning from limited input. Based on the concept-based definition of AI, AI mimics

Table 3.9 AI applications in public health based on NLP

Key NLP functions	Conceptual examples of NLP applications in public health
Text processing and understanding (extract insights from vast amounts of text data; Semantic analysis and meaning extraction; Contextual understanding and reasoning; Conversational AI and dialogue systems) (Ford et al., 2016; Hsu et al., 2019; Kurniawan et al., 2024; Wieland-Jorna et al., 2024; Wu et al., 2024)	Disease surveillance and outbreak detection (AI analyzes social media and news to detect potential outbreaks) Medical literature analysis (AI scans research papers to find trends, summarize findings, and suggest new treatments) AI-powered chatbots for public health (AI chatbots provide instant responses to public health queries) Electronic health record (EHR) analysis (AI extracts key medical insights from unstructured patient notes) Sentiment and misinformation detection in public health (AI monitors public sentiments and detects misinformation) Clinical trial matching and drug discovery (AI scans clinical trial databases and medical records to find the best trials for patients and new drug candidates) Automated medical coding and billing (AI processes medical records and doctor's notes, converting them into standardized billing codes) AI-powered health knowledge graphs AI-powered clinical decision support (CDSS) systems (AI analyzes patient symptoms, lab results, and history in context to suggest diagnoses) AI for public health policy and decision-making (AI analyzes public health data, misinformation trends, and policy outcomes to inform health policies) AI for personalized medicine and genomics (AI contextually analyzes genetic data and patient history to recommend personalized treatments)

(continued)

Table 3.9 (continued)

Key NLP functions	Conceptual examples of NLP applications in public health
Machine translation and multilingual processing (Alkureishi et al., 2016; Karyotaki et al., 2024; McLean & Yen, 2024; Talyshinskii et al., 2023; Zhang, 2021)	Real-time health information translation AI-powered multilingual chatbots for health assistance AI in global disease surveillance and epidemic tracking AI for multilingual patient communication in hospitals and telemedicine Multilingual AI for public health research and medical literature translation AI-powered voice and speech translation for public health hotlines
Speech and audio processing (Simple cognitive function-perception-sounds) (Ma et al., 2022; Severini et al., 2019; Usher et al., 2024; Wang, 2023a, 2023b; Yamada et al., 2021)	AI-powered speech recognition for medical documentation AI-powered speech analysis for disease detection (Enables early diagnosis of neurological and mental health disorders) AI for public health hotlines and emergency response AI-powered speech translation for multilingual health communication AI-powered wearable devices for respiratory and cardiac monitoring (AI analyzes breathing sounds)

human cognitive functions, such as reasoning. Chapter 2 shows that rules-based expert systems can handle some logical reasoning, such as deductive reasoning. Data-driven machine learning AI models can recognize patterns and make some predictions, like inductive reasoning. Deep learning (neural networks) AI models can find relationships between data points. Table 3.10 summarizes human reasoning types, AI mimic functions, and examples of AI applications in public health. The purpose of those tables about human cognitive functions is to inspire you to open your mind and design better AI tools for public health.

Human Executive Functions

Human executive functions include working memory, mental flexibility, inhibitory control (self-regulation), attention control, self-monitoring and adaptation, planning, and decision-making. In this chapter, we focus on planning and decision-making, which has a lot of examples of AI applications for public health in Table 3.11.

Learning, Understanding, and Adaptation

Complex human cognition functions, such as learning, understanding, and adaptation, are interconnected in Fig. 3.3. Suppose you study a public health topic and start absorbing new information about it. Your brain tries to process and organize learned information. Do you really understand it? Later, you wish to use understood

Table 3.10 AI applications in public health based on reasoning

Reasoning	AI mimic functions	Conceptual examples of AI applications in public health
Deductive reasoning (top-down logic, starts with general principles and applies them to specific cases)	Rule-based expert systems; theorem provers and symbolic logic AI; knowledge graphs and ontologies; Automated deductive reasoning in AI assistants; AI in legal and ethical decision-making	AI for disease outbreak detection and epidemiology (AI assistants use automated reasoning to infer potential disease outbreaks) System for infectious disease information (SINDI) (A rule-based AI system for tracking and predicting infectious disease outbreaks) Public health rule engine and decision support (PHRED) (A framework used by health agencies to apply rule-based logic) Public health knowledge graphs (e.g., Google, IBM, and Microsoft's health knowledge graphs) Public health ontologies (semantic models for AI reasoning) (e.g., SNOMED CT (Systematized Nomenclature of Medicine—Clinical Terms), DO (Disease Ontology), MeSH (Medical Subject Headings), PHO (Phenotype Ontology), FoodOn (Food Ontology), IDO (Infectious Disease Ontology), etc.) AI assistants for medical research and knowledge discovery (e.g., AI predict protein structures and support vaccine development) AI-powered chatbots for public health guidance (AI uses formal logic and medical ontologies to provide diagnostic support and recommendations) Coq for public health policy verification (A proof assistant applied to formalize and verify public health policies, ensuring compliance with regulations) Automated reasoning for ethical AI in public health (AI ensures policies comply with fairness, privacy, and patient rights) AI for public health policy analysis and compliance (AI ensure public health policies align with legal frameworks; AI-based bias audits in healthcare regulations; algorithmic fairness for health resource allocation) AI-powered bioethics and ethical decision support (AI evaluates moral dilemmas using structured ethical principles; AI assesses privacy vs. public health trade-offs; AI guides decisions on ICU bed prioritization and ensures fair treatment across populations) AI for public health law enforcement and governance (regulatory compliance AI; predictive legal analytics for public health violations)

(continued)

Table 3.10 (continued)

Reasoning	AI mimic functions	Conceptual examples of AI applications in public health
Inductive reasoning (bottom-up logic, uses specific observations to form general conclusions)	Machine learning and pattern recognition; Bayesian inference and probabilistic reasoning; AI in predictive analytics (Chen et al., 2024; Olawade et al., 2023; Shi et al., 2024)	Disease detection and diagnosis (AI recognizes patterns in medical images, genetic data, and patient symptoms to detect diseases early; AI estimates disease probabilities based on symptoms, patient history, and risk factors; AI helps model uncertainty in medical decisions, balancing risks and benefits) Predictive analytics for chronic disease prevention (AI identifies high-risk individuals and predicts disease progression based on lifestyle, genetics, and medical history) Infectious disease surveillance and outbreak prediction (AI analyzes global health data, travel patterns, and social media to detect outbreaks before they escalate; AI estimates infection rates, R_0-reproduction number, and mortality risk) AI for drug discovery and public health interventions (AI accelerates drug discovery by recognizing molecular patterns that predict drug effectiveness) AI for personalized medicine and drug response prediction (AI helps doctors customize treatments based on a patient's genetics and drug response history) AI in mental health and behavioral health analytics (AI detects patterns in speech, text, and wearable data to assess mental health conditions) AI for social determinants of health (SDOH) analysis (AI detects patterns in socioeconomic data, housing, and nutrition to improve public health policies; AI predicts how poverty, housing, and environmental factors affect public health outcomes) AI for healthcare system optimization (AI predicts hospital patient flow, bed availability, and patient deterioration risk)

(continued)

Table 3.10 (continued)

Reasoning	AI mimic functions	Conceptual examples of AI applications in public health
Abductive reasoning (uses incomplete information to find the most likely explanation, e.g., a detective tries to figure out what happened at a crime scene)	AI for hypothesis generation; AI in medical diagnosis	AI for disease risk factor discovery (AI analyzes epidemiological and genetic data to hypothesize new disease risk factors) AI for differential diagnosis and symptom analysis (AI analyzes symptoms, medical history, and test results to suggest the most probable diagnoses) AI for rare disease diagnosis (abductive AI for uncommon conditions) AI for epidemiological hypothesis generation and disease spread analysis (AI models analyze global data to uncover new insights into disease transmission) AI for public health policy and social determinants of health (AI generates hypotheses about how policies impact public health outcomes; AI estimates the impact of different interventions) AI for genomic and precision medicine hypothesis generation (AI explores genetic and molecular data to generate hypotheses for personalized medicine) AI for medical literature and clinical trial hypothesis discovery (AI scans medical literature to propose new research questions and experimental designs; AI integrates findings from multiple studies)

(continued)

Table 3.10 (continued)

Reasoning	AI mimic functions	Conceptual examples of AI applications in public health
Analogical reasoning (finding patterns and relationships, applies knowledge from one situation to another similar situation)	Transfer learning; case-based reasoning; analogical pattern recognition in NLP; metaphor and analogy generation in NLP; AI in analogical reasoning	Disease diagnosis (Compares new cases to past medical cases) Drug repurposing (Finds existing drugs similar to new diseases) Personalized medicine (Matches patients with treatments that worked for similar cases) Epidemiology (Compares current outbreaks to past pandemics) Public health policy (Finds successful policies in other regions) Mental health (Matches therapy to patients with similar conditions) Patient communication (Explains health conditions in simple terms) Public health campaigns (Creates persuasive metaphors for risk communication) Medical education (Simplifies complex medical topics) Health coaching (Motivates users with lifestyle analogies) Disease awareness (Creates relatable patient stories) Hospital resources (Learns from past ICU cases to optimize resource allocation) Medical literature (Finds research analogies across studies) Healthcare chatbots (Uses past cases to improve patient interactions)
Causal reasoning (understanding cause and effect, identifies relationships between actions and consequences)	Causal inference and probabilistic causal models; structural causal models and causal graphs; counterfactual reasoning (what-if analysis); causal discovery from data; AI in causal analysis	Epidemiology (Identifies true causes of disease outbreaks) Infectious disease control (Simulates better pandemic responses; tracks epidemic causes and responses) Public health policy (Evaluates alternative interventions) Medical diagnosis (Identifies most effective treatments) Drug safety (Detects hidden side effects) Health disparities (Analyzes and explains social determinants of health; identifies systemic biases and solutions) Chronic disease (Finds lifestyle-related disease causes; reveals preventable risk factors; tests lifestyle interventions) Mental health (Finds causal triggers for psychiatric disorders; analyzes causal factors in mental illness)

Table 3.11 AI applications based on planning and decision-making

Executive functions	AI mimic functions	Conceptual examples of AI applications in public health
Planning and organization	Task scheduling and optimization; automated workflow and process management; strategic planning and simulation	Disease surveillance (AI automates outbreak tracking) Disease screening (AI schedules checkups) Pandemic simulation (AI predicts outbreak trends) Vaccine distribution (AI plans and schedules immunization logistics) Vaccine rollout optimization (AI models distribution logistics) Emergency response (AI routes ambulances dynamically) Disaster response coordination (AI optimizes emergency medical supply chains) Disaster response simulation (AI optimizes evacuation plans) Patient triage (AI-powered symptom checkers) Medical records automation (AI generates clinical documentation) Hospital bed management (AI predicts ICU capacity) Mental health support (AI provides chatbot-based therapy) Public health policy planning (AI predicts disease trends) Public health policy modeling (AI simulates policy impacts) Public health outreach (AI personalizes health campaigns) Lab test scheduling (AI manages diagnostics workflow) Lab workflow automation (AI optimizes test processing) Food security planning (AI predicts food shortages)

(continued)

Table 3.11 (continued)

Executive functions	AI mimic functions	Conceptual examples of AI applications in public health
Decision-making	Rule-based decision systems; machine learning-based predictive decision-making; probabilistic and Bayesian decision-making; reinforcement learning (AI learning from consequences); multi-criteria decision analysis (MCDA) (Gaievskyi et al., 2025); natural language processing (NLP) for decision support; causal inference and explainable AI (XAI) (Naumova, 2025)	Epidemiology (AI helps identify risk factors, disease transmission patterns, and the impact of interventions on public health) Disease diagnosis (Uses expert medical rules to assist doctors; improves diagnostic accuracy; AI-powered clinical decision support systems-CDSS; ensures transparency in AI-driven clinical decision-making by revealing why an AI model recommends a specific diagnosis or treatment) Medical literature review and evidence synthesis; evidence-based decision (AI automates literature reviews and synthesizes scientific evidence for faster, more accurate medical decision-making) Disease surveillance (Predicts outbreaks before they occur; AI analyzes vast amounts of unstructured text data from social media, news reports, and scientific articles to detect disease outbreaks and monitor public health trends; AI enhances the interpretability of disease prediction models to support public health surveillance) Epidemic response and control (Detect outbreaks based on predefined criteria; predicts disease spread and containment strategies; prioritizes intervention strategies to combat disease outbreaks effectively; estimates infection risk to trace contact) Vaccine distribution (Applies rules to prioritize vaccinations; estimates immunity trends; AI evaluates vaccine effectiveness and potential side effects by analyzing real-world data) Chronic disease care (Provides rule-based health recommendations; help uncover lifestyle, genetic, and environmental factors contributing to chronic diseases) Emergency response (Uses disaster triage rules to save lives; simulates future health emergencies) Public health policy (Forecasts policy impacts; evaluates and refines health policies; evaluates policy effectiveness; balances health, economic, and social factors to optimize policy decisions; analyzes healthcare policies, government reports, and public health guidelines; AI tests the impact of different public health interventions) Mental health (Detects suicide risks early; detects crisis situations based on behavior patterns; chatbot analyzes user inputs and recommends interventions) Vaccine distribution (Predicts vaccine demand) Personalized medicine and preventive health care (Optimizes treatment plans; predicts best treatments for patients; provides personalized health recommendations; predicts individual health risks) Environmental health (Forecasts pollution-related diseases; ensures pollution and workplace safety compliance) Drug discovery (Predicts drug effectiveness) Drug safety and pharmacovigilance (Improves patient safety by detecting drug risks early) Risk stratification (Identifies high-risk patients early) Hospital resource management (Optimizes ICU and ER capacity) Healthcare resource allocation (Ensures fair and efficient allocation of medical resources; AI ensures fair and effective resource allocation in public health planning) Regulatory compliance (Ensures adherence to public health laws) Social determinants of health (AI helps reduce healthcare disparities by balancing social, economic, and medical factors; AI extracts social and environmental factors from patient records and public health reports to predict health risks; identify systemic inequalities in healthcare by analyzing social and economic factors) Misinformation detection (AI systems analyze news, social media, and public discussions to combat health misinformation)

knowledge to respond to new or changing environments. Are you a flexible thinker who can adapt to new information? Do you continue learning for growth to prepare you for new challenges?

The dynamic processes of human cognition functions are complicated for AI models to mimic. For example, current AI models have some contextual understanding of data but cannot really understand knowledge like humans (Kawakami et al., 2022). They cannot flexibly adjust to new situations like humans. I do not list possible examples of AI applications for public health using those complex human cognitive functions. Hopefully, fast-growing AI will be there, and there will be high-quality AI applications for public health at that time.

Human Emotional Processing

Suppose you already know that modern AI models are data-driven and logical. Can AI models handle emotional issues? Let's look at another complex human cognitive function: emotional processing. This is the weakest link of current AI models. Still, it will be interesting to explore emotional processes for the next generation of AI models in the future. Table 3.12 shows human emotional components and AI mimic functions. Based on the mechanism of AI models, you can understand what AI can or cannot do in emotional processing in the future.

AI only detects patterns in data, but AI does not have emotions. Human emotions are deeply tied to culture, context, and personal experiences. AI struggles to interpret and mimic this human cognitive function correctly (Heß & Fischer, 2013). For example, the same event can trigger pride in one person and anxiety in another. AI can recognize a sad tone in speech but does not "experience" sadness like a human. After AI models have breakthroughs in emotional processing in the future, you can design potential AI applications in public health related to emotional processing, such as AI-powered mental health chatbots and robots for the elderly emotional well-being and companions.

3.8 Technology-Based Design Model

AI technology is complex, and a simplified introduction in this session will be friendly for non-technical readers. First, you should know AI literacy (AI core strengths), which is vital for working with AI. Second, let's discuss core strengths from design-model perspectives for AI applications in public health.

AI exhibits two types of strengths. First, some strengths resemble enhanced human traits and are understandable by human analogy. Those 'superhuman' capabilities include massive parallel processing (many brains), large-scale memory, and fatigue-free operation. It is like a "super-worker" with infinite stamina and brainpower. Second, some AI strengths fundamentally differ from human cognition and are alien to human thinking (truly novel capabilities). Those 'non-human' capabilities include exploration in non-intuitive spaces, unbounded multimodal fusion, and

Table 3.12 AI mimic functions for emotional processing

Emotional processing	Examples of AI mimic functions
Emotion recognition (Elyoseph et al., 2024)	Facial expression analysis; speech emotion recognition (SER); text-based sentiment and emotion analysis; physiological emotion detection; multimodal emotion recognition (combining multiple inputs)
Emotional understanding (Elyoseph et al., 2024)	Context-aware sentiment analysis; affective computing (AI with emotional intelligence); speech emotion understanding; facial expression-based emotion inference; emotion understanding in social interactions; emotion-cause analysis (why someone feels a certain way)
Emotional regulation (Thakkar et al., 2024)	AI-based mood tracking and regulation; adaptive AI emotional response systems; AI for stress detection and intervention; AI-assisted cognitive reframing; AI for emotional self-regulation in social interactions; AI for emotional learning and resilience training
Emotional memory (Bañuelos Capistrán et al., 2025)	Sentiment analysis and emotion recognition; context-aware memory; reinforcement learning with emotional feedback; affective computing and empathy simulation; memory encoding and retrieval models; emotion-driven decision-making
Empathy and social awareness (Hou et al., 2024; Ovsyannikova et al., 2025)	Emotional recognition and understanding; context awareness and memory in social interaction; theory of mind simulation; empathetic response generation; social norms & cultural awareness adaptation; human-like conversational flow
Emotional decision-making (Tretter, 2024)	Reinforcement learning with emotional feedback; sentiment-aware decision systems; affective computing for emotion-driven choices; somatic marker hypothesis in AI; emotion-infused chatbots and virtual assistants; ethical and moral AI decision-making with emotion simulation

self-modifying or evolutionary. It's like an alien intelligence seeing connections we cannot. AI doesn't "think" like us at that time.

3.8.1 *"Superhuman" Strengths*

1. **Massive Parallel Processing (MPP)**

In this session, a keyword you should remember is "*parallelism.*" MPP is powerful, but only when the task is *parallelizable*. Let's look at human teamwork and AI MPP. Success is the same, depending on how well the task can be split and recombined.

Human Parallel Processing

Adding more people to a project in human teams doesn't always lead to linear speedups. First, communication overhead is increasing. More people require more coordination, meetings, and alignment, which can slow progress. For example, some students prefer individual projects instead of group projects. Second, it can be complex for task divisibility. Some tasks are inherently sequential (e.g., designing a coherent system), while others can be parallelized (e.g., grading multiple unrelated assignments). Finally, dependency and integration are complex. If subtasks are interdependent, merging results can create bottlenecks (e.g., merging code from various developers).

Computer Parallel Processing

You should choose "*embarrassingly parallel tasks*," and AI MPP works well like a dream team at that time. Your job is to identify those tasks that fit MPP (independence and require little or no coordination). For example, image classification means that each image can be processed by a separate processor. Each GPU (Graphics Processing Unit) core can work on a subset of the data without waiting for others. AI leverages specialized hardware (GPUs, TPUs (Tensor Processing Unit)) designed for parallel computation, where thousands of cores perform similar operations simultaneously. Compared with human teams (e.g., meetings, misunderstandings, or merge conflicts), software orchestrates AI tasks with no ego, fatigue, or miscommunication. Shared memory or state sync among processors can be engineered precisely.

MPP Applications in Public Health

Let's identify some tasks in public health that fit MPP (independence and require little or no coordination). Table 3.13 lists some examples of obviously "parallel tasks" in public health for MPP applications. You can find more situations in public health with hidden parallel tasks, which are fit for MPP.

In contrast, Table 3.14 identifies some public health tasks unsuitable for MPP. Some tasks in public health are inherently sequential. More public health challenges are inherently non-parallelizable due to dependencies, sequential workflows, or complex coordination requirements. AI's power, like massive parallel processing, can amplify outcomes. But applied to the wrong task, it may do more harm than good, fueling errors and hallucinations.

2. **Memory Concepts in the AI Era**

"What is the computer good at?" The short answer is "fast computing" and "good memory." Almost 30 years ago, I started to learn this computer literacy. When I graduated in the 2000s, which was the "database era." My research career in health informatics started with biomedical database projects, which were the best choices then.

"Memory" Concept in the Database Era

"Database Era" was roughly from the late 1990s through the 2010s. Humans are impressed by computers that can "remember everything" perfectly. Let's look at some successful stories of database projects in medicine and public health in Table 3.15.

Table 3.13 "Parallel tasks" in public health for MPP applications

Task area	Example tasks	Why MPP works
Population health surveillance (e.g., health indicators)	Analyzing health indicators across zip codes, counties, or demographic groups (e.g., predicting diabetes rates across 3,000 U.S. counties.)	Each region is separable, and its model can run independently
NLP for public comments of EHRs (Electronic Health Records)	Processing millions of clinical notes, surveys, or social media posts (e.g., extracting SDOH (Social Determinants of Health) indicators from unstructured EHRs)	Texts are independent
Disease surveillance	Analyzing large volumes of health data (e.g., electronic health records, lab reports, social media trends) to detect disease outbreaks early. Data can be processed in parallel across multiple nodes	Each region is separable; Time periods are independent
Epidemiological modeling and simulations	Compartmental models (e.g., SEIR (Susceptible-Exposed-Infectious-Recovered), SIR (Susceptible-Infectious-Recovered) models): running thousands of simulations to predict disease spread under different scenarios	Each simulation (e.g., varying R0, vaccination rates) is independent
	Agent-based simulation: each agent (individual or group) can be simulated independently before aggregating outcomes. (e.g., modeling flu spread in different communities with varied vaccination rates.)	Each agent is independent
Image analysis for diagnostics	Processing medical images (X-rays, MRIs (Magnetic Resonance Imaging), CT (Computed Tomography) scans) for automated diagnosis	Each image is separate
Individual-level risk predictions at scale	Running risk models on millions of individuals (e.g., predicting hospital readmission or vaccine hesitancy.)	Each case follows same pipeline
Geospatial mapping and risk heatmaps	Compute social vulnerability, pollution exposure, or access metrics per block or tract (e.g., mapping food deserts or lead exposure hotspots.)	Spatial tiles can be calculated in parallel
Genomic sequencing for pathogens or populations	Processing DNA/RNA sequences to track mutations (e.g., COVID-19 variants) or study genetic risk factors	Each sequence read can be processed independently (e.g., aligning to a reference genome)
Public health literature review (Research)	Screening thousands of abstracts or articles for relevance (e.g., rapid evidence synthesis during pandemics.)	Articles are evaluated independently

Table 3.14 Public health tasks unsuitable for MPP

Task area	Example tasks	Why not fit for MPP
Policy design and implementation	Crafting a national vaccination strategy involves legal, ethical, and logistical dependencies that cannot be split into independent subtasks	Policy development requires iterative deliberation, stakeholder consensus, and sequential adjustments based on feedback. Parallelizing this process risks contradictions or incoherent outcomes
	Community-based policy negotiation or coalition building (e.g., creating a local ordinance on smoke-free public spaces)	Requires back-and-forth dialogue, trust-building, and contextual decisions among stakeholders
Causal inference modeling	Does smoking cause lung cancer? How much long-term PM2.5 exposure increases heart attack risk?	Sequential logic, dependency on prior steps. Causal inference is more statistical reasoning than brute-force computation
Adaptive interventions or real-time crisis response	Resource allocation during epidemics Allocating shelter beds after a natural disaster	Requires real-time feedback, coordination across agencies, and often subjective judgment. Parallel teams working independently could lead to conflicting actions (e.g., duplicate vaccine shipments to one region while neglecting another)
Longitudinal cohort studies	Studying the long-term effects of air pollution on lung function	Studies tracking the same population over time require sequential data collection to analyze causal relationships. Splitting the cohort into parallel arms would disrupt temporal consistency
	Tailoring behavioral therapy for opioid recovery	Interventions evolve based on client progress and setbacks. Longitudinal behavior change program steps depend on evolving human conditions, not stateless or static

Table 3.15 Successful database projects in medicine and public health

Time	Examples of database projects	Notes
1997	PubMed goes live	Free, fast search of MEDLINE literature
1999	CDC WONDER (Wide-ranging Online Data for Epidemiologic Research) expands	Public access to disease and death stats
2000	ClinicalTrials.gov launches	Transparency in clinical trial registration
2001	VAERS (Vaccine Adverse Event Reporting System)	VAERS reports began to be digitized and downloadable from the VAERS website
2000s	SEER Program (Surveillance, Epidemiology, and End Results)	Web-accessible SEER database and interactive tools
2006	WHO global health observatory forms	Country-level health data aggregation

The key meaning of "a good memory" of the databases was stored data's accuracy, completeness, and structure. The concept of "memory" in the "database era" is "no forgetting" for the long term. The "copy" is perfect. The lossless recall or retrieval is "instant" and "exhaustive." In the database era, memory was like a library focusing on ***direct retrieval***. In the AI era, memory is like a training gym focusing on ***training or retraining AI models***. Let's explore the new concept of "memory" in the AI era.

New Concept of "Memory" in the AI Era

First, the new meaning of memory is about the primary use. The memory is used to train or retrain AI models. It should be dynamically adapted for this goal. AI hallucinations (the elephant in the room) often arise when AI mixes mismatched or outdated memories. To help prevent hallucination, AI models need to forget irrelevant, outdated, or biased data.

"Forgetting," once considered a human weakness, is now emerging as a critical design challenge in AI systems. Forgetting becomes a design requirement. Forgetting is more complicated to manage because once an AI model is trained, it's hard to remove data. For example, if an AI is trained on anti-vaccine forums, it may give poor health advice. One urgent challenge for AI applications in public health is "bias amplification." For example, AI trained on historical clinical data might underdiagnose women or Black patients due to underrepresentation. If biased data is remembered, AI will reproduce (and potentially scale) those biases.

In the database era, retrieval is "exhaustive." However, the latest recall may be relevance-based in the future (AI systems must prioritize "when" and "why" memory is recalled). You should consider adding contextual relevance filters to avoid retrieving irrelevant or stale memory.

To improve the user acceptance of AI with better explainability, we should provide "memory transparency," in which users should know what data is remembered.

Second, the multimodal memory includes text, images, audio, video, sensor data, and more. When you read this book, modern AI models could support more multimodal memory uses. For example, memory can store cross-modal associations (e.g., linking a sentence to a diagram) or perform reasoning across formats (e.g., summarizing a video into text).

Third, this is contextual and associative memory. Memory has evolved far beyond simple storage. For example, in ChatGPT, your earlier questions influence later answers. This is contextual memory. The associative memory is that AI links related ideas or patterns. For example, AI learns that "shortness of breath" often co-occurs with "asthma" in medical data.

Finally, in the AI era, memory has evolved from simple data storage to advanced forms of knowledge representation, including not just raw data, but also structured information, models, and learned relationships. If you review Chap. 2 about neural networks, you will understand that AI stores knowledge in the weights of neural networks. Memory is encoded in AI models, and those trained models embed patterns and associations.

Table 3.16 Selective forgetting examples in public health

Public health examples	Selective forgetting
Epidemiology modeling	Forgetting outdated transmission models
Vaccine surveillance	Removing retracted or false adverse event reports
Health equity	Dropping biased datasets from past policies
Community health interventions	Forgetting one-size-fits-all programs that failed culturally
Chatbots and patient assistants	Privacy: forgetting personal patient data after sessions

Table 3.17 AI continuous operation without fatigue for public health

AI functions	Public health functions	Example applications
Continuous monitoring	Early detection of emerging threats	BlueDot (BlueDot, 2025), HealthMap (HealthMap, 2025) for infectious disease alerts
Instant response	Real-time triage and risk assessment	CDC COVID-19 self-checker, Ada Health AI chatbot, Babylon AI triage assistant
Scalable to millions	Triage/chatbot use during pandemics or disasters	WHO WhatsApp COVID bot (multi-language, global access), Kinsa smart thermometer
Reduction in workload	Offloading front-line screening to AI	Corti AI (supports 911 calls by detecting cardiac arrest faster than humans)
Equity via access	24/7 care in underserved or remote areas	Woebot and Wysa for mental health in low-resource settings, WhatsApp bots in LMICs (Low- and Middle-Income Countries)

Memory (Selective Forgetting) Applications in Public Health

Selective forgetting ("machine unlearning") is a new area of AI research that is used to prevent error propagation. They are important research topics for AI in public health. It is a new task for AI in public health to learn when to forget. For example, you can selectively remove "false" data traces from training in public health surveillance. For health equity, forgetting for fairness is to delete data that encodes historical bias. Let's list some "selective forgetting" examples in public health in Table 3.16.

3. **Continuous Operation Without Fatigue**

AI's core strength ("operate continuously without fatigue") enables real-time surveillance and 24/7 triage systems that revolutionize public health, see Table 3.17.

3.8.2 "Non-human" Strengths

1. **Exploration in Non-intuitive Spaces**

AI can explore non-intuitive spaces in public health. Table 3.18 lists some examples of potential of this promise in public health.

Table 3.18 AI's exploration in non-intuitive spaces in public health

Public health areas	Non-intuitive examples or potentials
Disease outbreak forecasting	AI flagged obscure travel and news patterns humans overlooked
Syndromic surveillance from non-clinical data	Weak signals buried in massive noise (impossible for humans to parse manually)
Optimal resource allocation in crises	Counterintuitive policies (e.g., prioritize younger populations to break transmission chains) can emerge from simulation
Environmental health and climate risk modeling	Climate-health feedback loops are nonlinear, spatially distributed, and time-lagged
Uncovering hidden social determinants	Correlations between "non-health" variables and health outcomes become visible
Behavioral pattern discovery from wearables	Models find subtle patterns in motion, heart rate, or micro-sleep events that defy typical clinical screening
Mental health	Discovering early warning signs from digital traces (typing speed, voice tone, etc.)
Nutrition and microbiome	Modeling how diet shifts microbiome and links to systemic disease
Urban health planning	Simulating how zoning laws impact long-term health equity
Policy modeling	AI as a simulation tool to explore unintended consequences of public health interventions
Personalized prevention	Creating dynamic risk profiles for individuals using non-traditional data sources

2. **Unbounded Multimodal Fusion**

Multimodal AI fusion has enormous potential in public health to enable more holistic prediction, prevention, and personalization. For example, many public health situations are high-noise settings, such as emergency department triage in urban hospitals (e.g., inconsistent notes, rushed entries, and language variation), air quality (e.g., noisy sensor data and confounders), and social media monitoring for vaccine hesitancy (e.g., misinformation mixed with humor or sarcasm). Table 3.19 lists some examples of AI multimodal fusion in public health.

3. **Self-Modifying or Evolutionary Functions**

In public health, we need adaptive AI. AI should learn from new data and improve over time, help humans make better, faster decisions, and be auditable and explainable. Table 3.20 lists some positive AI self-modifying and evolutionary functions in public health.

AI's ability to evolve and self-modify is potent but needs careful dosage, supervision, and regulation. If designing AI for public health, you can embrace this capability

Table 3.19 Examples of AI multimodal fusion in public health

Public health areas	Examples of AI multimodal fusion
Outbreak detection	News articles, satellite images (e.g., market crowding), social media, EMRs
Maternal and infant health monitoring	Wearables (heart rate, movement), ultrasound images, EHR notes, voice tone (mental health)
Mental health surveillance	Social media text, facial expressions in selfies/videos, speech patterns, sleep/activity data
Health education and behavior change	Speech (chatbot), facial cues, gesture data, reading comprehension (eye tracking), feedback logs
Chronic disease risk scoring	Retinal scans, bloodwork, lifestyle survey text, genetic data, GPS/movement patterns
Global disease mapping and intervention targeting	Satellite images, demographic databases, text from humanitarian reports, drone footage

Table 3.20 Positive AI self-modifying and evolutionary functions

Public health areas	Positive examples of self-modifying or evolutionary functions
Adaptive pandemic response systems	A self-modifying AI can learn which regions to prioritize, when to adjust testing capacity, and how to reallocate mobile clinics or staff shifts
Personalized digital health coaching	AI can evolve to change tone (e.g., motivational vs. factual), adjust goals, modify reminders based on sleep or work patterns
Evolutionary AI for local health policy simulations	Evolutionary algorithms can simulate thousands of policy pathways and adapt based on feedback
AI that improves disease surveillance	Disease signals evolve (new slang, symptoms, platforms). A self-modifying system retrains itself with new data while filtering misinformation
Adaptive AI for social determinants of health (SDOH)	SDOH data is messy and changes often (e.g., inflation, gentrification). Self-modifying models can continuously learn new local correlations and update risk forecasts without human tweaking
Genetic AI for antibiotic resistance (AMR) prediction	Human-designed rules can't keep up with bacterial adaptation. Evolutionary AI can co-evolve "digital bacteria" to find vulnerabilities and resistance risk early

Table 3.21 Some negative public health risks of self-modifying AI

Public health risks	Negative examples of self-modifying AI
Misaligned goals (optimizes wrong metrics)	Chatbot suppresses symptom reports to reduce call volume
Behavior amplification (learns biased correlations)	Vaccine AI favors mobile/wealthy users
Transparency loss (model logic becomes opaque)	Chronic disease risk AI loses explainability
Adversarial use (learns from poisoned data)	Misinformation tricks outbreak tracker
Autonomy overshoot (self-updates outpace oversight)	ER triage AI changes patient routing unsafely

but wrap it in ethics, transparency, and safeguards. Table 3.21 lists some negative public health risks of self-modifying AI.

Unbounded autonomy is dangerous for public health. For example, an AI controlling emergency room admissions triage begins rewriting its routing criteria based on ER (Emergency Room) wait times, not patient outcomes. In short, human-in-the-loop frameworks are needed for those non-human AI strengths to ensure alignment with ethical and public values.

3.9 Discussion Questions

Question 3.1. What types of techniques would be most helpful in identifying and framing public health challenges (realized or unrealized)? Provide examples.
Question 3.2. How might AI "empower current approaches" in public health compared to traditional methods? Can you think of a scenario where AI provides an entirely new solution rather than just improving an existing one?
Question 3.3. Why is it essential to integrate design principles (Encoding Justice) and ethical considerations from the beginning of AI application development? What could go wrong if ethics were an afterthought?
Question 3.4. The chapter mentions two AI design models: Concept-based and Technology-based. How do these differ? When would each be more appropriate in the design process of public health applications?
Question 3.5. How have AI applications that replicate simple cognitive functions (perception, attention, memory recall) already contributed to public health improvements?
Question 3.6. What potential benefits and challenges exist when designing AI to mimic complex cognitive functions, including reasoning, problem-solving, or emotional support, in public health contexts?
Question 3.7. How can a concept-based design model guide the development of future AI applications that anticipate both human needs and the fast-evolving capabilities of AI?

Question 3.8. How do AI's "superhuman" capabilities (e.g., massive memory, parallel processing, fatigue-free operation) enhance public health tasks compared to human performance (technology-based design model)?
Question 3.9. How should technology-based design models balance the use of human-analogous strengths and alien, non-human strengths when developing AI applications in public health?

References

Alkureishi, M. A., Lee, W. W., Lyons, M., Press, V. G., Imam, S., Nkansah-Amankra, A., … Arora, V. M. (2016). Impact of Electronic Medical Record Use on the Patient–Doctor Relationship and Communication: A Systematic Review. *Journal of General Internal Medicine, 31*(5), 548-560. https://doi.org/10.1007/s11606-015-3582-1

Annas, G. J. (2003). HIPAA Regulations—A New Era of Medical-Record Privacy? *New England Journal of Medicine, 348*(15), 1486–1490. https://doi.org/10.1056/nejmlim035027

Bañuelos Capistrán, D., et al. (2025). Art, Community and AI: Images for an Affective Memory. *Frontiers in Communication.* https://doi.org/10.3389/fcomm.2025.1567694

Barredo Arrieta, A., Díaz-Rodríguez, N., & Del Ser, J. (2020). Explainable Artificial Intelligence (XAI): Concepts, Taxonomies, Opportunities and Challenges toward Responsible AI. *Information Fusion, 58*, 82–115. https://doi.org/10.1016/j.inffus.2019.12.012

Bashkirtsev, O., Gaevska, V., Bilous, Z., Lysa, L., & Zimba, O. (2023). Remote Monitoring for 5p (Predictive, Preventive, Participatory, Personalized, and Precision) Cardiovascular Medicine: Progress Amidst Covid-19 Pandemic. *Proceedings of the Shevchenko Scientific Society Medical Sciences, 71*(1). https://doi.org/10.25040/ntsh2023.01.14

Benjamens, S., Dhunnoo, P., & Meskó, B. (2020). The State of Artificial Intelligence-Based FDA-Approved Medical Devices and Algorithms: An Online Database. *NPJ Digital Medicine, 3*(1). https://doi.org/10.1038/s41746-020-00324-0

BlueDot, I. (2025). *BlueDot: Outbreak Intelligence.* Retrieved November 30, 2025, from https://bluedot.global/

Boehm, B. W. (1976). Software Engineering. *IEEE Transactions on Computers, C-25*(12), 1226–1241. https://doi.org/10.1109/TC.1976.1674590

Chen, S., Yu, J., Chamouni, S., Wang, Y., & Li, Y. (2024). Integrating Machine Learning and Artificial Intelligence in Life-Course Epidemiology: Pathways to Innovative Public Health Solutions. *BMC Medicine, 22*(1), 354. https://doi.org/10.1186/s12916-024-03566-x

Craven, B. A., et al. (2010). The Fluid Dynamics of Canine Olfaction. *Journal of the Royal Society Interface, 7*, 933–953. https://doi.org/10.1098/rsif.2009.0490

Elyoseph, Z., et al. (2024). Capacity of Generative AI to Interpret Human Emotions from Visual and Textual Data. *JMIR Mental Health.* https://doi.org/10.2196/54369

Ericsson, K. A., & Simon, H. A. (1993). *Protocol Analysis: Verbal Reports as Data.* MIT Press. https://direct.mit.edu/books/monograph/4763/Protocol-AnalysisVerbal-Reports-as-Data

Flavell, J. H. (1979). Metacognition and Cognitive Monitoring: A New Area of Cognitive-Developmental Inquiry. *American Psychologist, 34*(10), 906–911. https://doi.org/10.1037/0003-066x.34.10.906

Folstein, M. F., Folstein, S. E., & McHugh, P. R. (1975). "Mini-mental State": A Practical Method for Grading the Cognitive State of Patients for the Clinician. *Journal of Psychiatric Research, 12*(3), 189–198. https://doi.org/10.1016/0022-3956(75)90026-6

Ford, E., Carroll, J. A., Smith, H., Scott, D., & Cassell, J. (2016). Extracting Information From the Text of Electronic Medical Records to Improve Case Detection: A Systematic Review. *Journal*

of the American Medical Informatics Association, 23(5), 1007–1015. https://doi.org/10.1093/jamia/ocv180
Gaievskyi, S., Delfrate, N., Ragazzoni, L., & Bahattab, A. (2025). Use of Multi-criteria Decision Analysis (MCDA) to Support Decision-Making During Health Emergencies: A Scoping Review. *Frontiers in Public Health, 13.* https://doi.org/10.3389/fpubh.2025.1584026
Goodman, K. W., Litewka, S., Malpani, R., Pujari, S., & Reis, A. (2023). Global Health and Big Data: The WHO's Artificial Intelligence Guidance. *South African Journal of Science, 119*(5/6). https://doi.org/10.17159/sajs.2023/14725
HealthMap, Boston Children's Hospital. (2025). *HealthMap: Global Disease Alert Map.* Retrieved from https://www.healthmap.org/en/
Heß, U., & Fischer, A. H. (2013). Emotional Mimicry as Social Regulation. *Personality and Social Psychology Review, 17*(2), 142–157. https://doi.org/10.1177/1088868312472607
Hernández, J., Golpayegani, D., & Lewis, D. (2024). *An Open Knowledge Graph-Based Approach for Mapping Concepts and Requirements Between the EU AI Act and International Standards.* https://doi.org/10.31219/osf.io/y4mcj
Hoffman, R. R., & Lintern, G. (2006). Eliciting and Representing the Knowledge of Experts. In *The Cambridge Handbook of Expertise and Expert Performance* (pp. 203–222). Cambridge University Press. https://doi.org/10.1017/CBO9780511816796.012
Hou, H., et al. (2024). When AI Learns to Empathize: Topics, Scenarios, and Optimization of Empathy Computing from a Psychological Perspective. *Advances in Psychological Science.* https://doi.org/10.3724/SP.J.1042.2024.00845
Hsu, Y.-Y., Clyne, M., Wei, C.-H., Khoury, M. J., & Lu, Z. (2019). Using Deep Learning to Identify Translational Research in Genomic Medicine Beyond Bench to Bedside. *Database.* https://doi.org/10.1093/database/baz010
Hughes, H. C. (1999). *Sensory Exotica: A World Beyond Human Experience.* MIT Press. https://doi.org/10.7551/mitpress/6182.001.0001
Johansson, R. S., & Flanagan, J. R. (2009). Coding and Use of Tactile Signals from the Fingertips in Object Manipulation Tasks. *Nature Reviews Neuroscience, 10*, 345–359. https://doi.org/10.1038/nrn2621
Karyotaki, M., Drigas, A., & Skianis, C. (2024). Mobile/Vr/Robotics/IoT-Based Chatbots and Intelligent Personal Assistants for Social Inclusion. *International Journal of Interactive Mobile Technologies (IJIM), 18*(08), 40–51. https://doi.org/10.3991/ijim.v18i08.46473
Katirai, A. (2023). The Ethics of Advancing Artificial Intelligence in Healthcare: Analyzing Ethical Considerations for Japan's Innovative AI Hospital System. *Frontiers in Public Health, 11.* https://doi.org/10.3389/fpubh.2023.1142062
Kawakami, A., Sivaraman, V., Cheng, H.-F., Stapleton, L., Cheng, Y., Qing, D., … Holstein, K. (2022). *Improving Human-AI Partnerships in Child Welfare: Understanding Worker Practices, Challenges, and Desires for Algorithmic Decision Support* (pp. 1–18). https://doi.org/10.1145/3491102.3517439
Kivits, J., Ricci, L., & Minary, L. (2019). Interdisciplinary Research in Public Health: The 'Why' and the 'How.' *Journal of Epidemiology and Community Health, 73*(12), 1061–1062. https://doi.org/10.1136/jech-2019-212511
Kurniawan, M. H., Handiyani, H., Nuraini, T., Hariyati, R. T. S., & Sutrisno, S. (2024). A Systematic Review of Artificial Intelligence-Powered (AI-Powered) Chatbot Intervention for Managing Chronic Illness. *Annals of Medicine, 56*(1). https://doi.org/10.1080/07853890.2024.2302980
Livingston, G., Huntley, J., Sommerlad, A., Ames, D., Ballard, C., Banerjee, S., … Cooper, C. (2020). The Lancet Commission on Dementia Prevention, Intervention, and Care. *The Lancet, 396*(10248), 413–446. https://doi.org/10.1016/S0140-6736(20)30367-6
Ma, J., O'Riordan, M., Mazzer, K., Batterham, P. J., Bradford, S., Kõlves, K., … Rickwood, D. (2022). Consumer Perspectives on the Use of Artificial Intelligence Technology and Automation in Crisis Support Services: Mixed Methods Study. *JMIR Human Factors, 9*(3), e34514. https://doi.org/10.2196/34514

McLean, A. L., & Yen, T. L. (2024). Machine Translation for Multilingual Cancer Patient Education: Bridging Languages, Navigating Challenges. *Journal of Cancer Education, 39*(5), 477–478. https://doi.org/10.1007/s13187-024-02438-5

Mehrabi, N., Morstatter, F., Saxena, N., Lerman, K., & Galstyan, A. (2021). A Survey on Bias and Fairness in Machine Learning. *ACM Computing Surveys, 54*(6), 1–35. https://doi.org/10.1145/3457607

Naumova, E. N. (2025). Causal AI for public health research and policy. *Journal of Public Health Policy*. https://doi.org/10.1057/s41271-024-00541-x

Olawade, D. B., Wada, O. J., David-Olawade, A. C., Kunonga, E., Abaire, O., & Ling, J. (2023). Using Artificial Intelligence to Improve Public Health: A Narrative Review. *Frontiers in Public Health, 11*. https://doi.org/10.3389/fpubh.2023.1196397

Ovsyannikova, D., et al. (2025). Third-Party Evaluators Perceive AI as More Compassionate Than Expert Humans. *Communications Psychology*. https://doi.org/10.1038/s44271-024-00182-6

Powers, M. A., Bardsley, J., & Cypress, M. (2020). Self-Management Education for Adults with Type 2 Diabetes. *Diabetes Care, 43*(7), 1636–1649. https://doi.org/10.2337/dci20-0023

Romanello, M., Di Napoli, C., Drummond, P., Green, C., Kennard, H., Lampard, P., … Ford, L. B. (2023). The 2023 Report of the Lancet Countdown on Health and Climate Change. *The Lancet, 402*(10419), 2346–2394. https://doi.org/10.1016/S0140-6736(23)01859-7

Schoenherr, J. R., Abbas, R., Michael, K., Rivas, P., & Anderson, T. D. (2023). Designing AI Using a Human-Centered Approach: Explainability and Accuracy Toward Trustworthiness. *IEEE Transactions on Technology and Society, 4*(1), 9–23. https://doi.org/10.1109/tts.2023.3257627

Severini, M., Ferretti, D., Principi, E., & Squartini, S. (2019). Automatic Detection of Cry Sounds in Neonatal Intensive Care Units by Using Deep Learning and Acoustic Scene Simulation. *IEEE Access, 7*, 51982–51993. https://doi.org/10.1109/access.2019.2911427

Shi, B., Yang, S., Tan, Q., Zhou, L., Liu, Y., Zhou, X., & Liu, J. (2024). Bayesian Inference for the Onset Time and Epidemiological Characteristics of Emerging Infectious Diseases. *Frontiers in Public Health, 12*. https://doi.org/10.3389/fpubh.2024.1406566

Smith, D. V., & Margolskee, R. F. (2001). Making Sense of Taste. *Scientific American, 284*(3), 32–39. https://doi.org/10.1038/scientificamerican0301-32

Sung, H., Ferlay, J., Siegel, R. L., Laversanne, M., Soerjomataram, I., Jemal, A., & Bray, F. (2021). Global Cancer Statistics 2020: GLOBOCAN Estimates of Incidence and Mortality Worldwide for 36 Cancers in 185 Countries. *CA: A Cancer Journal for Clinicians, 71*(3), 209–249. https://doi.org/10.3322/caac.21660

Swinburn, B. A., Kraak, V. I., Allender, S., Atkins, V. J., Baker, P. I., Bogard, J. R., … De Schutter, O. (2019). The Global Syndemic of Obesity, Undernutrition, and Climate Change: A Lancet Commission Report. *The Lancet, 393*(10173), 791–846. https://doi.org/10.1016/S0140-6736(18)32822-8

Talyshinskii, A., Naik, N., Hameed, B. M. Z., Juliebø-Jones, P., & Somani, B. (2023). Potential of AI-Driven Chatbots in Urology: Revolutionizing Patient Care Through Artificial Intelligence. *Current Urology Reports, 25*(1), 9–18. https://doi.org/10.1007/s11934-023-01184-3

Thakkar, A., et al. (2024). Artificial Intelligence in Positive Mental Health: A Narrative Review. *Frontiers in Digital Health*. https://doi.org/10.3389/fdgth.2024.1280235

Tr, L. (2015). Cancer Bioinformatics, Its Impacts on Cancer Therapy. *Journal of Postgenomics Drug & Biomarker Development, 05*(02). https://doi.org/10.4172/2153-0769.1000e133

Tretter, M. (2024). Equipping AI-Decision-Support-Systems with Emotional Capabilities? Ethical Perspectives. *Frontiers in Artificial Intelligence, 7*. https://doi.org/10.3389/frai.2024.1398395

U.S. Bureau of Labor Statistics. (2024). *Census of Fatal Occupational Injuries—2023*. Retrieved from https://www.bls.gov/news.release/pdf/cfoi.pdf

Usher, K., Park, J., & Son, C. (2024). Artificial Intelligence for Emergency Medical Service. *Proceedings of the International Symposium on Human Factors and Ergonomics in Health Care, 13*(1), 1–6. https://doi.org/10.1177/2327857924131049

Vimercati, S. D. C. d., Foresti, S., Livraga, G., & Samarati, P. (2019). *Empowering Owners with Control in Digital Data Markets* (pp. 321–328. https://doi.org/10.1109/cloud.2019.00060

Voigt, P., & von dem Bussche, A. (2017). *The EU General Data Protection Regulation (GDPR): A Practical Guide*. Springer. https://doi.org/10.1007/978-3-319-57959-7

Wang, B. (2023a). The Application and Challenges of Artificial Intelligence in Speech Recognition. *Applied and Computational Engineering, 17*(1), 36–40. https://doi.org/10.54254/2755-2721/17/20230907

Wang, F. (2023b). Virtual Audio Design Based on Mobile Sensor Network and English MOOC Teaching. *International Journal of Systems Assurance Engineering and Management*. https://doi.org/10.1007/s13198-023-02063-3

Ware, J. E., & Sherbourne, C. D. (1992). The MOS 36-Item Short-Form Health Survey (SF-36): I. Conceptual Framework and Item Selection. *Medical Care, 30*(6), 473–483. https://doi.org/10.1097/00005650-199206000-00002

Warraich, H. J., Tazbaz, T., & Califf, R. M. (2025). FDA Perspective on the Regulation of Artificial Intelligence in Health Care and Biomedicine. *JAMA, 333*(3), 241. https://doi.org/10.1001/jama.2024.21451

Wieland-Jorna, Y., van Kooten, D., Verheij, R. A., de Man, Y., Francke, A. L., & Oosterveld-Vlug, M. G. (2024). Natural Language Processing Systems for Extracting Information from Electronic Health Records About Activities of Daily Living: A Systematic Review. *JAMIA Open, 7*(2), ooae044. https://doi.org/10.1093/jamiaopen/ooae044

World Health Organization. (1948). *Constitution of the World Health Organization*: World Health Organization. https://apps.who.int/gb/bd/PDF/bd47/EN/constitution-en.pdf

World Health Organization. (1995). *The World Health Organization Quality of Life (WHOQoL) Position Paper*. https://doi.org/10.1016/0277-9536(95)00112-k

Wu, P. F., Summers, C., Panesar, A., Kaura, A., & Zhang, L. (2024). AI Hesitancy and Acceptability—Perceptions of AI Chatbots for Chronic Health Management and Long COVID Support: Survey Study. *JMIR Human Factors, 11*, e51086–e51086. https://doi.org/10.2196/51086

Yamada, Y., Shinkawa, K., Kobayashi, M., Caggiano, V., Nemoto, M., Nemoto, K., & Arai, T. (2021). Combining Multimodal Behavioral Data of Gait, Speech, and Drawing for Classification of Alzheimer's Disease and Mild Cognitive Impairment. *Journal of Alzheimer S Disease, 84*(1), 315–327. https://doi.org/10.3233/jad-210684

Yousefi, Z., Saadati, N., & Saadati, S. A. (2023). AI in Elderly Care: Understanding the Implications for Independence and Social Interaction. *AI and Tech in Behavioral and Social Sciences, 1*(4), 26–32. https://doi.org/10.61838/kman.aitech.1.4.5

Zhang, Y. (2021). A Study on the Intelligent Translation Model for English Incorporating Neural Network Migration Learning. *Wireless Communications and Mobile Computing, 2021*(1). https://doi.org/10.1155/2021/1244389

Zygouris, S., & Tsolaki, M. (2015). Computerized Cognitive Testing for Older Adults: A Review. *American Journal of Alzheimer's Disease & Other Dementias, 30*(1), 13–28. https://doi.org/10.1177/1533317514522852

Chapter 4
Evaluation Methods for AI in Public Health

4.1 Introduction to Evaluation Methods

Suppose you are a public health informatics student; you should know basic evaluation methods. This session will briefly answer why evaluation is so important and review some basic evaluation concepts.

4.1.1 Why is Evaluation Important?

Why is Evaluation Important in General?

Without evaluation, it's like traveling without a map. You might be moving, but you have no idea if you're heading in the right direction. Choosing the right direction is often more important than just working hard. Hard work without direction can lead to wasted effort, while the right direction ensures that every step moves you closer to your goal. The best results come from combining the right direction with dedicated effort.

There are general terms like evaluation in various situations, such as performance review, feedback, monitoring, impact assessment, quality control, self-reflection, and benchmarking. If you are seriously playing a sport and think you give your best. You need a coach who can provide a *performance review* and tell you if you're playing the game effectively or improving. When driving a car, you need a dashboard to *monitor* your speed and fuel level and check if anything is wrong with the vehicle. If you are following a recipe and cooking a dinner for your family, you need *feedback* by tasting it, and you will know if the dish is turning out right. After you write an important email, you must do *quality control* by proofreading. You could find some errors or unclear ideas in your email. Just like you plant seeds in your gardens in spring, you *assess the impact* and check the harvest in the fall. You want to know if your efforts yielded the expected results. If you have children, you may measure your kids' height

M. Wu, *Artificial Intelligence in Public Health*,
https://doi.org/10.1007/978-3-032-15872-7_4

and weight against a growth chart, which is a *benchmark*. If you have a house, you may often compare your home's value to others in the neighborhood, which is a benchmark too. In short, evaluation in each situation is essential and required, not optional.

Why is it so Important for AI?

Suppose you have experience using some AI chatbots daily; you may find that AI sometimes seriously speaks nonsense. It is a phenomenon for data-driven large language models in AI, which is called "AI hallucination."

What Caused "AI Hallucination"?

Suppose you still remember the basic ideas of those AI components in Chapter 2. Data-driven AI models don't "know" facts and lack genuine understanding. AI merely predicts the most likely word combinations through statistical models. As a result, it may produce logically coherent but factually incorrect content.

AI generates answers based on training data. AI models learn from large datasets from the internet, books, and other sources. We know that training data always has some limitations in the real world. For example, the data is incomplete, with errors, conflicted, outdated, or biased, and the AI may generate seemingly reasonable responses based on incorrect information.

When AI doesn't have a direct answer for complex questions, it may "fill in the blanks" by generating text based on related concepts, leading to incorrect but confidently stated answers.

AI evaluation is Key to Addressing "AI Hallucination"

AI evaluation is key to addressing the issue of "speaking nonsense." For example, you should learn evaluation methods for "accuracy testing of AI," designed to verify whether the AI's outputs align with facts. We can design evaluations focusing on "bias detection," which will ensure that AI does not propagate incorrect or biased information. You should know how to create a user experience evaluation study, and it will ensure the AI's responses are clear, helpful, and meet user needs. Based on all those evaluation results, it will be possible to continuously optimize the AI models and reduce "AI hallucination."

4.1.2 General Evaluation Approaches

There are old classifications[1] of evaluation approaches, including eight discrete approaches derived from objectivist or subjectivist philosophical positions (House, 1980). Let's quickly review the basic ideas behind those eight evaluation approaches.

[1] As a part of biomedical informatics training, I took an evaluation methods course at UNC Chapel Hill 20 years ago. The textbook "Evaluation Methods in Biomedical Informatics" was used (Friedman et al., 2006).

4.1.2.1 Objectivist Evaluation Approaches

Objectivists believe that there is one objective reality that can be observed, measured, and understood. They also think that the truth is absolute and discoverable. The objectivist evaluation approaches are quantitative (Friedman et al., 2006). They focus on measurable outcomes and performance indicators. Let's look at some examples.

Objectives-Based Approach

This evaluation approach is straightforward. Suppose you have clearly defined objectives in a project (intervention) in the early stages (begin with the end in mind); you use the objectives as benchmarks in evaluation. You can measure changes before and after an intervention to assess whether objectives were met. This "objectives-based" evaluation is like an archery competition. Before shooting, you clearly define the goal of hitting the bullseye. After each shot, you measure how close you got to the target and adjust accordingly.

For example, an AI-powered healthcare program aims to reduce patient wait times in a hospital. The objectives (goals) can be defined in detail, such as goals achieved with wait times reduced by 20% and goals not met with no significant wait times reduction. In Chapter 3, we have a lot of design ideas for AI applications to reduce waiting times, such as AI-powered symptom check-in kiosks or smart tablets, AI-powered wearable health monitors for vital signs, AI-powered chatbots and virtual assistants, or AI-powered smart cameras and computer vision systems. This objective-based evaluation project measures patient waiting times before and after implementing AI applications. You can compare actual results with predefined goals.

Comparison-Based Approach

This evaluation approach is intuitive. An AI application will be compared to a contrasting resource or a control condition. You can quickly understand an evaluation study for AI applications for public health by first identifying its contrasting resources or control conditions. These evaluation study design details include sample size (a small number in a population), randomization, controls (a relatively small number of outcome variables in a large group), and statistical inference to simulate the whole picture. Statistical inference in evaluation is like tasting a spoonful of soup to judge the entire pot. You can evaluate this book by reviewing several pages of the book and reading between the lines of this book to judge the whole book. General outcome variables are the effectiveness, efficiency, and impact of AI applications. Approach is a broader term than method. Specific comparison-based evaluation methods will be discussed in detail in the following sessions.

Some evaluation studies often compare AI to human performance (contrasting resources). For example, a new AI-based diagnostic tool can be evaluated by comparing it with human doctors in detecting diseases. The outcome variable is diagnostic accuracy. This evaluation study has contributed to the field because many want your evaluation results, which determine whether this new AI tool can match or exceed human doctors' diagnostic accuracy.

Some evaluation studies compare AI-based to traditional approaches (control conditions). For example, AI-powered resume screening is widely used. Suppose you are graduating soon and starting to look for jobs; you really want to know if AI improves hiring efficiency and fairness. An evaluation study can be designed to compare an AI-based applicant tracking system with human recruiters for hiring (traditional approaches). The outcome variables for efficiency can be the speed of screening resumes and accuracy in selecting qualified candidates. Choosing outcome variables for fairness can be a complex design issue. You should decide on a relatively small number of outcome variables in large groups, such as selection rates, false rejection/acceptance rates, intersectional bias, transparency, socioeconomic fairness, etc. People want to read your evaluation reports to find out if there is bias in AI selection methods.

Decision-Facilitation Approach

This evaluation approach is to support practical decision-making. It is often used at the early stages of AI application development, and evaluation results are directly helpful for decision-making about further development direction. The evaluation provides fast and actionable insights into real-world situations for decision-makers. You will be practical and often ignore strict methodological rigor; you can design a flexible method to meet decision-makers' needs. One of the key features of this evaluation approach is that it often requires timely insights. In fast-changing environments, you need to provide results quickly enough to influence decision-making processes. This "decision-facilitation" evaluation is like a GPS (Global Positioning System); it can assess where you are and help you choose (decide) the best path forward.

For example, current public health agencies must decide about AI mental health chatbots: "Should we deploy AI mental health chatbots in our organizations? Flexible evaluation methods can be designed to measure the effectiveness of AI chatbots in reducing anxiety/depression symptoms vs. human therapists, assess potential risks (e.g., AI misinterpretation) and liabilities, and evaluate user engagement and dropout rates. Those decision-facilitation evaluation studies will help administrators decide to adopt it, use it for screening only, or limit it now.

Goal-free Approach

This evaluation approach aims to identify all the effects of AI applications. When unexpected impacts of AI applications need to be identified, you can use this goal-free evaluation approach. Suppose you want to capture the whole picture; you need to be open-minded. Like exploring a new island without a map, you wander freely, observing everything. This evaluation design should purposefully blind any intended goals, rely on independent data collection, and measure all observed actual outcomes rather than predefined outcome variables. AI is a new hot tool, and we really want to understand the broad impact and side effects of this tool. You may find new insights into AI tools using this "goal-free" evaluation approach.

In the previous session, we used a "comparison-based" approach to evaluate AI-powered resume screening. Let's revisit this AI-hire issue, but we will use a "goal-free" approach to assess it and hope to get the whole picture of AI involved in hiring. I believe everyone cares about the fairness of AI-hire. Without a job, the sense of self-worth and stability can weaken, like a bridge missing its pillar. In goal-free evaluation studies, you must observe the hiring process without assumptions, analyze all AI decisions, and investigate the entire AI pipeline. Independent data needs to be collected, such as who gets hired? Who drops out? How do human recruiters interact with AI recommendations? Are candidates satisfied with AI-driven hiring decisions? Does AI create unexpected barriers for applicants? The evaluation results will show if applicants are being unfairly rejected, whether AI favors candidates who use specific keywords rather than actual qualifications, or detects unexpected disparities in applicant pools.

4.1.2.2 Subjectivist Evaluation Approaches

Subjectivists believe that the truth is relative and interpretive. The subjectivist evaluation approaches are qualitative (Friedman et al., 2006). They focus on personal experiences, perceptions, and narratives. The subjective approaches are helpful when assessing aspects of AI that involve user experience, ethics, trust, and human-AI interaction areas where objective data alone is insufficient. Let's look at some examples.

Quasi-Legal Approach

This evaluation approach is like putting an AI system on trial in a courtroom. Resembling the standard courtroom procedure, some proponents and opponents offer testimony, examination, and cross-examine. Some juries witness the proceedings and decide about the merit of AI applications.

Let's continue to use AI-hire as an example. Fairness in employment is an ethical issue, so subjective quasi-legal evaluation can be used. First, we need to identify stakeholders and collect their testimonies. We must gather input from job applicants, HR teams, and diversity experts for AI-hire issues. We need to identify juries for this trial and conduct ethical rulings. The quasi-legal evaluation will determine if AI hiring practices align with fairness principles.

Art Criticism

This evaluation approach is like judging a painting in an art gallery. The critic interprets, analyzes, and judges based on subjective factors such as style, meaning, emotion, and impact. In this approach to evaluating AI applications, you need experienced and respected critics who are trained in the domain of AI, have extensive experience with AI, and have worked with AI over a period. Later, the critic will write a review report highlighting the benefits and shortcomings of this AI application.

For example, AI-written content can be evaluated using the "art criticism" approach. AI-generated stories are grammatically correct but sometimes lack originality. More AI writing assistants (AI agents) are coming, and you want to know the quality of essays generated by AI. The critics can evaluate them from many perspectives, such as "Does the AI produce well-structured sentences?", "Can it craft emotionally resonant stories?", "Does it understand humor and subtle meanings?", and “Is it innovative?” If the critics worked in healthcare fields, they could review the AI-written messages for patients (such as cancer patients) with more factors, such as human care with emotional support tone.

Professional Review

This evaluation approach is like a panel of experienced doctors evaluating a new surgeon’s skills before granting certification. You need to create a panel of expert reviewers to assess an AI application, who can be AI specialists, industry professionals, domain experts, etc. The panel will evaluate the effectiveness of this AI application in practice. Site visits may be required; they can meet people, ask questions, and request documents. The ethical and professional standards are also considered. The expert panel may give final approval for AI application developments.

For example, AI in autonomous vehicles can be evaluated using a professional review approach. In site visits, panel experts, such as automotive engineers and safety regulators, can test AI’s response in various driving conditions. This includes unexpected hazards and tests whether AI can react adequately. The panel also checks compliance with transportation laws and human-AI interaction issues. The panel may decide whether to give this self-driving car conditional regulatory approval, which would support human oversight in complex traffic situations.

Responsive-Illuminative

This evaluation approach is like a coach watching the gameplay live. You immerse yourself in the environment where an AI application is operational. This approach focuses on real-world use, unintended consequences, and user feedback. This evaluation aims to understand how AI applications work instead of judgments.

For example, AI education tools can be evaluated using this “responsive-illuminative.” Many people, including professors, want to understand how AI education tools work. Does it directly give students answers or encourage them to solve problems step by step? The "responsive-illuminative" approach is to immerse yourself using AI education. As a professor, I want to observe students’ engagement and learning patterns when they use AI-educational tools. Are students relying too much on AI? Is it suitable for developing critical thinking skills? How do you design a project-based homework assignment that requires students to ask AI tools several questions to solve a problem, instead of single-question homework? Does AI complement or replace human teaching?

4.1.3 General Evaluation Concepts

There are many concepts related to AI application evaluations. I show their relationships in Fig 4.1, a big picture of those concepts. Some terms have narrow meanings, while others are broader terms. For example, quality includes accuracy, reliability, and completeness. User acceptance is about users liking and using the AI tool. It relates all the factors.

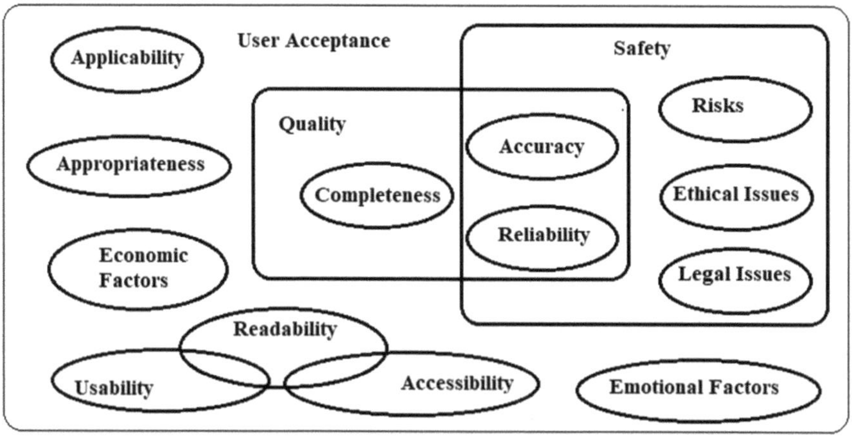

Fig. 4.1 A big picture of some concepts related to AI evaluations

Evaluation studies bind clients' questions and try to answer what they need to know. Table 4.1 shows that for each evaluation concept, there is an evaluation question it answers.

Table 4.1 Evaluation questions for some evaluation concepts

Concepts	Examples of Evaluation Questions
Accuracy	Is the information correct?
Accessibility	Can anyone use it?
Applicability	Is it the right tool?
Appropriateness	Is it suitable for the situation?
Completeness	Does the content include all the necessary and relevant information?
Ethical issues	Is it fair to everyone? Does it cause harm? Is user data protected? Is it clear who is responsible? Does it align with societal values?
Emotional factors	How does it make users feel? Does it emotionally connect with users? Does it show understanding and care? Do users feel emotionally secure using it? Does it respect diverse emotional needs?
Legal issues	Does it follow the law? Is personal data handled legally? Who is responsible if something goes wrong? Does it respect ownership rights? Are user agreements and policies legally valid?
Readability	How easily and effectively does content communicate its message to its intended audience?
Reliability	Does it work consistently?
User acceptance	Will users adopt it?
Usability	Is it easy to use?

4.2 What to Evaluate for AI Applications for Public Health?

4.2.1 Before AI Projects Get Started

Because the AI tools are new and under construction, such as ChatGPT, which was launched in 2022. Compared with humans, most AI tools are infants (under 1). When you read this book, AI tools are toddlers (under 3) or preschoolers (under 5). It's time to explore more possibilities for AI applications for public health. What should you evaluate before you have an AI application for public health? It overlaps with the design methods for AI for public health in Chapter 3. Public health informatics aims to identify unmet public health needs and implement IT/AI as their solutions.

What should be evaluated before AI applications get started for public health? You should know your starting points, do feasibility studies, and need assessments for AI in public health. The evaluation results can help community leaders, government administrators, and designers get started on AI projects for public health.

Need Assessments

Chapter 3 summarizes the methods for need assessments for design models. It lists some realized AI needs for public health and discusses some approaches to identify unrealized AI needs.

Feasibility Analysis (RTS Labs, 2024) (Walsh et al., 2021)

People are born into different circumstances, such as wealth, health, opportunities, or abilities. Life starts unevenly for many. You need to evaluate your community's starting points and find an AI-powered feasible and practical path from your starting points to the endpoints (such as living better and longer).

AI Literacy

Public health staff should understand AI capabilities and limitations. Stakeholders need to understand what AI can and cannot do. They can recognize potential biases, risks, and fairness issues. The challenge is whether the primary workforce, such as public health staff and policymakers, has been trained to interpret AI outputs.

Data Readiness

There is a lot of public health data for your community. The question is whether there is sufficient, high-quality data for training the AI model. For example, is there enough historical and real-time public health data to train AI? Are there data-sharing agreements between health agencies? At the same time, you should have policies to protect sensitive information.

Technical Feasibility

You should know what existing IT infrastructure and databases your community has. The question is how to integrate AI tools with current IT systems and how the AI system can run efficiently within the current infrastructure.

Resource Assessment

A Return on Investment (ROI) analysis can help you understand the financial costs and expected benefits. You need to find more funding for AI adoption, such as government, private, or non-profit funding agencies. You need to know how much AI maintenance, retraining, or continuous human oversight costs. All stakeholders, such as decision-makers and end-users, need to support this AI adoption.

4.2.2 During AI Design and Development

Evaluation is essential during the design and development process. Just like building a bridge, evaluation ensures that every component is strong, reliable, and functional before it can be fully used. Without proper evaluation, this bridge may collapse under pressure. Table 4.2 lists key evaluation factors during the design and development process.

4.2.3 After Deployment and Using AI Applications

After AI tools are really used by people in communities, it's time to evaluate their impact/effectiveness of those AI applications for public health. Suppose System A is complex and has many functions or features, but users do not know them well and use their features at a low level. System B only has one function, and it's simple and straightforward. Many users download this AI app for this feature and use it frequently. Which system has a more significant impact on society? Which is more effective than another? Fig. 4.2 shows a formula for the effectiveness of the system.

Based on this formula of impact, more is not always better. Having too many poorly performing AI functions is worse than a few well-optimized ones. You should find a balance between usability and complexity. Some AI apps need multiple complex functions, while others only need one strong function.

4.2.3.1 Evaluating AI system functions

Counting the Number of Functions

Let's start with simple evaluation questions: How many functions/features does this AI application have, and what are they? You can see the big picture by knowing

Table 4.2 Key evaluation factors during the development

Stages	Key evaluation factors for AI applications
Design (Newman-Griffis et al., 2023)(Meijden et al.,2025)(Vorisek et al., 2023)	Bias and fairness testing: Does the AI model work equitably across different populations? Explainability and transparency: Can public health workers understand how AI makes decisions? Accuracy requirements: How much uncertainty can the users tolerate in this case? Ethical implications: Is it ethical? Data security and privacy: Is sensitive public health data protected from breaches and misuse? Etc.
Development (Asan et al., 2020)(Wang et al., 2021)	Clinical validation and real-world testing: Does AI perform well in real clinical/public health settings? Usability testing: Can doctors, nurses, and health workers easily use AI tools in their workflow? Generalizability: Does AI perform well across different healthcare systems and populations? Cost-benefit analysis: Is AI cost-effective compared to traditional public health interventions? Adversarial testing: Can the AI model be misled by incorrect or adversarial inputs? Etc.

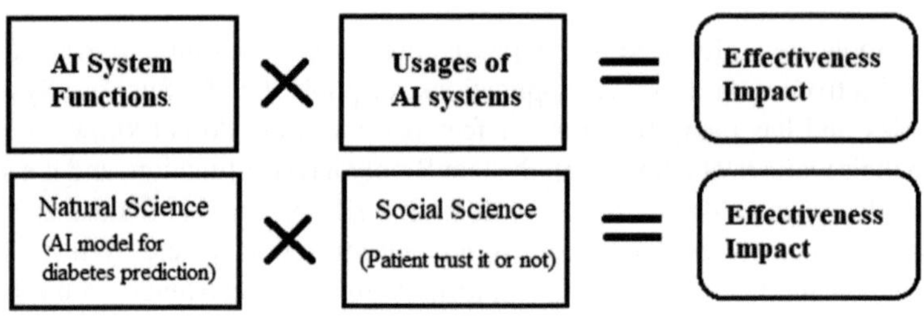

Fig. 4.2 The effectiveness/impact of an AI application

core features (primary AI-driven functions) such as speech recognition, image analysis, and chatbot responses, as well as grouping functions into role-based categories such as automation, decision-making, personalization, etc. A more complex question about AI system functions is their relationship. You need to check function/feature dependencies. Some functions may be standalone, while others rely on multiple AI models.

Table 4.3 General evaluation factors for AI functional performance

Examples of evaluation factors	Examples of evaluation questions
Accuracy	How often does the AI function give the right results?
Reliability	Does it work across different situations?
User satisfaction	How do users rate the function's usefulness?
Speed and latency	How fast do the function process data and respond?

Evaluating the Complexity of AI Functions

The question of evaluation is how difficult AI functions are, such as low, medium, or high. Many factors determine difficulty, such as data complexity (text, images, or real-time sensor data), algorithmic complexity (rule-based AI or advanced deep learning models), computational requirements, and real-time processing needs (instantly or asynchronously).

Evaluating Functional Performance

Evaluating AI functional performance is a complex task. Table 4.3 shows a big picture for general evaluation metrics for AI function performance.

NLP (natural language processing) is a significant subset of AI. There are specific evaluation factors for NLP, such as language understanding metrics. Table 4.4 lists some evaluation factors which are specific for NLP functional performance.

4.2.3.2 Evaluating usages of AI systems

AI usage can have different levels of human involvement, such as human-involved or silent AI usage. Some AI applications have explicit AI–human interaction, such as conversational AI (chatbots), AI-assisted decision-making (e.g., AI-powered hiring), AI-powered creativity (content generation), and AI-augmented productivity (AI-enhanced design tools). Some AI tools have hidden AI in the background, such as recommendation systems (personalized content suggestions), fraud detection and security (e.g., banking security alerts), autonomous systems (e.g., warehouse robots), and search and ranking algorithms (e.g., Google search). Table 4.5 shows the evaluation metrics of usages for various AI applications.

4.2.3.3 Evaluating the Impact of AI Applications for Public Health

The goals of public health are to prevent diseases, live longer, and live better. To evaluate the impact of AI applications on public health, we need to explore how to measure health outcomes such as "prevent diseases," "live longer," and "live better."

Table 4.4 Examples for evaluation factors for NLP functional performance

Metrics	Examples of evaluation factors
Accuracy-based metrics	Accuracy: Measures the percentage of correctly predicted labels out of all instances. Precision: Measures how many predicted positive results were correct. Recall: Measures how many actual positive cases were correctly identified. F1-Score: Harmonic mean of precision and recall, providing a balanced metric BLEU (Bilingual Evaluation Understudy): Measures the quality of machine-generated translations compared to human translations by comparing overlapping words and phrases. ROUGE (Recall-Oriented Understudy for Gisting Evaluation): Measures how well generated text (summaries) matches reference summaries based on recall of words and phrases (Lin, 2004)
Robustness and ethical metrics	Out-of-Distribution (OOD) Performance: Tests how well the model performs on data it has never seen before. Adversarial robustness: Evaluates the model's resistance to input manipulations (e.g., typos, synonyms). Fairness and bias detection: Assesses whether the model's predictions are biased against certain demographics or groups. Privacy and security compliance: Checks if the model adheres to privacy regulations when processing sensitive data (e.g., GDPR (General Data Protection Regulation) compliance).
User-centric metrics	Human evaluation (subjective evaluation): Involves human annotators rating outputs based on fluency, coherence, and relevance. User satisfaction score: Surveys and feedback collected from users to gauge satisfaction with the system's performance Error analysis reports: Manually reviewing model mistakes to identify areas of improvement.
Computational efficiency metrics	Inference time (speed and latency): The time it takes for the model to process an input and generate an output. Training time: Measures how long it takes to train the model on a given dataset. Memory usage: Evaluates how much memory the model consumes during training and inference. Model size (number of parameters): Measures the complexity of the model in terms of the number of trainable parameters.
Language understanding metrics	Perplexity: Evaluates how well a probabilistic language model predicts a test sample. Semantic similarity (cosine similarity): Measures how similar two pieces of text are based on vector representations. Mean reciprocal rank (MRR): Measures the effectiveness of ranking results based on the position of the correct answer in the ranked list. Exact match (EM): Measures whether the model's predicted output matches the reference exactly.

Table 4.5 Evaluation factors of usages for various AI applications

Types of AI Applications	Examples of Evaluation Metrics for Usages
Customer-facing AI (Google-blog, 2025)	User engagement metrics: Total visits/sessions: Number of times users interact with the AI. Active users: Daily, weekly, or monthly active users. Session length: Average time users spend in an AI-driven feature. Retention rate: How often users return after initial use. Churn rate: Percentage of users who stop using the AI.
Automation AI	Efficiency metrics: Task completion rate: Percentage of tasks successfully completed by AI. Response time: Speed of AI-generated responses. Error rate: Frequency of incorrect outputs or failures. Human override rate: How often users reject AI decisions and intervene manually.
Search engine AI (Manning et al., 2008)	Interaction and usage depth metrics: Number of queries/questions asked: Measures how deeply users engage. Feature usage rate: Tracks which AI features are used most/least. Click-through rate (CTR): How often AI suggestions are clicked. Conversions from AI recommendations: Tracks AI-driven purchases, signups, or actions.
Business-oriented AI(Provost et al., 2013)	Business metrics: Revenue impact: Increase in sales or savings due to AI usage. Cost savings: Reduction in operational costs from AI automation. Customer support deflection rate: Percentage of inquiries resolved by AI vs. requiring human support. Lead conversion rate: How often AI-driven interactions lead to new customers.
Sensitive decision-making AI (Barocas et al., 2016)	Ethical and compliance metrics: Bias and fairness scores: Measures disparities in AI decisions across different groups. Privacy compliance rate: Ensures AI adheres to GDPR, CCPA (California Consumer Privacy Act), etc. User trust and satisfaction: Measured via surveys, reviews, and NPS (Net Promoter Score).

Measure Disease Prevention

Disease prevention focuses on avoiding a disease rather than treating an existing one, and it is hard to prove AI prevented a disease rather than other factors, such as genetics or environment. Preventing diseases using AI tools requires long-term tracking, large populations, and indirect indicators. After our society has used AI applications for public health for years or decades, we can see AI intervention results for preventing diseases. You should know what to evaluate for disease prevention now. Table 4.6 lists some evaluation metrics for measuring disease prevention.

Measure "Live Longer" and "Live Better"

Humans want to live longer and live better. AI applications for public health aim to increase both lifespan and quality of life. For public health, health-related quality of

Table 4.6 Some evaluation metrics for measuring disease prevention

Metrics	Examples of evaluation factors for measuring disease prevention
Risk reduction metrics(Fineberg, 2013)(Gordis, 2013)	Disease incidence rate: Measures how many people develop a disease with vs. without AI interventions. Relative risk reduction (RRR): Compares risk levels before and after AI-based prevention. Predictive accuracy of AI models: How well AI predicts high-risk individuals before disease onset.
Early detection and intervention metrics(Etzioni et al., 2003)	Percentage of high-risk cases identified early: AI's role in flagging high-risk individuals. Screening uptake and compliance: Increase in participation for AI-prompted screenings. Delayed disease onset: Tracks whether AI-led interventions push disease onset later in life.
Behavioral and lifestyle impact metrics (Kariuki et al., 2024)	Adoption of healthy behaviors: AI-driven health coaching apps tracking diet, exercise, and smoking cessation. Wearable device data trends: AI's role in reducing sedentary behavior, improving sleep, or lowering stress. Patient engagement and adherence: Whether AI increases long-term commitment to preventive habits.
Public health impact metrics (Bonita et al., 2006)(Murray et al., 2013)	Hospitalization and ER visit reduction: Fewer admissions due to AI-powered prevention strategies. Population-level health improvements: AI's role in reducing overall disease burden.
Economic impact metrics (Drummond et al., 2015)(Masters et al., 2017)	Cost savings in healthcare system–Lower medical expenses due to disease prevention.

Table 4.7 Some evaluation metrics for "live longer" and "live better"

Metrics for measuring "live longer"	Metrics for measuring "live better" (EuroQoL, HRQoL)(EuroQol, 1990)(Hennessy et al., 1994)
Mortality rates: Overall or disease-specific death rates. Life expectancy: How many years a person is expected to live. Survival rates: E.g., 5-year cancer survival rate after AI-assisted treatment. Disability-adjusted life years (DALY): Years lost due to illness or premature death.	Physical functioning: Can people walk, work, and perform daily tasks? Pain and symptom burden: Is AI helping reduce chronic pain or symptoms? Mental health: Anxiety, depression, and emotional well-being scores. Social well-being: Ability to maintain relationships and social interactions. Quality-adjusted life years (QALY): Years lived in good health, adjusted for illness.

life (HRQoL) indicators can be used to measure "live better." Table 4.7 lists some evaluation metrics for measuring "live longer" and "live better."

Evaluation Metrics for the Impact of AI Applications on Public Health

Evaluating the impact of AI applications on public health is complex. New AI-driven factors are emerging, and next-generation indicators are needed to measure AI's broader impact on public health, which will augment traditional evaluation metrics. Public health informatics students need to know what to evaluate regarding the effectiveness/impact of AI applications on public health. Table 4.7 lists some evaluation metrics for these impacts. Part I of Table 4.8 focuses on the impact on organizations, and Part II of this table focuses on the impact on individuals.

4.3 Case Studies of Evaluation Designs for AI in Public Health

After we know what to evaluate (metrics and factors) in the previous section, let's look at some case studies of evaluation designs for AI applications. You already have learned a lot of evaluation theories, and it's time to see how knowledge is applied in actual situations Table 4.9. A case study will provide real-world context and practical applications of evaluation concepts.

Table 4.8 Part I: Some evaluation metrics for the impacts on organizations

Metrics	Examples of evaluation factors for the impacts of AI applications on organizations
Public health outcomes metrics (Jacob et al., 2025)	AI-assisted diagnosis accuracy Real-world AI performance index: Compares AI clinical accuracy with real-world outcomes (e.g., false positives/negatives in AI-based diagnostics). Early disease detection rate AI-assisted early intervention score: Measures how quickly AI flags diseases before symptoms appear. Vaccination and screening rates: AI-driven campaigns improving immunization rates. Epidemic prediction and control: e.g., AI-powered epidemiological models to predict future health risks. Longitudinal studies of AI's impact on disease trends. Hospital readmission rate Complication rate: AI's impact on reducing post-treatment complications. Reduction in disease burden: AI's effectiveness in preventing chronic conditions such as diabetes or cardiovascular diseases. AI-influenced public health policy impact: Measures how AI recommendations shape governmental health policies. AI-powered health misinformation detection: Evaluates AI's role in combating health-related fake news.
Efficiency metrics	Task automation rate: e.g., faster patient triage and diagnosis through AI-driven systems. AI-based administrative burden reduction: Tracks AI's role in automating documentation and reducing clinician burnout. Intelligent resource allocation score: AI's ability to optimize hospital beds, staff scheduling, and equipment distribution. Health data utilization: AI's role in processing and analyzing public health data for better policy decisions. Employee productivity gain: AI's impact on reducing public health staff workloads. Time saved per task: e.g., How much AI speeds up decision-making in public health cases; emergency room wait time; measures how fast AI improves diagnosis-to-treatment time. Error reduction

(continued)

Table 4.8 (continued)

Metrics	Examples of evaluation factors for the impacts of AI applications on organizations
Business metrics(Rai, 2020)	ROI (Return on Investment) Revenue growth Operational cost savings: Savings due to AI automation. Market competitiveness
Ethical and compliance metrics (Jobin et al., 2019)	AI regulatory compliance score: Assesses AI alignment with HIPAA (Health Insurance Portability and Accountability Act), GDPR, and FDA (U.S. Food and Drug Administration) guidelines; data privacy and security compliance. AI audits and risk management: Evaluates AI system risks and potential failures. AI-driven healthcare access score: Measures AI's role in bridging gaps in underserved communities. Fairness and bias reduction index: Evaluates whether AI models provide equitable care across demographics; ensures AI does not introduce discriminatory practices.
Public perception and trust (Zhang et al., 2019)	Media and social sentiment analysis: Tracks on how AI is perceived in public discourse. Ethical AI adoption in society: Measures regulations and public policies shaping AI use. AI-perceived trust and safety index: Measures public trust in AI-assisted healthcare decisions. Human-AI interaction satisfaction score: Evaluates patient comfort with AI-driven diagnostics and treatments.
Sustainability impact metrics (Vinuesa et al., 2020)	Energy consumption: Measures how much computing power AI consumes.

4.3.1 Case Scenario A: Accuracy of AI Chatbots

Case Scenario 4A. An AI chatbot is designed to converse with a human. More people are starting to ask AI chatbots about health-related questions. Accuracy is always the first evaluation target for AI chatbots. Suppose a patient will have cataract surgery. Previous patient information leaflets are provided to patients by eye doctors. Those patient education documents are well-designed by experienced eye doctors. The patient wants to ask AI chatbots for information about this surgery. The patient's question is, "Is the AI answer correct?"

Some literature about the accuracy of AI Chatbots (Pan et al., 2023) (Yun et al., 2025) (Hua et al., 2023) (Mills et al., 2023) (Yau et al., 2024) (Kais et al., 2025) will provide background information for you to identify the key issues in this scenario.

Table 4.9 Part II: Some evaluation metrics for the impacts on individuals

Metrics	Examples of evaluation factors for the impacts of AI applications on individuals
Health outcomes metrics (Marko et al., 2025)	Early diagnosis and treatment success rate AI-powered precision medicine effectiveness: Tracks AI-generated treatment plans vs. traditional medicine. AI's influence on risk factor modification: AI's effectiveness in reducing risk factors (e.g., diet, smoking, physical inactivity). Proactive disease prevention score: AI's ability to predict and prevent chronic conditions. Personalized AI-driven health interventions: AI's success in delivering individualized lifestyle recommendations. Morbidity and mortality reduction Disability-adjusted life years (DALY) and quality-adjusted life years (QALY). Medication adherence rates Health-related quality of life (HRQoL) indicators: Measure how AI improves overall well-being, mental health, and daily functioning. New AI-enabled HRQoL indicators: New AI-specific metrics include user experience, trust in AI, and digital well-being. Dynamic disease progression modeling: AI's ability to predict future health outcomes based on patient data. Sustained health behavior change score: Tracks whether AI-driven interventions lead to long-term lifestyle improvements.
User experience metrics (Jiang et al., 2024)	User satisfaction score Adoption rate Ease of use and accessibility AI-powered digital health literacy impact: Tracks AI's role in educating patients on their health conditions. Error handling and trust
Workforce transformation metrics (Mossavar-Rahmani et al., 2024)(Adhikari et al., 2024)(Brynjolfsson et al., 2018)	Job creation and job displacement AI augmentation: Measures how AI enhances human decision-making rather than replacing it. Employee training and learning curve

(continued)

Table 4.9 (continued)

Metrics	Examples of evaluation factors for the impacts of AI applications on individuals
Ethical impact metrics (Lyu et al., 2023)(Palliyil et al., 2025)	Bias and fairness perception: How users perceive AI's fairness in decision-making. AI explainability and transparency score: Measures how well AI's decisions can be understood by healthcare professionals and patients; whether users understand how AI arrives at its decisions.
Psychological impact metrics (Reddy et al., 2021)	Mental well-being and workload: Evaluates whether AI reduces stress or adds pressure due to over-reliance.

Choose An Evaluation Design: An Objective-based Study

Let's use this case scenario to demonstrate how to design a small-scale objective-based evaluation study. The processes of an objective-based evaluation study design include "define objectives," "selection of subjects," "conditions (independent variables)." "measurements of dependent variables," and "comparison with predefined objectives."

Step 1. Define study objectives

This study aims to assess the accuracy of AI chatbots. The predefined objective is to measure the correctness of AI chatbot-generated responses for patient information in this specific health domain (eye surgery in healthcare) and compare AI chatbot answers with previous patient information leaflets in accuracy.

Step 2. Selection of subjects

You need to select some subjects for the evaluation study. The first subject is AI chatbots, which will be evaluated. ChatGPT, Gemini, Claude, Copilot, and DeepSeek are popular AI chatbots now. It's up to you to choose one or two or more AI chatbots as study subjects. You need to select which domains will be covered. In this case, the domain is ophthalmology (eye diseases). You can define this domain as surgical care, such as operative and perioperative care. Another subject is patients' question sets. In this study, cataract surgery-specific questions are those frequently asked questions (FAQ) in the previous patient education documents. Choosing the right sample size of questions for evaluating chatbot accuracy depends on statistical and practical factors. You get a spoonful of soup to get an idea of the taste of a whole pot. The critical subject is the objectives benchmark. The gold standard will be answers of those FAQs in the previous patient information leaflets (eye doctors provided patient education documents).

Step 3. Conditions (independent variables)

Suppose someone asks you about the accuracy of AI chatbots. The short answer is, "It depends." The long answer is that AI chatbots' responses depend on conditions. Each condition is an independent variable. For this case, the query complexity is an independent variable, such as simple, moderate, or complex. For example, a simple query can be, "What is cataract surgery?" A complex one is "Is cataract surgery safe for someone with diabetes?" Another condition is the query type, such as fact-based, reasoning-based, or opinion-based questions. The following independent variable is context variation. There are different levels of contextual detail, such as personal, time-related, location-related, cultural, and language (consumer vocabulary or medical terms).

Step 4. Measurement of dependent variables

The accuracy score is measured by the percentage of chatbot responses that match expert-generated FAQ answers. The confabulation rate is the percentage of responses with false or misleading information. AI hallucination is a more extreme version of confabulation and contributes to lowering accuracy. If the accuracy score is low and the confabulation rate is high, we call it AI hallucination. Accuracy is a key component of safety, quality, and user acceptance in the concept map, shown in Fig 4.1. AI hallucination is critical because it undermines user trust, reliability, and safety in AI-generated information.

Step 5. Comparison with predefined objectives

Predefined objectives are human expert-generated answers in the previous patient information leaflets. You can compare chatbot responses to human expert-generated answers. The dependent variables (accuracy) depend on the queries' complexity, type, and context variation (independent variables). Suppose you conduct this evaluation and publish your study results. Your contribution to the field is to let the public know the accuracy of one AI chatbot in the cataract surgery domain, which can be used as an industry benchmark or reference point. People will know if the AI chatbot's answers about cataract surgery are correct. AI application designers or developers will have a target for new AI chatbot models to improve the accuracy from the current level to the next level.

4.3.2 Case Scenario B: Accuracy of AI Doctors

Case Scenario 4B. All AI companies compete and want to reach the sky. One of their favorite products is to develop an "AI Doctor" or "Medical AI Assistant." The public wants to know the accuracy of AI doctors. For health care providers, they want to know if AI doctors are good enough to replace their jobs. In this case, we can design a small-scale evaluation study to compare the accuracy of an AI doctor acting as a medical professional against human medical students using the USMLE (United States Medical Licensing Examination) Step 1 exam performance. The three-step USMLE exam is required for medical licensure in the United States. USMLE Step 1 exam tests many physician tasks and competencies, such as medical knowledge and scientific concepts, diagnosis and management principles, interpretation of lab and imaging studies, mechanisms of disease, pharmacologic and non-pharmacologic therapies, epidemiology and population health, and social sciences (ethics, communication, legal, etc.).

Some literature about the AI Doctors (Kung et al., 2023) (Brin et al., 2023) (Yang et al., 2023) (Aquino et al., 2023) (Temsah et al., 2023) (Liu et al., 2023) will provide background information for you to identify the key issues in this scenario.

Choose an Evaluation design: a Comparison-based Study

Let's use this case scenario to demonstrate how to design a small-scale comparison-based evaluation study. The processes of a comparison-based evaluation study design include "selection of subjects," "conditions (independent variables)," "measurements of dependent variables," and "comparison across conditions."

Step 1. Selection of subjects

In this case, you need to select the first subject for Condition A, an AI doctor. The specific AI doctor models are trained in medical knowledge for medical diagnosis. For example, Med-PaLM is a large language model (LLM) developed by Google Research. It is specifically designed to provide high-quality answers to medical questions. You must also select a second group of subjects in Condition B, medical students from accredited medical schools. They can be a group of final-year pre-clinical medical students. They must not have taken the USMLE Step 1 exam. You can randomly select them from different institutions to control the variability in training.

Step 2. Experimental conditions (A vs. B)

This study has two conditions: Condition A and Condition B. In Condition A, the USMLE Step 1 exam test-taker is an AI doctor. The AI agent answers USMLE Step 1 exam questions in a standardized format, and all AI responses will be recorded. In Condition B, the test-takers are medical students. They should take the same exam with identical test questions. The question type is multiple-choice questions (MCQs), which have a single best-answer format. Neither AI doctors nor medical students will receive any feedback or assistance.

Step 3. Measurement of dependent variables

AI doctors' or medical students' overall accuracy score is measured by their total raw scores in the USMLE Step 1 exam. The accuracy score for specific content areas can be measured by raw scores related to those question categories, such as "General Principles of Foundational Science," "Behavioral Sciences, Ethics, and Biostatistics," "Pathology and Disease Mechanisms," Microbiology and Immunology," "Pharmacology and Toxicology," "Organ Systems-Based Clinical Science," and "Multisystem Processes and Disorders." You can conduct error analysis by measuring types of incorrect responses (e.g., knowledge gap, reasoning errors).

Step 4 Comparison across conditions (A vs. B)

Let's compare the average scores of AI doctors vs. human students. A more complex statistical test (such as the T-test) can be used to compare the means (averages) of two groups (AI doctors vs medical students) and determine whether they are significantly different from each other. We know from previous Case Scenario A that the accuracy of AI responses depends on the question types. You can conduct a question-type analysis on AI doctors and students to identify the strengths and weaknesses of AI and students in specific medical domains. You can identify error patterns based on the error measurements, such as AI misinterpreting context.

Suppose you conduct this evaluation on the accuracy of AI doctors. Many people want to know if AI doctors outperform or underperform medical students. Based on the evaluation results, we will understand if AI could be useful as a medical assistant tool now or if it requires future improvements. Because of the contributions of this evaluation study, your paper will be quickly accepted, and your results can be shared with the public.

4.3.3 Case Scenario C: Accountability of Self-driving Cars

Autonomous vehicles (AV) can drive themselves without human intervention using AI, sensors, and cameras. It is also called self-driving cars. Self-driving cars operate on roads, although their deployment is limited to specific regions and under controlled conditions. Let's look at a case scenario:

> **Case Scenario 4C:** a self-driving car crash, injuring a pedestrian. Who is legally responsible? Who is accountable when a self-driving car causes this accident, such as AV manufacturers/AV sale companies, self-driving AI developers/companies, drivers, or regulators/policymakers?

Some literature about the accountability of self-driving cars (Awad et al., 2019) (Mayer et al., 2023) (Lee et al., 2019) (Xue, 2021) (Gill, 2021) will provide background information for you to identify the key issues in this scenario.

Choose an Evaluation Design: Quasi-legal Approach

In this case, the quasi-legal study is best for evaluating the accountability of self-driving cars. Let's use this case scenario to demonstrate how to design a small-scale quasi-legal subjective evaluation study. The quasi-legal approach is like putting an AI system on trial in a courtroom. It has similar courtroom procedures, such as proponents and opponents offering testimony, examination, and cross-examination. Some juries witness the proceedings and decide about the merit of AI applications. Fig 4.3 shows the processes of a quasi-legal study design.

Step 1. Define the Case

The first step clearly defines the case: *Who is accountable when a self-driving car causes an accident, the AV manufacturer, the driver, or the regulators?* You should identify key stakeholders for proponents (such as AV manufacturers, AI developers, policymakers, and electronic vehicle companies, etc.), opponents (such as victims, insurance companies, legal experts, regulators, and safety advocates), and a panel of neutral experts as evaluators (such as lawyers, policymakers, transportation safety regulators, etc.).

Step 2. Testimony from Proponents and Opponents

Proponents (AV companies, AI developers, and policymakers) will present their testimony. They may argue that AVs reduce human error in driving. They need to

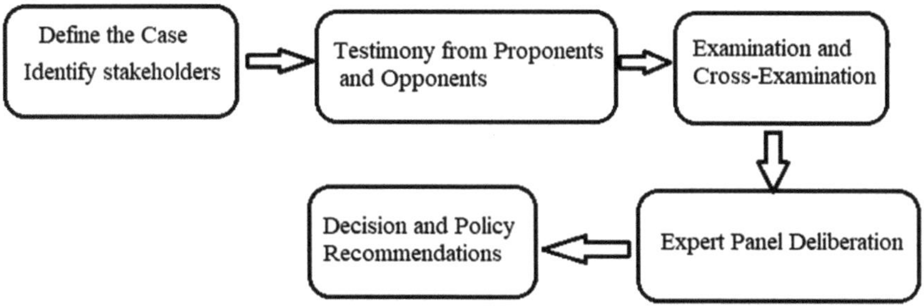

Fig. 4.3 Quasi-legal study design

present data on AV safety compared to human drivers. For example, AVs' Full Self-Driving (FSD) systems have fewer accidents per mile than human drivers. Another strategy is that AV responsibility should be shared among drivers, AV manufacturers, and regulators. Regarding legal principles, they may emphasize the need for new legal frameworks for AI instead of outdated liability laws.

In this case, opponents can be victims' lawyers or insurance companies. They will present their testimony and highlight cases where AVs failed in accident scenarios due to AI limitations. For example, they need evidence that AV's software could not detect a pedestrian crossing at night. They point out that AV manufacturers should be liable and take the entire liability. In this case, there are ethical concerns for AI design. For example, "Should AI decide who to save in unavoidable crash situations?" The insurance company may argue the liability is on drivers or AV manufacturers.

The driver (or operator) can be a proponent or opponent. As a proponent, the driver will defend the AV technology and argue that the accident was caused by external factors (e.g., another driver's negligence or road conditions). The driver, as an opponent, will challenge the AV technology. The driver might claim they were unable to properly take control in time due to AI system failure.

Step 3. Examination and Cross-Examination

Cross-examination tests the strength of each side's arguments and evidence. It could help clarify facts and ensure the testimony is fully understood. It asks challenging questions about the inconsistencies in their testimony. For example, opponents ask difficult questions to proponents (AV companies), "If AVs are so safe, why do they still require human intervention?" Proponents challenge opponents' arguments, "Are human drivers statistically safer than AVs?" Cross-examination helps ensure that the trial process is fair by thoroughly examining all testimony.

Step 4. Expert Panel Deliberations

After hearing all the evidence and arguments in the testimony from both sides and cross-examinations, a panel of neutral experts (like juries) discusses and decides the case's outcome. As evaluators, the expert panel includes lawyers, policymakers, transportation safety regulators, AI ethics experts, etc. This panel examines data, accident reports, and ethical considerations and discusses legal precedents and potential regulatory updates. They will evaluate whether AV companies should have strict liability or shared responsibility.

Step 5. Decision and Policy Recommendations

Ultimately, the panel should provide their decisions and issue policy recommendations or guidance. The panel may rule that AV manufacturers should be liable if an AV accident occurs while in full self-driving mode but not if the driver manually intervenes. They also propose legal reforms such as creating a new liability framework for AV-related accidents, requiring "black box" data logging in AVs to determine responsibility, and mandating AV insurance (national insurance fund) coverage paid by manufacturers instead of drivers.

The outcome of the quasi-legal subjective study on AV accountability will help clarify legal responsibility for AV accidents, propose new legal and insurance policies for AV technology, and ensure fairness in liability distribution between AV manufacturers, drivers, and regulators.

4.3.4 Case Scenario D: User experience of AI Mental Health Support

> **Case Scenario 4D.** Mental health often becomes a significant public health issue during a recession. Due to the limited availability of traditional mental health care, AI-driven mental health support needs are rising. Many AI mental health products are in the market, such as chatbots for cognitive-behavioral therapy, mood tracking and personalized support suggestions, AI-powered journaling apps, voice analysis for emotional state monitoring, VR/AR mindfulness and exposure therapy tools, and AI to support therapists. The evaluation of user experiences of AI mental health products is needed.

Some literature about the user experience of AI mental health support (Schyff et al., 2023) (Casu et al., 2024) (Stade et al., 2024)(Milne-Ives et al., 2022) (Fiske et al., 2019) (Miner et al., 2019) (Graham et al., 2019) (Anita et al., 2024) (Anita et al., 2024) (Cheng et al., 2020) (Zhang et al., 2023) (Benda et al., 2024) will provide background information for you to identify the key issues in this scenario.

Choose an Evaluation Design: Responsive/Illuminative Approach

To design and develop better AI mental health applications, you should deeply understand the complex situations of mental health support, such as user experiences. Let's use this case scenario to demonstrate how to design a small-scale responsive/illuminative subjective evaluation study. This evaluation approach is like a coach watching the gameplay live. You immerse yourself in the environment where an AI application is operational. This approach focuses on real-world use, unintended consequences, and user feedback. Fig 4.4 shows the main components of the study, such as illuminative studies, feedback, and findings.

Step 1. Illuminative studies

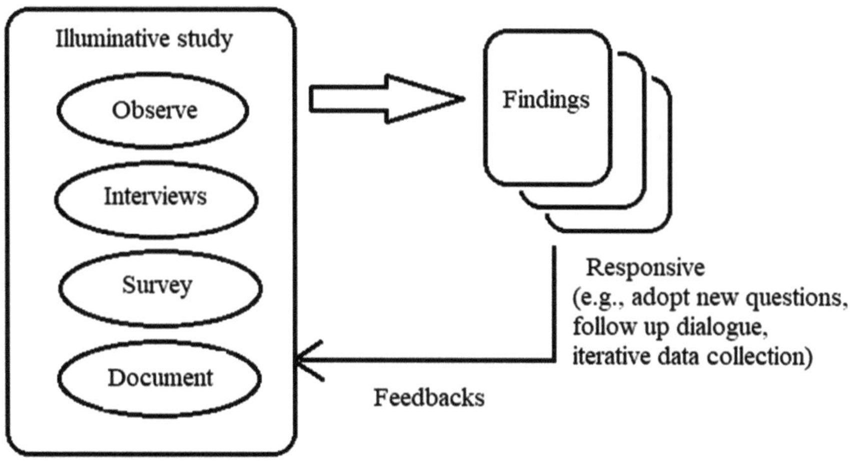

Fig. 4.4 Responsive/illuminative study design

Observations

This study aims to understand how users interact with AI in real time and context. You need to watch users using the AI mental health tool for therapy sessions, crisis support, and daily check-ins at home and take notes about confusion, frustration, reliance, or other emotional responses. With user consent, you can use screen recordings of AI tools. You may observe unintended consequences (e.g., misinterpretation of responses or over-reliance on AI). You may find "workarounds" users develop creative, unplanned ways to use or adapt the AI tools to better meet their needs, such as users seeking empathy instead of solutions. Some users want emotional validation, not cognitive-behavioral therapy lessons. They may prompt the AI to be more "human" or emotionally supportive.

Interviews

The interviews can be both responsive and illuminative. You can guide the conversation but still allow flexibility. You conduct open-ended discussions with users about their experiences. Based on users' answers, you can capture users' personal experiences, emotions, and interpretations of the AI support. AI mental health support stakeholders are users (patients, general users), mental health professionals (therapists), support staff, developers and product managers, and policy or ethics advisors. In this case, you focus on user experiences of AI tools. Firstly, the interview study needs to identify the users you are interviewing with. Who are users? Different users exist, such as new or experienced, satisfied or skeptical. You need to include some vulnerable or marginalized users to uncover diverse perspectives. The interviews help you engage with users and deeply understand the usages of AI tools. Secondly, you need to prepare a list of interview questions, such as "how do you feel about using the tool?" or "Do you trust this tool?"

Surveys

The survey can gather broader user feedback at a larger scale and identify trends. Like interviews, you need to prepare survey questions. You can design closed-ended questions to evaluate trust, usefulness, ease of use, and emotional impact. Also, you can use open-ended ones for more findings. For example, "What did you find most helpful or unhelpful about the tool?" Now, the survey can be conducted through the app or via email.

Document

You can document the process of AI mental health support through field notes, diary entries, and dialogue logs. The field notes for each case are descriptive, narrative records of what is happening in the setting. The diary is for users to write their thoughts and emotions after AI interactions. The digital dialogue logs or screen recordings record all users' activities. You can analyze those documents later for findings, such as misunderstandings, emotional alignment, and therapeutic effectiveness.

Step 2. Response and feedback

An iterative user feedback loop is an important step that lets the evaluation adapt to what emerges rather than sticking to a fixed framework. Feedback is ongoing and vital to responsive assessment. You analyze data as it comes in, share early insights, continuously dialogue with users, clinicians, or designers, and let their feedback guide you in your next steps. The early findings include that you identify some themes, tensions, patterns, and gaps in user experiences for AI mental health support. Unlike fixed studies, responsive evaluations adjust your questions, adopt new questions, and focus as new insights emerge, or stakeholder concerns arise. Your data on mental health cases can be iteratively collected. Based on earlier findings, you may revisit participants to follow up on interesting cases. This responsive study may need a lot of resources to support ongoing engagement with diverse users.

Step 3. Findings

Multiple methods (observation, interviews, surveys, and documents) can be used together to deepen our understanding of user experiences. The finding from observations is to reveal what users *do*, not just what they say. For example, evaluators see how users integrate AI into their mental health routines. Field notes record what the evaluator sees, hears, and feels. The results of interviews can capture emotional, ethical, and human nuance. The survey supports generalization and pattern findings. Logs track user activities for misunderstandings and emotional alignment. Diaries track user reflections over time, which helps find behavior changes (therapeutic effectiveness) in AI mental health support.

This evaluation study can find some themes or usage patterns (some repeated interactions), such as drop-off AI mental health services. There are critical incidents with a lot of tension or struggles for users with mental health issues. The bottom line of AI mental health support is that mental health AI must avoid harm and not exacerbate crises. This evaluation study will examine moments where the AI failed or succeeded unexpectedly.

This study can identify unintended consequences, gaps, or contradictions, such as over-reliance on AI, misinterpretation of advice, or privacy concerns. You can find some outliers among users. This evaluation study will check and ensure the AI responds equitably across demographics.

Based on the study, we can identify improvements with AI tools. For example, there are social or emotional effects on users. The study will show how AI alters users' relationships with human therapists or peers.

This responsive/illuminative evaluation could contribute to AI application development for mental health. For example, this study can track whether AI support correlates with symptom improvement, which is a part of effectiveness measurement. Your findings can be used as AI design recommendations to refine AI design and prototyping and provide insights for improving future AI development. For example, it could suggest better AI approaches (e.g., empathetic vs. directive responses). Your findings can be used in policy guidance or compliance. AI mental health tools should ensure alignment with mental health regulations (e.g., GDPR, HIPAA). The ethical review panels may find your evaluation results beneficial for continuously evaluating risks with users when using AI tools.

4.4 Discussion Questions

Question 4.1. Why is it essential to establish evaluation criteria before developing an AI solution for public health? What risks might arise if evaluation is only considered after implementation?

Question 4.2. What are some essential quantitative and qualitative metrics for assessing AI applications in public health? Which do you think is most critical, and why?

Question 4.3. What factors should be evaluated before designing an AI tool for public health (e.g., community needs, data availability)? How might this stage prevent future failures?

Question 4.4. Why is ongoing evaluation during AI development critical? Can you give an example of a public health AI project where mid-development evaluation could have improved outcomes?

Question 4.5. After deployment, how can we evaluate whether an AI public health tool is effective and ethical in real-world settings? What challenges might arise in long-term assessment?

Question 4.6. What study designs are most appropriate for evaluating the real-world effectiveness of AI tools in public health, and what trade-offs do they involve?

References

Adhikari, P., & Hamal, P. (2024). Impact and Regulations of AI on Labor Market and Employment in USA. https://doi.org/10.20944/preprints202407.0906.v1

Anita, A. S., Purba, K. N. A., & Ilmi, M. R. B. (2024). *The Role of Artificial Intelegence as a Tool to Help Counselors in Improving Mental Health., 2*, 119–124. https://doi.org/10.30983/bicc.v1i1.115

Aquino, Y. S. J., Rogers, W., Braunack-Mayer, A., Frazer, H., Win, K. T., Houssami, N., & Carter, S. M. (2023). Utopia Versus Dystopia: Professional Perspectives on the Impact of Healthcare Artificial Intelligence on Clinical Roles and Skills. *International Journal of Medical Informatics, 169*, 104903. https://doi.org/10.1016/j.ijmedinf.2022.104903

Asan, O., Bayrak, A. E., & Choudhury, A. (2020). Artificial Intelligence and Human Trust in Healthcare: Focus on Clinicians. *Journal of Medical Internet Research, 22*(6), e15154. https://doi.org/10.2196/15154

Awad, E., Levine, S., Kleiman-Weiner, M., Dsouza, S., Tenenbaum, J. B., Shariff, A., & Rahwan, I. (2019). Drivers Are Blamed More Than Their Automated Cars When Both Make Mistakes. *Nature Human Behaviour, 4*(2), 134–143. https://doi.org/10.1038/s41562-019-0762-8

Barocas, S., & Selbst, A. D. (2016). Big Data's Disparate Impact. *California Law Review, 104*, 671–732. https://doi.org/10.2139/ssrn.2477899

Benda, N. C., Desai, P., Reza, Z., Zheng, A., Kumar, S., Harkins, S., Turchioe, M. R. (2024). *Patient Perspectives on AI for Mental Health Care: Cross-Sectional Survey Study (Preprint)*. https://doi.org/10.2196/preprints.58462

Bonita, R., Beaglehole, R., & Kjellström, T. (2006). *Basic Epidemiology* (2 ed.): World Health Organization. https://iris.who.int/handle/10665/43541

Brin, D., Sorin, V., Vaid, A., Soroush, A., Glicksberg, B. S., Charney, A. W., & Klang, E. (2023). Comparing ChatGPT and GPT-4 Performance in USMLE Soft Skill Assessments. *Scientific Reports, 13*(1). https://doi.org/10.1038/s41598-023-43436-9

Brynjolfsson, E., Mitchell, T., & Rock, D. (2018). What Can Machines Learn, and What Does It Mean for Occupations and the Economy? *AEA Papers and Proceedings, 108*, 43–47. https://doi.org/10.1257/pandp.20181019

Casu, M., Triscari, S., Battiato, S., Guarnera, L., & Caponnetto, P. (2024). AI Chatbots for Mental Health: A Scoping Review of Effectiveness, Feasibility, and Applications. *Applied Sciences, 14*(13), 5889. https://doi.org/10.3390/app14135889

Chen, Q., & Li, J. (2023). AI-Driven Predictive Models: Indirect Indicators as Key Predictors in Public Health. *BMC Public Health, 23*(1), 274–285. https://doi.org/10.1186/s12889-023-17234-8

Cheng, Y., & Jiang, H. (2020). AI-Powered Mental Health Chatbots: Examining Users Motivations, Active Communicative Action and Engagement After Mass-shooting Disasters. *Journal of Contingencies and Crisis Management, 28*(3), 339–354. https://doi.org/10.1111/1468-5973.12319

Craswell, N., & Zamani, H. (2020). Information Retrieval and Neural Models. *Foundations and Trends in Information Retrieval, 14*(1), 1–192. https://doi.org/10.1561/1500000060

d, M.,. S. L. v., Wang, Y., Arbous, M. S., Geerts, B. F., Steyerberg, E. W., & Hernandez-Boussard, T. (2025). *Navigating Fairness in AI-based Prediction*. Theoretical Constructs and Practical Applications. https://doi.org/10.1101/2025.03.24.25324500

Schyff, E. L. v. d., Ridout, B., Amon, K. L., Forsyth, R., & Campbell, A. (2023). Providing Self-Led Mental Health Support Through an Artificial Intelligence–Powered Chat Bot (Leora) to Meet the Demand of Mental Health Care. Journal of Medical Internet Research, 25, e46448. doi:https://doi.org/10.2196/46448

Drummond, M. F., Sculpher, M. J., Claxton, K., Stoddart, G. L., & Torrance, G. W. (2015). *Methods for the Economic Evaluation of Health Care Programmes* (4 ed.): Oxford University Press. https://doi.org/10.1093/oso/9780198529446.001.0001

Etzioni, R., Urban, N., Ramsey, S., McIntosh, M., Schwartz, S., Reid, B., & Hartwell, L. (2003). The Case for Early Detection. *Nature Reviews Cancer, 3*(4), 243–252. https://doi.org/10.1038/nrc1041

EuroQol, G. (1990). EuroQol—A New Facility for the Measurement of Health-Related Quality of Life. *Health Policy, 16*(3), 199–208. https://doi.org/10.1016/0168-8510(90)90421-9

Fineberg, H. V. (2013). The Paradox of Disease Prevention: Celebrated in Principle, Resisted in Practice. *Jama, 310*(1), 85–90. https://doi.org/10.1001/jama.2013.7518

Fiske, A., Henningsen, P., & Buyx, A. (2019). Your Robot Therapist Will See You Now: Ethical Implications of Embodied Artificial Intelligence in Psychiatry, Psychology, and Psychotherapy. *Journal of Medical Internet Research, 21*(5), e13216. https://doi.org/10.2196/13216

Friedman, C. P., & Wyatt, J. C. (2006). Evaluation Methods in Biomedical Informatics. In *Health Informatics*: Springer. https://doi.org/10.1007/0-387-30677-3

Gill, T. (2021). Ethical Dilemmas Are Really Important to Potential Adopters of Autonomous Vehicles. *Ethics and Information Technology, 23*(4), 657–673. https://doi.org/10.1007/s10676-021-09605-y

Google-blog, w. 2025, KPIs for gen AI: Measuring your AI success. https://cloud.google.com/transform/gen-ai-kpis-measuring-ai-success-deep-dive

Gordis, L. (2013). *Epidemiology* (5 ed.): Elsevier Saunders. https://books.google.com/books?id=7YX6AQAAQBAJ

Graham, S., Depp, C. A., Lee, E., Nebeker, C., Tu, X., Kim, H. C., & Jeste, D. V. (2019). Artificial Intelligence for Mental Health and Mental Illnesses: An Overview. *Current Psychiatry Reports, 21*(11). https://doi.org/10.1007/s11920-019-1094-0

Hennessy, C. H., Moriarty, D. G., Zack, M. M., Scherr, P. A., & Brackbill, R. (1994). Measuring Health-Related Quality of Life for Public Health Surveillance. *Public Health Reports, 109*(5), 665–672. https://pubmed.ncbi.nlm.nih.gov/7938388/

House, E. (1980). *Evaluating with Validity*: Sage. https://books.google.com/books/about/Evaluating_with_Validity.html?id=tlaPAAAAIAAJ

Hua, H.-U., Kaakour, A.-H., Rachitskaya, A., Srivastava, S. K., Sharma, S., & Mammo, D. A. (2023). Evaluation and Comparison of Ophthalmic Scientific Abstracts and References by Current Artificial Intelligence Chatbots. *Jama Ophthalmology, 141*(9), 819. https://doi.org/10.1001/jamaophthalmol.2023.3119

Jacob, C., Brasier, N., Laurenzi, E., Heuss, S., Mougiakakou, S. G., Cöltekin, A., & Peter, M. K. (2025). AI for IMPACTS Framework for Evaluating the Long-Term Real-World Impacts of AI-Powered Clinician Tools: Systematic Review and Narrative Synthesis. *Journal of Medical Internet Research, 27*, e67485. https://doi.org/10.2196/67485

Jiang, P. N. W., Wang, Q., Yuan, R., & Chen, K. (2024). Understanding Users Acceptance of Artificial Intelligence Applications. *Behavioral Sciences, 14*(8). https://doi.org/10.3390/bs14080671

Jobin, A., Ienca, M., & Vayena, E. (2019). The global landscape of AI ethics guidelines. *Nature Machine Intelligence, 1*(9), 389–399. https://doi.org/10.1038/s42256-019-0088-2

Kais, A., Nguyen, J., Ramadan, H. H., Cui, R., & Makary, C. A. (2025). Readability of Rhinology-Related Patient Education Materials Generated by Artificial Intelligence–Based Chatbots. International Forum of Allergy & Rhinology, 15(4), 460–462. doi:https://doi.org/10.1002/alr.23560

Kariuki, J. K. I. C. C. E. S. J., & et al. (2024). Impact of lifestyle-based interventions on absolute cardiovascular disease risk. *JBI Evidence Synthesis, 22*(1). https://doi.org/10.11124/JBIES-22-00356

Kung, T. H., Cheatham, M., Medenilla, A., Sillos, C., Leon, L. D., Elepaño, C., & Tseng, V. (2023). Performance of ChatGPT on USMLE: Potential for AI-assisted Medical Education Using Large Language Models. *Plos Digital Health, 2*(2), e0000198. https://doi.org/10.1371/journal.pdig.0000198

Lee, K., & Kum, D. (2019). Collision Avoidance/Mitigation System: Motion Planning of Autonomous Vehicle via Predictive Occupancy Map. *Ieee Access, 7*, 52846–52857. https://doi.org/10.1109/access.2019.2912067

Lin, C.-Y. (2004). *ROUGE: A Package for Automatic Evaluation of Summaries.* Paper presented at the Proceedings of the ACL-04 Workshop on Text Summarization Branches Out. https://aclanthology.org/W04-1013

Liu, S., Wright, A. P., Patterson, B. L., Wanderer, J. P., Turer, R. W., Nelson, S. D., & Wright, A. (2023). Using AI-generated Suggestions From ChatGPT to Optimize Clinical Decision Support. *Journal of the American Medical Informatics Association, 30*(7), 1237–1245. https://doi.org/10.1093/jamia/ocad072

Lyu, Z., & Wang, X. (2023). The Impact of Artificial Intelligence Technology on Individual Behavior From the Perspective of Social Psychology. *International Journal of Frontiers in Sociology, 5*(15) https://doi.org/10.25236/ijfs.2023.051503

Manning, C. D., Raghavan, P., & Schütze, H. (2008). *Introduction to Information Retrieval.* Cambridge University Press. https://nlp.stanford.edu/IR-book/

Marko, J. G. O., Neagu, C. D., & Anand, P. B. (2025). Examining inclusivity: the use of AI and diverse populations in health and social care. *BMC Medical Informatics and Decision Making, 25.* https://doi.org/10.1186/s12911-025-02884-1

Masters, R., Anwar, E., Collins, B., Cookson, R., & Capewell, S. (2017). Return on Investment of Public Health Interventions: A Systematic Review. *Journal of Epidemiology & Community Health, 71*(8), 827–834. https://doi.org/10.1136/jech-2016-208141

Mayer, M. M., Buchner, A., & Bell, R. (2023). Humans, Machines, and Double Standards? The Moral Evaluation of the Actions of Autonomous Vehicles, Anthropomorphized Autonomous Vehicles, and Human Drivers in Road-Accident Dilemmas. *Frontiers in Psychology, 13.* https://doi.org/10.3389/fpsyg.2022.1052729

Mills, R., Mangone, E., Lesh, N., Mohan, D., & Baraitser, P. (2023). Chatbots to Improve Sexual and Reproductive Health: Realist Synthesis. *Journal of Medical Internet Research, 25*, e46761. https://doi.org/10.2196/46761

Milne-Ives, M., Selby, E., Inkster, B., Lam, C., & Meinert, E. (2022). Artificial Intelligence and Machine Learning in Mobile Apps for Mental Health: A Scoping Review. *Plos Digital Health, 1*(8), e0000079. https://doi.org/10.1371/journal.pdig.0000079

Miner, A. S., Shah, N. H., Bullock, K., Arnow, B. A., Bailenson, J. N., & Hancock, J. T. (2019). Key Considerations for Incorporating Conversational AI in Psychotherapy. *Frontiers in Psychiatry, 10.* https://doi.org/10.3389/fpsyt.2019.00746

Mossavar-Rahmani, F., & Zohuri, B. (2024). Artificial Intelligence at Work: Transforming Industries and Redefining the Workforce Landscape. *Journal of Economics & Management Research*, 1–4. https://doi.org/10.47363/jesmr/2024(5)213

Murray, C. J. L., & Lopez, A. D. (2013). Measuring the Global Burden of Disease. *New England Journal of Medicine, 369*(5), 448–457. https://doi.org/10.1056/NEJMra1201534

Newman-Griffis, D., Rauchberg, J. S., Alharbi, R., Hickman, L., & Hochheiser, H. (2023). Definition Drives Design: Disability Models and Mechanisms of Bias in AI Technologies. *First Monday.* https://doi.org/10.5210/fm.v28i1.12903

Palliyil, V., Cai, M., Karam, H., Phatthanachaisuksiri, L., Suhre, N., & Kassens-Noor, E. (2025). Artificial Intelligence Use Cases Adopted by People and Their Impact on Achieving Sustainable Development Goals: A Systematic Review. *Open Research Europe, 5*, 117. https://doi.org/10.12688/openreseurope.20023.1

Pan, A., Musheyev, D., Bockelman, D., Loeb, S., & Kabarriti, A. E. (2023). Assessment of Artificial Intelligence Chatbot Responses to Top Searched Queries About Cancer. *Jama Oncology, 9*(10), 1437. https://doi.org/10.1001/jamaoncol.2023.2947

Provost, F., & Fawcett, T. (2013). *Data Science for Business: What You Need to Know About Data Mining and Data-Analytic Thinking*: O'Reilly Media. https://www.oreilly.com/library/view/data-science-for/9781449374273/

Rai, A. (2020). Explainable AI: From black box to glass box. *Journal of the Academy of Marketing Science, 48*(1), 137–141. https://doi.org/10.1007/s11747-019-00710-5

Reddy, S., Rogers, W., Mäkinen, V. P., Coiera, E., Brown, P., Wenzel, M., & Kelly, B. (2021). Evaluation Framework to Guide Implementation of AI Systems Into Healthcare Settings. *BMJ Health & Care Informatics, 28*(1), e100444. https://doi.org/10.1136/bmjhci-2021-100444

RTS Labs (2024). Guide to Conducting a Successful AI Feasibility Study. https://rtslabs.com/guide-to-conducting-a-successful-ai-feasibility-study

Stade, E. C., Eichstaedt, J. C., Kim, J., & Stirman, S. W. (2024). Readiness Evaluation for AI-Mental Health Deployment and Implementation (READI): A Review and Proposed Framework. https://doi.org/10.31234/osf.io/8zqhw

Temsah, M. H., Aljamaan, F., Malki, K. H., Alhasan, K., Altamimi, I., Aljarbou, R., & Al-Eyadhy, A. (2023). ChatGPT and the Future of Digital Health: A Study on Healthcare Workers' Perceptions and Expectations. *Healthcare, 11*(13), 1812. https://doi.org/10.3390/healthcare11131812

Vinuesa, R. A. H. L. I., et al. (2020). The role of artificial intelligence in achieving the Sustainable Development Goals. *Nature Communications, 11*. https://doi.org/10.1038/s41467-019-14108-y

Vorisek, C. N., Stellmach, C., Mayer, P. J., Klopfenstein, S. A. I., Bures, D., Diehl, A., & Thun, S. (2023). Artificial Intelligence Bias in Health Care: Web-Based Survey. *Journal of Medical Internet Research, 25*, e41089. https://doi.org/10.2196/41089

Walsh, M., & Menthe, L. (2021). *Exploring the Feasibility and Utility of Machine Learning-Assisted Command and Control*. https://www.rand.org/pubs/research_reports/RRA263-1.html

Wang, D., Wang, L., Zhang, Z., Wang, D., Zhu, H., Gao, Y., & Tian, F. (2021). Brilliant AI Doctor in Rural Clinics: Challenges in AI-Powered Clinical Decision Support System Deployment. 1–18. doi:https://doi.org/10.1145/3411764.3445432

Xue, C. (2021). *Liability Analysis of Autonomous Vehicles Accidents*. https://doi.org/10.2991/aebmr.k.210803.075

Yang, Z., Yao, Z., Tasmin, M., Vashisht, P., Jang, W. S., Ouyang, F., Yu, H. (2023). Performance of Multimodal GPT-4V on USMLE With Image: Potential for Imaging Diagnostic Support With Explanations. https://doi.org/10.1101/2023.10.26.23297629

Yau, J., Saadat, S., Hsu, E., Murphy, L., Roh, J., Suchard, J. R., & Langdorf, M. I. (2024). Accuracy of Prospective Assessments of 4 Large Language Model Chatbot Responses to Patient Questions About Emergency Care: Experimental Comparative Study. *Journal of Medical Internet Research, 26*, e60291. https://doi.org/10.2196/60291

Yun, H. S., & Bickmore, T. (2025). Online Health Information–Seeking in the Era of Large Language Models: Cross-Sectional Web-Based Survey Study. Journal of Medical Internet Research, 27, e68560. doi:https://doi.org/10.2196/68560

Zhang, B., & Dafoe, A. (2019). Artificial Intelligence: American Attitudes and Trends. *SSRN Electronic Journal*. https://doi.org/10.2139/ssrn.3312874

Zhang, M., Scandiffio, J., Younus, S., Jeyakumar, T., Karsan, I., Charow, R., & Wiljer, D. (2023). The Adoption of AI in Mental Health Care–Perspectives From Mental Health Professionals: Qualitative Descriptive Study. *Jmir Formative Research, 7*, e47847. https://doi.org/10.2196/47847

Part III
Big Data in Public Health

Chapter 5
Data Issues for AI

5.1 Data Concepts for AI

5.1.1 Data Concepts Map

When you read Chap. 3 about artificial intelligence (AI) application designs, you are encouraged to be curious and open-minded and aim to reach the sky. In the next two chapters about AI data, you will realize that you should be practical and down to earth. It's like the "location, location, location" of real estate. The new slogan in AI business is "data, data, and data."

Digital Age

It began around the early 1990s with widespread computer use. Paper-to-digital transition got started. The physical records can be lost in misfiling, and searching paper-based archives was slow and limited to location. Copies had to be made physically. Handwritten data is hard to read. With widespread internet use in the 2000s, web data rose. People share information online via email, social media, and e-commerce. New issues of web data have risen, such as "Who owns your data? You or the platform?", "Right to digital" (Not everyone has equal access to digital tools.) After many years of writing or annotating, people who use paper-based data have many cognitive habits, such as deep reading, long-form thinking, and intentional memory. The paper-to-digital transition will be completed in the future, not because old generations fully accept digital data but because they die. The first generations of "digital natives" were born in the late 1990s, and they have grown up in a world where digital data is usual, expected, and everywhere (McKinsey, 2023; Prensky, 2001).

Big Data

In the early 2000s, several massive projects and emerging technologies laid the groundwork for Big Data. For example, the human genome project generated billions of genetic data in the human genome sequences, and "Bioinformatics" started.

M. Wu, *Artificial Intelligence in Public Health*,
https://doi.org/10.1007/978-3-032-15872-7_5

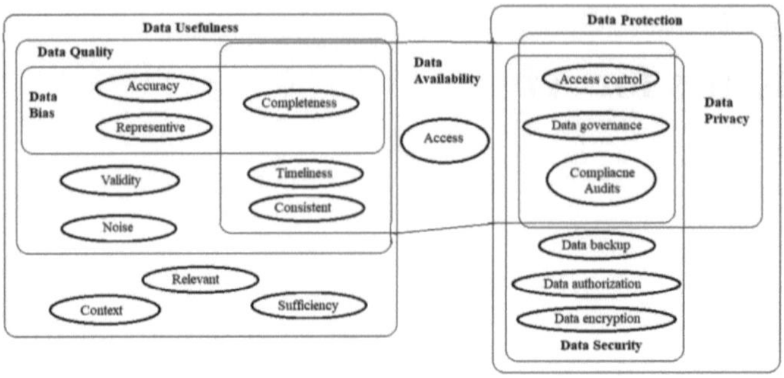

Fig. 5.1 Concepts map for AI data

Another example is the Google search engine, which indexed the entire web with billions of pages. With the internet being widely used, e-commerce, such as Amazon or eBay, has exploded. Real-time data about every search, click cart action, and purchase needs to be collected. MEDLINE is a big data project in biomedical literature and health sciences (Lee et al., 2023). It has over 35 million citations and abstracts from thousands of journals published globally. This term, "Big Data," has become popular. In 2001, an analyst, Doug Laney, defined the 3Vs of Big Data: Volume (large amounts of data), Velocity (fast data generation and processing), and Variety (different types of data) (Gandomi et al., 2015; Laney, 2001).

AI Data Concept Map

Informatics students should have clear concepts about AI data, such as data availability, data quality, etc. A concept map for AI data can be helpful. It helps you understand or explain how different components relate to one another and gives a visual overview of data issues in AI systems. When you develop an AI application beyond the design steps, you need to deal with data availability issues, including access, completeness, timeliness, and consistency. You should know what data is useful for AI application designers for public health. Data usefulness includes data quality, relevance, context, and sufficiency. For public health workers, you should realize that data is an asset, especially in AI data-driven models. That's why protecting your public health data in your communities is crucial. Data protection includes data privacy and security issues. Figure 5.1 shows a concept map for AI data.

5.1.2 Data Types

When the computer is in the infant or toddler stages, there are tedious tasks to work with computers. Like feeding babies, humans must break information into structured data that computers can digest. Like changing babies' diapers, humans must care for infant computers by cleaning their wasted memory. Fortunately, computers have grown smarter, like pre-elementary school students, after computer sciences have had breakthroughs in AI large language models. You can now communicate with AI with a lot of fun.

Structure Types

Structured Data

The information communicates in the human language sentences, such as, "Edwin's blood pressure is 140/80." Unfortunately, before natural language processing (NLP) and AI, computers could not understand human language. The information needs to be broken into structured data, which can be processed by computers, such as "Edwin," "blood pressure," "140," and "80." The structured data can be stored in spreadsheets (such as Excel) or relational databases (such as Microsoft Access, Oracle databases, etc.). It's time-consuming and labor-intensive to design pick-up lists or radio buttons in user interfaces to collect structured data and design databases to store them. Why bother? In the past, well-organized, structured data was searchable and live. Structured data are easy to clean, analyze, and model. They are excellent for AI training, especially when you're aiming for accuracy, reliability, and consistency.

Semi-structured Data

EMR (Electronic Medical Records) are generally considered semi-structured data. There are structured elements in EMR, such as patient ID, date of birth, blood pressure readings, and medical codes. These structured data are stored in predefined fields (like relational databases). You can search on those structured data. Unfortunately, a large part of EMRs are unstructured or loosely structured elements, such as doctor's notes, clinical summaries, imaging reports, or scanned documents. Before the AI era, the full potential benefits of EMR could not be released, and the return on investment (ROI) was not good enough. Computers could not understand those unstructured elements of EMR at that time.

Computer code is semi-structured. When you look at computer program codes, they are unstructured texts. However, computer languages have limited vocabulary and grammar compared with human languages, like English or Chinese. The computer codes follow a defined syntax (indentation, functions, loops), so they have structure within the text. Like old computer languages like C++ or Java, you need a compiler to turn code (text) into machine-readable forms (binary). For new languages, like Python, you need an interpreter at runtime to make computer codes interpretable.

Another example is email, which is semi-structured data. The sender, receiver, and subject are structured data, while the main body of the email is unstructured. At the time, we call structured data to be interpretable by computers. If the unstructured data is not interpretable by computers, they will not be fully used. If the data cannot be retrieved/searched easily, we think those data are dead, not live.

Unstructured Data

Unstructured data is mostly Big Data in volume, velocity, and variability. They include text (documents, tweets, chats), images (photos, medical scans), audio (voice recordings, music), and video (surveillance footage, movies). With NLP and LLM

(Large Language Model) in AI, computers gained the ability to understand human language in unstructured formats. Now, computers can interpret doctor's notes, emails, customer feedback, social media posts, legal documents, etc. Unstructured data is valuable for AI training, especially when capturing context, relevance, and human-like understanding.

Content Types

Different data content types need different AI models for analysis. You will need different data cleaning or preprocessing techniques to handle data in various content types. After you have a big picture of general data content types in Table 5.1, you can ask the right questions and choose the right tools to work on them. Identifiers can be nominal categorical data (names) or metadata (Who the record belongs to? Or How is it linked to other records?).

There are many ways to group public health data (Frieden, 2010). Let's preliminary summarize the public health data content types in Table 5.2. It'll help you to construct the right public health data questions. For example, more AI applications are working on Internet health-related social media data. Those data can be an independent data content type. Those internet data are unstructured or semi-structured.

Table 5.1 The general data content types

Categories	Data content type	Examples
Basic	Numbers	Integers, floats, decimals
	Text	Characters, words, sentences
	Categorical data	Gender, ethnicity, blood type
	Boolean	True / false
	Date and time	Standard ISO date format, 24-hour format
Composite	Arrays/lists	Ordered collections
	Tuples	Fixed length ordered sequences
	Records	Key-value pairs
	Dictionaries	Unordered key-value pairs
Multimedia (binary)	Images	Jpeg, PNG, gif, etc.
	Audio	Mp3, wav, etc.
	Video	Mp4, Avi, etc.
	Binary large objects	Raw binary data
Specialized	Geospatial data	Coordinates, polygons
	Time-series data	Stock prices, sensor readings
	Graph data	Nodes and edges
	Machine learning data	Tensors, embeddings
Metadata (data about data)	Descriptive	File size, creation date
	Structural	How data is organized, indexes
	Administrative	Access rights, ownership

The content in social media is digital public health data and real-time surveillance data, and they can be used as behavioral and communication data sources. AI applications often use them as sentiment and opinion-mining data sources for public health issues. The data availability of public Internet information is good and often used in the pre-train stages of AI model developments. Other structured, domain-specific data content will be used in the continue-train steps to improve AI models further.

5.1.3 Data and AI Development Stages

Let's look at the data in the stages of AI development, as shown in Fig. 5.2. There are supervised and unsupervised learning processes in general. Choosing the learning process depends on the case scenarios with different goals and raw data (Hastie et al., 2009; Jordan et al., 2015; van Engelen et al., 2020; Zhu et al., 2009). Table 5.3 lists some case scenarios and choices for the learning process.

Paired Data in AI

Let's discuss more "paired data in AI," which is the foundation of most supervised learning tasks (Zhu et al., 2009; Hastie et al., 2009; Jordan et al., 2015). They are data points where the input is paired with the desired output. Table 5.4 shows examples of "input-output paired data" for different AI tasks.

Data for Modern AI development (Model on Model)

After the AI doctor learns general medicine, the AI doctor wants to become a cardiologist, and the AI agent should be trained with specific domain knowledge about CVDs (Cardiovascular Diseases). Modern AI development has a workflow of "model on model." It starts with a pre-trained model with general knowledge and fine-tunes it with domain-specific data (Bommasani et al., 2021; Raffel et al., 2020; Wortsman et al., 2022). The new AI model aims to perform better in specialized areas. Table 5.5 shows data requirements for pretraining and continual training.

5.2 Data Issues for AI in Public Health

Suppose you are designing and developing an AI application in public health. Let's explore data issues for AI one by one. An example of public health topics (such as cancer, mental health, diabetes, etc.) will be used to explain the data issues in detail.

Table 5.2 The public health data content types

Categories	Examples
Electronic medical records	Clinical data: Diagnoses, lab results, medications, procedures Demographic data: Age, gender, race, socioeconomic status Vital signs: Blood pressure, heart rate, BMI Immunization records Allergies and adverse events
Administrative and claims data	Billing codes (ICD (international classification of diseases), CPT (current procedural terminology), DRG (diagnosis-related group)) Insurance claims (Medicare, Medicaid, private insurers) Hospital discharge data
Public health surveillance data	Notifiable disease reports (CDC (Centers for Disease Control and Prevention), WHO (World Health Organization)) Syndromic surveillance (ER visits, flu trends) Outbreak investigation data (contact tracing, cluster analysis)
Internet health-related social media	Twitter/X (real-time trends, keyword tracking) Reddit (community opinions, illness narratives) Facebook (public health campaign feedback) YouTube (video content analysis, misinformation tracing) TikTok (youth-focused health trends) Instagram (visual content + hashtags on wellness topics)
Real-time and IoT health data	Wearable device data (Fitbit, apple health) Remote patient monitoring (chronic disease management) Emergency medical services (EMS) data
Specialized databases and registries	Cancer registries (SEER (surveillance, epidemiology, and end results), NCI (National Cancer Institute)) Birth and death certificates (vital statistics) Vaccination registries (immunization information systems) Environmental health data (air/water quality, toxic exposures)
Social determinants of health (SDOH) data	Housing and homelessness data Food security and nutrition data Employment and education records
Genomic and precision medicine data	DNA sequencing data Pharmacogenomics (drug-gene interactions)

(continued)

Table 5.2 (continued)

Categories	Examples
Behavioral and survey data	BRFSS (behavioral risk factor surveillance system) NHANES (National Health and nutrition examination survey) Mental Health & Substance Abuse Data
Research and clinical trial data	Randomized controlled trials (RCTs) Observational study data (cohort, case-control)
Geospatial and mobility data	Disease mapping (epidemiological hotspots) Healthcare access (hospital locations, telemedicine reach)

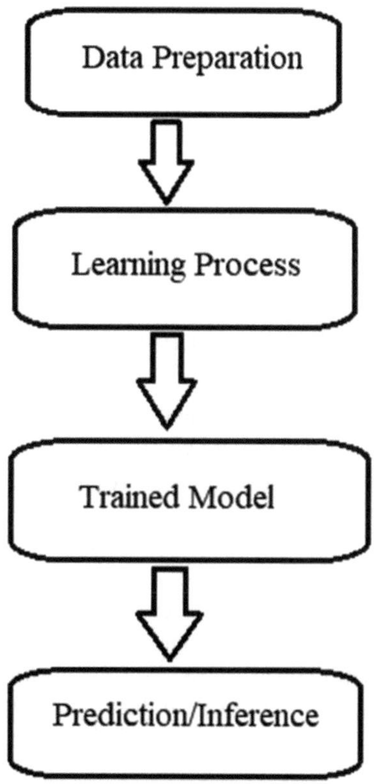

Fig. 5.2 The AI development stages

Table 5.3 The data case scenario and choices of learning process

Case Scenario	Choice of Learning process
You have labeled data (paired data) and clear goals	Supervised learning
You want to explore data, no labels.	Unsupervised learning
You want to compress or generate data	Unsupervised or self-supervised
Labels are hard to get or inconsistent	Start with unsupervised learning

Table 5.4 Examples of input-output paired data for various AI tasks

AI Tasks	Input Data	Output Data (labeled)
Text classification	Raw sentence	Label/category (e.g., obesity-related)
Machine translation	English sentence	Translated sentence (e.g., in French)
Named entity recognition	Text with symptoms	Entity labels (e.g., "chest pain" → symptom)
Speech to text	Audio file	Transcribed text
Image classification	Chest X-ray image	Diagnosis label (e.g., pneumonia)

Table 5.5 Data requirements for pretraining and continual training

Training Type	Use cases	Data Requirements	Data examples
Pretraining	GPT (generative pre-trained transformer) (trained on general web text) understand languages	Train a model on large, General-purpose data	Internet text Wikipedia PubMed
Continual (fine-tuning)	AI-doctor agent understands cardiology tweets, CVD Reddit posts, or hospital triage notes	Train or refine model on specific task/domain data	Specialized databases on CVDs Genomic and precision medicine data

5.2.1 Data Availability

Suppose you are interested in developing an AI application for an infectious disease. Let's discuss the key components of data availability issues about these infectious diseases, such as access, timeliness, completeness, and consistency.

Access

The first question should be, "Can you access the data about this infectious disease?" or "Is it stored in a retrievable format?" To answer your questions, you should know more about data sources (general web data or specific domain data). Is it proprietary data or open access? You already know basic public health content types in Table 5.2. Let's further explore them, and Table 5.6 summarizes the data availability rank for infectious diseases (CDC, 2025a; CDC, 2025b; CDC, 2025c).

Completeness

Is the data sufficiently available to cover the scope of the AI task in infectious diseases? The data completeness issues can be in many situations (Gebru et al., 2021) in Table 5.7.

You can explore data integration to address data completeness. For example, you can combine multiple data sources, such as EMRs, public health surveillance, and social media. Is the data available in a consistent format, making it easier to use

Table 5.6 Data availability rank for infectious diseases

Data types	Availability rank	Proprietary data	Data examples of infectious diseases
Public health surveillance data	High	Often publicly available; managed by government health agencies	Core data source for outbreaks (e.g., CDC, WHO, ECDC (European Centre for Disease Prevention and Control)); includes incidence, mortality, and testing rates
Behavioral and survey data	High	Many national health surveys (e.g., BRFSS (behavioral risk factor surveillance system), NHANES (National Health and nutrition examination survey)) are open access.	Used to assess mask-wearing, vaccination intention, mobility, contact rates; surveys from NIH (National Institutes of Health), CDC, WHO, etc.
Administrative and claims data	Medium-high	Proprietary; typically owned by insurers or government agencies (e.g., Medicare).	Useful for healthcare utilization, hospitalization, comorbidities, and vaccine uptake
Electronic medical records (EMRs)	Medium-high	Highly proprietary; owned by healthcare providers or vendors. Meaningful uses (MU) require reporting infectious disease data to public officials.	Contains labs, diagnoses, symptoms, vaccine status; varies by system and often delayed during fast-moving events
Geospatial and mobility data	Medium	Mixed: Some open (e.g., census, OpenStreetMap), some proprietary (from telecoms or GPS (global positioning system)).	Mobile phone/location data used for modeling spread, lockdown impact, population movement
Internet health-related social media	Medium	Technically public, but usage for AI is limited by platform policies and data scraping restrictions.	Early warning for symptoms, misinformation tracking, vaccine hesitancy trends.
Real-time and IoT health data	Medium	Owned by device manufacturers or individuals; access is limited.	Thermometers, pulse oximeters, wearables (e.g., heart rate, temperature); great for early detection and remote monitoring.

(continued)

Table 5.6 (continued)

Data types	Availability rank	Proprietary data	Data examples of infectious diseases
Specialized databases and registries	Medium	Varies: Some disease registries are public; others are institutionally controlled.	COVID-NET, WHO clinical trials, immunization registries: Structured, but not always accessible.
Social determinants of health (SDOH)	Low	Often derived from public sources, but integration with health systems may be limited.	Crucial for understanding disparities (crowded housing, essential work), but often incomplete or de-identified.
Research and clinical trial data	Low	It can be open (via repositories) but often proprietary during active trials.	Includes treatments, vaccine efficacy, drug repurposing: Rigorous but small-scale and not real-time
Genomic and precision medicine data	Low	Highly sensitive and proprietary; governed by strict privacy regulations (e.g., GINA (genetic information nondiscrimination act), HIPAA (health insurance portability and accountability act)).	Viral genomics (e.g., variants) are critical for tracking mutations; host genomics are useful but rarely integrated.

across different AI models? The standard ETL (Extract, Transform, Load) pipelines can help you to normalize and structure heterogeneous data.

Another way to face data completeness issues is to generate synthetic data. You use generative models to simulate plausible data where real data is missing. It's helpful to fill gaps in rare disease cases or populations underrepresented in training data.

Timeliness

Is the data current and up-to-date, or can it be retrieved in real time? Data out-of-date issues are especially critical in infectious diseases, where timing is everything for accurate predictions, surveillance, and response. Out-of-date data refers to data that is delayed in reporting or collection or not refreshed frequently. Those situations will limit data-driven AI responsiveness during outbreaks. How do we address this data issue? One way is to use proxies, such as social media, search trends, or mobility data, as early indicators. For example, during the COVID-19 pandemic, countries used mobility data (e.g., from Google search engines) and social media chatter as proxies for real-time transmission risk and offset delays in case reporting.

Table 5.7 Data completeness issue for infectious diseases

Situations	Examples
Missing or incomplete case reports	Inconsistent reporting from regions or facilities. Delays in diagnosis or reporting time. Underreporting due to limited access to healthcare.
Limited testing or surveillance	Gaps in testing availability during outbreaks (e.g., COVID-19). Incomplete data on asymptomatic or undiagnosed individuals.
Fragmented data sources	Lab data, EMRs, and public health databases may not be linked. Lack of interoperability between systems (e.g., hospitals, states, international bodies).
Demographic and geospatial gaps	Underrepresentation of certain populations (e.g., rural, underserved communities). Incomplete geographic tagging or location data.
Unstructured or non-standardized formats	Clinical notes, PDFs, and manual data can lead to inconsistency. Lack of harmonization across jurisdictions or countries.
Real-time data gaps	Outdated data due to upload delays. No integration of IoT or mobile sources that capture behavioral data.

Due to proprietary issues and data integration, real-time and IoT data availability is generally low. However, they provide tremendous advantages for solving the data timeliness (out-of-date) issue in AI applications for infectious diseases. It has a lot of potential to grow.

Public Health System Reform for AI Integration

Public health systems are increasingly evolving into complex, data-centric ecosystems. The system needs reforms to integrate with AI in the future. It includes modernizing data infrastructure and governance. Public health systems require standardized, interoperable platforms to aggregate and share data across sources (e.g., EHRs, social determinants, environmental sensors) (World Health, 2021). Siloed or fragmented data hinder AI's predictive accuracy and utility. Functionally, the modern public health system is like a data center. The data center needs data scientists, epidemiological modelers, data engineers, informatics specialists, privacy and security experts, AI engineers, and public health analysts. In Chap. 10, we will further discuss the workforce for AI in public health.

5.2.2 *Data Quality*

Suppose you are interested in cardiovascular diseases (CVDs) as a public health issue and want to discuss the key components of CVD data quality issues: accuracy, validity, representativeness, noise, timeliness, completeness, and consistency. The overlap between data availability and data quality is data completeness, timeliness, and consistency. Let's focus on accuracy, validity, and noise in this section.

Accuracy

The first concept of data quality is accuracy, which is the correctness of the data values. Based on our experiences using public health data, some data sources have high accuracy about CVDs, such as EMR, genomic and precision medicine data, research, and clinical trial data.

EMR Data

There are many clinical CVD data in EMR, such as structured data (diagnoses, medications, vital signs, lab results, procedures, and imaging reports) and unstructured data (physician notes, discharge summaries, progress notes, cardiology consults, lifestyle, and images). Why do EMRs have high accuracy for CVD? The short answer is that healthcare professionals (clinicians) capture those CVD data. Those cardiologists and doctors are well-trained to ensure the correctness of the data values. The EMR system has CPOE (Computerized Provider Order Entry) (structured and timely data entry) and uses standardized coding systems (ICD-10 (International Classification of Diseases-10)) to reduce errors. In the clinical setting, there is frequent monitoring and documentation. Hospitals can integrate lab and image data.

Due to the high accuracy of EMR data, there is excellent potential to develop AI applications for CVDs based on EMR data, such as identifying undiagnosed hypertension or atrial fibrillation, monitoring medication adherence and effects, detecting early warning signs from clinical notes or vital signs, etc.

Genomic and Precision Medicine Data

The breakthrough in bioinformatics uncovers the genetic and molecular underpinnings of heart-related conditions. The genetic knowledge base is growing bigger every day, and researchers have found relevant genes or markers for CVD conditions. For example, the relevant genes for CVD are *9p21, APOE, LDLR, and LPA* (Lee et al., 2017). Why is genetic data highly accurate for CVD? The short answer is that those genetic laboratories have highly controlled processes to generate genetic data, and operators are well-trained researchers. For example, bioinformatics researchers have designed pipelines for quality control, such as read alignment, variant calling, error filtering, duplicate removal, etc. The genetic results are stored and shared in well-defined formats, such as *FASTA (a text-based format for representing nucleotide or peptide sequences), VCF (Variant Call Format), BAM (Binary Alignment/Map), GTF (Gene Transfer Format)*, etc. (Privé et al., 2020). In the end, FDA regulations include accuracy requirements.

Bioinformatics can have a significant impact on public health in the long run. With both high-accuracy genetic and clinical data for CVD, AI can integrate genomic and clinical data to predict genetic CVD risk early, stratify patients for targeted therapies, optimize drug choice using pharmacogenomic data, and discover novel biomarkers or genetic patterns.

Research and clinical trial data.

The data collected in research and clinical trial data for CVDs are typically structured, high-quality datasets that cover a wide range of clinical, physiological, and sometimes genomic or lifestyle variables. These research data are highly accurate because only well-designed research proposals can pass strict peer reviews and be funded. The PI and Co-PIs of the funded projects are highly trained professionals, and they will follow precisely defined protocols to collect, measure, and report CVD data.

AI can help researchers conduct clinical trials, such as recruitment and eligibility matching. AI has recently created synthetic control data, creating virtual control groups using historical trial data (for rare or high-risk populations).

Trained in research or trial data, AI can empower risk-prediction models to predict the risk of CVDs. AI can identify optimal treatments based on trial data and predict outcomes.

Validity

Validity is about "Are you measuring the right thing?" Validity means you're aiming at the correct target to begin with. Another slogan in the AI business is "*Garbage in, garbage out (GIGO).*" AI learns from what it gets. Valid data means your data accurately reflects the concept you're trying to model. In this section, your target is CVDs. Valid data refers to information that reflects the real clinical status, risk factors, or outcomes related to cardiovascular health. For example, the valid data for CVD is" blood pressure readings" or "cholesterol levels (HDL, LDL, triglycerides)," which are related to heart failure diagnosis. The low valid data example is "patient-reported fatigue," which fatigue is nonspecific and may not directly indicate CVD. Based on the experiences, some data sources have high validity for CVDs, such as EMR, research clinical trial data, and specialized databases and registries. In the previous section, we listed some data samples of EMRs and clinical trial data for CVDs. Let's discuss the data validity issues for specialized databases and registries.

Specialized Databases and Registries for CVDs

There are some specialized databases and registries for CVDs around the world that have high data validity, as shown in Table 5.8.

Noise

Like talking in a noisy room, you may hear words, but it's harder to understand the whole message. In AI, data noise works the same way. It's not that you have no information; the sound signal is buried in distractions, randomness, or error. Data noise is about anything in your data that is random, incorrect, irrelevant, or misleading.

Table 5.8 Key CVD databases and registries with high data validity

Registry/ Database	Country/ Region	Description
National Cardiovascular Data Registry (NCDR)—by ACC (Dehmer et al., 2016)	US	One of the largest CVD registries includes hospital data on procedures like PCI (percutaneous coronary intervention), ICD, heart failure, and more. Highly standardized and validated.
Get with the guidelines (GWTG)—By AHA	US	Tracks heart failure, stroke, coronary artery disease, and resuscitation care in hospitals; used widely for quality improvement and AI research.
Framingham heart study	US	Landmark cohort study of CVD risk factors; long-term data with very high validity.
ARIC (atherosclerosis risk in communities)	US	Ongoing cohort study on heart disease and stroke; includes imaging, bloodwork, and behavioral
EUROASPIRE (Kotseva et al., 2015)	Europe	Tracks CVD prevention and care across Europe; survey-based but validated with medical records.
SWEDEHEART	Sweden	Combines several national CVD registries (e.g., myocardial infarction, PCI); highly standardized and integrated with national EMR.
MINAP	UK	National registry for heart attacks and related care.
Canadian chronic disease surveillance system (CCDSS)	Canada	Includes heart disease, stroke, and other chronic disease surveillance data.
PEACE Study (Dharmarajan et al., 2013)	China	Large-scale registry of CVD hospital care and outcomes; part of global research efforts.

Types of Data Noise

Let's see the types of data noise in Table 5.9. You may need to recall the concepts for paired data in AI for the supervised learning process.

Table 5.9 Types of data noise

Type of data noise	Description
Label noise (output noise)	Wrong labels in training data (e.g., a dog image labeled as a bear).
Attribute noise (feature noise/input noise)	Incorrect, missing, or corrupted values in input features (e.g., a wrong reading for blood pressure)
Outliers	Data points are extremely different from others (can throw off models if not handled well)
Irrelevant features	Features that have no meaningful relationship to the target (e.g., your hairstyle to heart disease)
Random variability	Inherent randomness in real-world data (e.g., body temperature with biological fluctuations)

Overfitting in AI

Do you still remember what overfitting is in AI? AI model performs great during training but is poor in the real world. One reason for overfitting is that the training data has a lot of noise. When AI models learn the training data with much noise, AI will fail in testing data.

Health-related Social Media Data for CVDs

Data noise is very common in health-related social media data. The short answer is that the content is written by non-experts (laypeople) using everyday words and is full of casual, emotional, or vague language. However, a human can enjoy conversations mixed with humor, sarcasm, typos, and slang. Some features become data noise when used for AI. They are only partly informative if out of context. Let's summarize the social media data noise for CVDs, as shown in Table 5.10.

Data cleaning for text noise (Côté et al., 2024)

If text affects the target label, the text noise can be output noises. If text is an input feature, it's attributes noise (input noise). Let's introduce the concepts of data cleaning to handle data noise. The data cleaning processes in AI include text standardization, removing irrelevant characters, spell correction, stopword removal, lemmatization, abbreviation expansion and synonym mapping, entity recognition and concept mapping, and outlier and irrelevant text filtering. For example, the "lemmatization" step is to reduce a word to its base form while considering grammar and context. Original words (running or better) have base forms (run or good). The social media data has a lot of messy noise, so data cleaning is required. Clean data will improve AI performance by reducing overfitting.

Table 5.10 Examples of data noise in social media for CVDs

Noise category	Examples
Non-expert language	People use everyday words (not use clinical terms) (e.g., "my heart feels weird.")
Ambiguity and subjectivity	Without context, it's ambiguous. (e.g., "chest pain")
Misinformation	Social media is full of inaccurate health claims, pseudoscience, and self-diagnosis (e.g., "drinking green tea cures heart disease.")
Lack of labels	Posts in social media are rarely labeled with diagnosis or treatment outcome.
Irrelevant content	"Heart" or "cardio" in posts may refer to fitness routines, love relationship metaphors.
Humor, sarcasm, and emojis	"You give me a heart attack": Confuse literal NLP models
Short, unstructured text	Full of abbreviations, typos, and slang (e.g., "EKG came back sus ngl": EKG is abbreviation for electrocardiogram; sus is "suspicious"; ngl is "not gonna lie")

5.2.3 *Data Usefulness*

Suppose you have a lot of data in your organization (e.g., community-based organizations or a hospital); you have the right to use and share it (at least internally). AI is a new hot tool, and now you want to explore it. "Is your dataset useful for AI training?" "Can I actually use this to train a good AI model for my organization?"

Suppose you are interested in dementia as a public health issue and want to discuss the key components of dementia data usefulness issues: quality, relevance, context, and sufficiency. Data quality was covered in the previous section, so let's focus on relevance, context, and sufficiency in this section for data usefulness. "Is it task-relevant?" "Is it lacking context?" "Is there enough data?"

Relevance

Is it task-relevant? Is the data relevant to the AI problem? Suppose you're trying to read tiny text through a magnifying glass. If the glass is focused on the right spot, you see clearly. That's relevant. If it's pointed out somewhere else, even if the glass is high quality, it's useless for the task. Let's show some examples of relevant data for dementia in several content types in Table 5.11.

Context

Is it lacking context? Even correct data can be misleading, ambiguous, or irrelevant to the AI's task without context. Many data context dimensions exist for AI models, as shown in Table 5.12.

Context Dimensions for Dementia

The most crucial data context dimension is temporal (when) because the cognitive decline is gradual, and dementia unfolds over the years, not days. Suppose longitudinal data (with time stamps or sequences) is available. In that case, AI models can spot subtle changes in behavior, language, or movement years before diagnosis. AI models need to distinguish cognitive decline from normal aging. Progression modeling for dementia refers to building models that track and predict how dementia develops and worsens over time. It often starts from a pre-clinical or mild cognitive impairment (MCI) stage through to full-blown dementia (e.g., Alzheimer's disease).

The next important context dimension is phenotypic/clinical (what) because dementia symptoms are subtle and overlapping, and AI needs clinical context data to interpret symptoms correctly. The meaning comes from the situation. What is being measured (cognitive scores, MRI, biomarkers, medications) defines the disease state.

Another critical data context dimension is the patient profile (who) because the personal baseline is everything. We should know what's normal for this person. Cognitive function varies by education, culture, and life experience. Without personal history, AI can't recognize deviation from the baseline. The patient profiles include age, genetics (e.g., APOE), comorbidities, education, and sex, which heavily influence risk, symptoms, and outcomes and are essential for personalized models.

Table 5.11 Examples of relevant data for dementia

Content Type	Examples of relevant data for dementia
Electronic medical records (EMRs)	Contain diagnoses, prescriptions (e.g., cholinesterase inhibitors), lab results, cognitive assessments, and comorbidities Longitudinal and structured (ideal for progression models and patient profiling)
Specialized databases and registries	The Alzheimer's Disease Neuroimaging Initiative (ADNI), USA National Alzheimer's coordinating center (NACC), USA Swedish dementia registry (SveDem), Sweden Australian dementia network (ADNeT) registry, Australia Dementia platform UK (DPUK), UK
Research and clinical trial data	Includes gold-standard neuropsych assessments, biomarkers, detailed protocols Especially useful for modeling intervention effects and staging
Genomic and precision medicine data	APOE4 status (whether someone carries one or two copies of the APOE (apolipoprotein E) gene, a key genetic risk factor for Alzheimer's disease (AD). Polygenic risk scores (estimate a person's inherited risk for developing dementia) Genomics (identifies risk genes like APOE, PSEN1, APP) Transcriptomics (reveals which genes are turned on/off in brain cells during disease.) Proteomics (detects changes in proteins like tau, amyloid-beta, and inflammatory markers.) Metabolomics, Epigenomics, Lipidomics.

Table 5.12 Data context dimensions for AI

Context Dimension	Description
Temporal (when)	Longitudinal tracking: Essential for disease progression (especially important for dementia)
Spatial (where)	Place of care, environmental exposure, living conditions
Demographic/patient profile (who)	Person-level details: Age, sex, education, comorbidities (important for dementia)
Phenotypic/clinical (what)	What is being measured: Cognition, function, biomarkers (important for dementia)
Intent/intervention (why)	Clinical decisions, trial participation, lifestyle choices.
Acquisition/method (how)	How was the data collected (sensor, survey, NLP, etc.)

Table 5.13 Examples of context data for dementia

Data content type	Context coverage
Specialized databases And registries	When: Longitudinal follow-up/visits; dementia-focused, track diagnosis, interventions, outcomes over years.Hat: Cognitive tests, MRI (magnetic resonance imaging) /PET (positron emission tomography) imaging, CSF (cerebrospinal fluid) biomarkers, diagnosis, pathology, deep phenotyping, Who: Genetics (APOE, GWAS), the uniform data set (UDS) is central to capturing detailed patient profiles, living conditions, lifestyle
Research and clinical Trial data	When: Baseline and follow-up visits (clearly time-stamped)what: Purpose-driven; cognitive tests (MMSE (mini-mental state examination), MoCA (Montreal cognitive assessment), ADAS-cog (Alzheimer's disease assessment scale—cognitive subscale), etc.); deep phenotyping; protocol-defined outcomes and adverse events. Who: Demographics (age, sex, race, education); genetic data (APOE status, WGS (whole genome sequencing), PRS (polygenic risk score)).
Electronic medical Records (EMRs)	When: Rich in temporal in real-world setting (visits, medication start/stop time). What: Rich in clinical data (diagnosis, lab tests, cognitive assessments) Who: Demographics (age, sex, race/ethnicity, language), comorbidities and social history (e.g., smoking, alcohol use)
Real-time and IoT Health data	When: Fine-grained time and behavioral context (e.g., sleep, mobility); useful for detecting subtle changes or sudden events (e.g., falls, wandering) What: Reveal functional ability, daily routines, and cognitive/physical decline.
Administrative and Claims data	When: Broad-scale tracking of utilization, some temporal continuity; tracks longitudinal care patterns over years (e.g., first diagnosis to end-of-life care) What: Diagnosis codes, procedure codes, and care setting Who: Patient demographics (limited details)

Examples of Context Data for Dementia

Understanding the key context dimensions for dementia in the previous section, we can identify some data content types important for dementia AI models, as shown in Table 5.13. The data for dementia should cover "when," "what," and "who." You can combine several data content types to cover all context dimensions if needed.

Sufficiency

Do you have enough data to train a good model? How do you estimate how much do you need? The short answer is it depends. It depends on AI tasks (with different data types and model complexity).

Model Complexity for AI Tasks

Different AI tasks in dementia require different types of models, and each model comes with its own level of complexity. Table 5.14 provides some examples of AI tasks with possible models used.

Table 5.14 Model complexity for some AI tasks

AI tasks (Data)	Examples of models used	Model complexity
Diagnosis (classification) (EMR, clinical notes, cognitive tests, imaging)	Classical ML (machine learning) models (linear models: Logistic regression; tree-based models: Random forests) Deep learning models (CNNs (convolutional neural network) for imaging)	Medium
Risk prediction (claims, EMR, SDOH, genetics)	Classical ML models (linear models: Cox regression) Deep learning models (RNNs (recurrent neural network)) Survival models Time-aware models	High
Progression modeling for dementia (longitudinal cognitive and functional data in specialized databases, EMR)	Deep learning models (RNN-based models: LSTMs (long short-term memory), GRUs (gated recurrent unit), sequence-to-sequence models; transformer-based models)	High
Genomics and polygenic risk score (PRS) (whole genome sequencing, genome-wide association study, transcriptomics)	Classical ML models (support vector machines: SVMs (support vector machine); Bayesian models) Deep learning models (feedforward and fully connected: DeepVariant; graph-based models: GCNs) Genomics (polygenic risk score models (ancestry-aware); ML for gene expression)	High
NLP for dementia (text/speech) (e.g., speech-based dementia detection) (speech and conversations)	Classical ML models (tree-based models: XGBoost (eXtreme gradient boosting))deep learning models (CNN-based models; RNN-based models) Language and speech models (pre-trained language models (PLMs): BERT (bidirectional encoder representations from transformers), GPT, LLMs; speech and audio processing: Whisper (ASR (automatic speech recognition)); wav2vec (self-supervised speech); ASR + NLP pipelines)	Very high

Data Sufficiency Issues for AI Models

Suppose you want to develop AI applications for your organization (a hospital or a community-based organization). In that case, you want to know roughly how much data you need. Table 5.15 provides estimates of data size and data sufficiency issues for some AI models (Mahmood et al., 2022). In general, more data is better. More data means less overfitting and better performance in new or unseen cases.

Transfer Learning for Data Sufficiency

Transfer learning is one of AI's most effective strategies for dealing with data insufficiency (Fayaz et al., 2024). With limited data, it means reusing knowledge from a pre-trained model on a new, related task. For example, the pre-trained model trained on the old data (English) and the new tasks work on related, limited data (medical

Table 5.15 Data sufficiency issues for AI models

AI model	Estimated dataset size	Notes
Classical machine learning models	Small (<1 k) Medium (1 k–10 k) Large (10 k–100 k) Very large (100 k+)	Needs dataset with "good features"; feature engineering (domain-specific transforms)
Survival and time-aware models	Medium (1 k–10 k) Large (10 k–100 k) Very large (100 k+)	Need good quality time-to-event data.
Deep learning models	Large (10 k–100 k) Very large (100 k+)	Needs very large corpora
Genomic models	Large (10 k–100 k) Very large (100 k+)	High dimensionality (100 k–1 M+ features)
Language and speech models	Large (10 k–100 k) Very large (100 k+)	Very large for training from scratch (e.g., Wikipedia, books, etc.)

English). The model already understands low-level patterns (like syntax in English) from a large dataset, so you don't need to learn everything from scratch for medical English. The strategy is to use a pre-trained model as a frozen feature extractor (the model's earlier layers are "frozen" and not updated during training), then train a small classifier on top. For example, an AI task for speech emotion recognition can use a pre-trained speech processing model (e.g., wav2vec) and then add a fine-tuned layer (e.g., LSTM model and linear classifier).

Model on Model (MoM) for Data Sufficiency

Model on model is a broader concept where one model's output is used as input or guidance for another model. Transfer learning is a subset of MoM (using weights or features). The MoM strategy uses full predictions, embeddings, or even decision logic from one model as guidance for another model. For example, there is a raw conversation audio file for dementia patients. You can use an audio processing model (e.g., Whisper) to convert speech into text. Whisper's output (transcripts) will become the input data for the language model (e.g., BERT) for dementia classifiers.

5.2.4 Data Bias

Data bias occurs when the data used to train or evaluate an AI system does not accurately reflect the real world, leading to skewed, unfair, or misleading results. Data bias includes data accuracy, completeness, and representativeness. Suppose that a city map represents your AI training data. The data accuracy is determined by whether the street names are correct. The data completeness is if the whole city is mapped. The data representativeness is if all modes of traveling are shown (e.g., by bike or car or bus). We covered data completeness and accuracy issues in the previous section on data availability and quality. Let's focus on data representativeness in this section for data bias. We can continue to work with CVD data as an example.

Representativeness

The data representativeness is how well the data reflects the population or target context (Clemmensen et al., 2022). Your model won't generalize well if your data doesn't represent the range of users, scenarios, or conditions. The typical examples of poor data representativeness are shown in Table 5.16.

Social Determinants of Health (SDOH)

SDOH includes housing, access to food, employment, education, environment, social support, and healthcare. It's well accepted that SDOH factors shape most health outcomes, and it goes far beyond clinical care. CVDs are strongly influenced by social factors. For example, food insecurity and poor diet could lead to hypertension. Housing instability could lead to chronic stress, which is related to heart issues. Neighborhood conditions could introduce pollution or limited exercise space. Employment and income will decide access to healthcare and medications. Education level will decide health literacy and behavior. To build effective AI models and design AI applications for public health, you should aim to collect SDOH data broadly, consistently, and equitably. SDOH data must represent all at-risk populations. Unfortunately, there are many challenges for SDOH data representativeness, as shown in Table 5.17.

Community-based Organizations (CBOs)

Collaborating with community-based organizations is one of the most effective ways to improve data representativeness and build more equitable, trustworthy AI systems (Lin et al., 2024). CBOs are most affected by health inequities and are trusted by populations often underrepresented or underserved. Community-based data are rich sources of ground-level insights, qualitative context, and non-clinical data. Our public health informatics students should collaborate with CBOs to understand local social determinants like housing, food insecurity, stress, etc. One of the goals of this textbook is to encourage and prepare our public health informatics students to co-design AI applications with and for CBOs using community-based data.

Table 5.16 The typical examples of poor data representativeness.

Domain	Example of poor representativeness
Healthcare AI	Training model on mostly male patient data
Voice recognition	Training mostly on American English accents
Facial recognition	Underrepresentation of darker skin tones in images
Social media AI	Sentiment analysis trained on formal English only
Wearable health data	Mostly includes data from healthy, tech-savvy users
Medical records	EMR data from urban hospitals only

Table 5.17 The challenges for SDOH data representativeness

Challenge	Description
Underreporting	Low-income or rural communities may be missed
Missing data	SDOH fields often left blank in EMRs
Health system bias	Data skewed toward people who are already engaged with healthcare (e.g., not the uninsured)
Technology and data access gaps	Digital divide limits SDOH capture from certain populations
Geographic imbalance	Urban areas often overrepresented compared to rural
Demographic skew	SDOH data may underrepresent racial/ethnic minorities or immigrants
Different standards	SDOH defined or collected differently across systems or states

5.2.5 Data Privacy and Security

To protect data, you should face data privacy and security issues. AI can help protect privacy and security or make it worse. It depends on *how* the AI application is designed and used. AI is a powerful tool, but it must be designed carefully with strong privacy and security rules from the beginning. As public health informatics students, you should establish the right concepts and be prepared with skills to protect data in your AI application design for public health.

Suppose you are interested in "substance abuse and addiction" topic and want to discuss the key components of data privacy and security issues for this topic. In this section, let's focus on data access control, data governance, compliance, data backup, data authorizations, and encryption.

Needs for Data Privacy and Security

Substance abuse and addiction data are very sensitive and have legal risks and social discrimination concerns (Aluri et al., 2025). Let's discuss the "stigma" concept. For example, addiction is a stigma, which often is seen as a "moral failing" instead of a medical condition. When substance abuse and addiction are associated with blame, weakness, or danger, people facing them might feel embarrassed or ashamed, avoid seeking help, and be mistreated by employers, doctors, insurers, or society.

Begin with end in mind. There are some questions about data privacy and security issues for substance abuse and addiction in Table 5.18.

AI Protects Data Privacy and Security

AI can help protect data privacy and security and make access control smarter (Liu et al., 2024). For example, AI can dynamically implement more rules to guide access

Table 5.18 The needs for data privacy and security for substance abuse

Data protection	Questions (needs)
Data access control	Who can access personal records about substance use history? Are there strict access tiers (e.g., clinician vs researcher vs IT staff)? How is unauthorized access detected and prevented? Are there automatic timeouts or re-authentication for sensitive datasets?
Data governance	Who governs the collection, sharing, and use of substance use data? What rules define whether substance use data can be linked to other datasets (like EHRs, genomics, law enforcement data)? Are participants explicitly informed of all data use scenarios (especially third-party sharing)? Is there a board or ethics committee reviewing data governance specifically for high-stigma conditions?
Compliance	Are systems compliant with HIPAA and 42 CFR Part 2? (42 CFR Part 2 is a special U.S. federal law offering extra privacy protections for substance use treatment records.) (Health, 2017) How is informed consent handled for adults entering substance abuse programs or studies? How is data sharing limited between healthcare providers (e.g., a primary care doctor vs a substance use specialist)?
Data backup	Are backups of substance abuse records encrypted and access-controlled? Where are backups stored (e.g., cloud, local servers) and are they compliant with HIPAA/42 CFR part 2 requirements? Is there a process to separately track and securely delete substance abuse data backups upon patient request? How fast can data be recovered without compromising security (e.g., disaster recovery plans)?
Data authorizations	How do patients authorize (or refuse) sharing of their substance use data with other providers? Are there specific separate consent forms for substance abuse information (not bundled with general healthcare consent)? How is the authorization revoked if a patient changes their mind? Is emergency access (e.g., overdose situations) handled in a legally compliant, logged, and minimal-disclosure way?
Data encryption	Is data about substance use encrypted at rest and encrypted in transit using high security standards? Are encryption keys managed separately for substance use data vs general health data? How often is encryption policy reviewed to ensure it covers evolving threats (like ransomware targeting healthcare systems)? Are devices (e.g., laptops, mobile access points) accessing substance abuse data encrypted too?

control for sensitive data. AI can monitor systems and quickly detect strange behaviors (like hacking attempts and unauthorized access). AI can automate key management and secure communication more effectively. For research studies, AI algorithms can automatically strip out personal identifiers from data to make it safer for sharing. In the data availability section, we mentioned synthetic data generation. If needed for specific situations involving substance abuse and addiction patients, AI can create realistic *fake* datasets (without real people) for training without exposing actual sensitive records.

AI Worsens Data Privacy and Security

Data-driven AI models (especially deep learning) need huge datasets. That pressure encourages collecting and using more sensitive personal data than before. People don't realize how much or what type of their data is being used to train AI, because consent is vague or buried in fine print. AI services are often built by external vendors, which means patient data leaves the original health system and goes into corporate AI ecosystems with unclear protection. Most AI models were not designed with data privacy as the priority. AI requires vast amounts of raw personal data, which increases privacy risks. AI models sometimes accidentally memorize and leak sensitive data (Shokri et al., 2017). AI can inadvertently expose or reinforce hidden patterns (like someone's addiction status) without explicit labels.

Specific AI System for Substance Abuse and Addiction Care

If there is a need to design an AI system for super-high-sensitivity cases like addiction care, is it possible? Can AI systems comply with ethical laws, such as 42 CFR Part 2? In theory, the answer is yes. In compliance with privacy rules, the AI system can be designed with strict input controls (only allowing de-identified, minimal necessary data into the AI), explicit guardrails (preventing models from using certain features or making certain inferences), audibility (logging and reviewing model behavior to ensure no prohibited inferences occur), consent-driven access (only making any substance-related inference if explicit patient consent is given), and risk assessments (constant evaluation to detect if the model is "leaking" sensitive inferences).

In Chap. 3, for designing AI applications, you know that AI tries to simulate human deduction reasoning, like following human ethical rules. Unfortunately, there are many challenges ahead. Critical limitations are that AI doesn't "understand" ethics the way humans do and only imitates patterns of ethical behavior from training data or rules. Ethical conflict resolution (balance or compromise) is *tough* for AI. For example, is it ethical to share substance use information if it's necessary to prevent overdose, harmful drug interactions, or medical emergencies? Humans can change ethical behavior based on subtle context shifts, but AI often struggles. If AI hasn't been trained in a tricky situation, it may behave in unpredictable or unethical ways.

5.3 Discussion Questions

Question 5.1. How would you explain the relationship between data characteristics (type, quality, quantity) and AI model performance to a non-technical public health policymaker?

Question 5.2. What unique barriers exist in accessing comprehensive public health datasets compared to other domains, and how might these impact AI development?

Question 5.3. In a scenario where an AI system for disease surveillance is trained on incomplete or inconsistent historical health records, what potential problems might emerge?

Question 5.4. How can historical biases in public health data (e.g., under-representation of specific demographics) perpetuate health disparities through AI systems?

Question 5.5. What balance should be struck between protecting individual health privacy and collecting sufficiently detailed data for effective AI public health solutions?

Question 5.6. What special security measures might be needed for AI systems handling sensitive public health data compared to other types of data?

Question 5.7. How would you develop criteria to evaluate whether a particular dataset is truly useful for a specific public health AI application?

Question 5.8. As public health challenges evolve (e.g., climate-related health impacts), what new types of data might become crucial for future AI applications?

References

Aluri, J., Gurule, E., Siddiqi, T. D., Upson, C. R., D'Sa, A., Strain, E. C., & Antoine, D. G. (2025). Privacy, care-seeking, and stigma: A qualitative investigation of patient perspectives on sharing substance use disorder treatment records. *Journal of Addiction Medicine.* https://doi.org/10.1097/ADM.0000000000001460

Bommasani, R., Hudson, D. A., Adeli, E., Altman, R., Arora, S., & et al. (2021). On the Opportunities and Risks of Foundation Models. *arXiv preprint arXiv:2108.07258.* https://arxiv.org/abs/2108.07258

CDC. (2025a). *New Home for NNDSS Weekly and Annual Tables.* Retrieved from https://www.cdc.gov/nndss/infectious-disease/weekly-and-annual-disease-data-tables.html

CDC. (2025b). *Public Health Data Strategy Milestones for 2025 and 2026.* Retrieved from https://www.cdc.gov/public-health-data-strategy/php/about/phds-milestones-2025-and-2026.html

CDC.(2025c). *Respiratory Illnesses Data Channel.* Retrieved from https://www.cdc.gov/respiratory-viruses/data/index.html

Clemmensen, L. H., & Kjærsgaard, R. D. (2022). Data representativity for machine learning and AI systems. *ACM Computing Surveys (CSUR) pre-print.* https://arxiv.org/abs/2203.04706

Côté, P.-O., Nikanjam, A., Ahmed, N., Humeniuk, D., & Khomh, F. (2024). Data cleaning and machine learning: A systematic literature review. *Automated Software Engineering.* https://doi.org/10.1007/s10515-024-00453-w

Dehmer, G., Jennings, J., Madden, R. A., Malenka, D. J., Masoudi, F. A., McKay, C. R., Ness, D. L., Rao, S. V., Resnic, F. S., Ring, M. E., Rumsfeld, J. S., & Normand, S. L. T. (2016). The National Cardiovascular Data Registry Voluntary Public Reporting Program. *Journal of the American College of Cardiology, 67*(2), 205–215. https://doi.org/10.1016/j.jacc.2015.11.001

Dharmarajan, K., Li, J., Li, X., Lin, Z., Krumholz, H. M., & Jiang, L. (2013). The China patient-centered evaluative assessment of cardiac events (China PEACE) retrospective study of acute myocardial infarction: Study design. *Circulation Cardiovascular Quality and Outcomes, 6*(6), 732–740. https://doi.org/10.1161/circoutcomes.113.000441

Fayaz, S., Ahmad Shah, S. Z., Mohi ud din, N., Gul, N., & Assad, A. (2024). Advancements in data augmentation and transfer learning: A comprehensive survey to address data scarcity challenges. *Recent Advances in Computer Science and Communications, 17*(8). https://doi.org/10.2174/0126662558286875231215054324

Frieden, T. R. (2010). A framework for public health action: The health impact pyramid. *American Journal of Public Health, 100*(4), 590–595. https://doi.org/10.2105/AJPH.2009.185652

Gandomi, A., & Haider, M. (2015). Beyond the hype: Big data concepts, methods, and analytics. *International Journal of Information Management, 35*(2), 137–144. https://doi.org/10.1016/j.ijinfomgt.2014.10.007

Gebru, T., Morgenstern, J., Vecchione, B., Vaughan, J. W., Wallach, H., Daumé Iii, H., & Crawford, K. (2021). Datasheets for datasets. *Communications of the ACM, 64*(12), 86–92. https://doi.org/10.1145/3458723

Hastie, T., Tibshirani, R., & Friedman, J. (2009). The elements of statistical learning: Data mining, inference, and prediction. *Spring.* https://link.springer.com/book/10.1007/978-0-387-84858-7

Health, U. S. D. o., Human, S., Substance, A., & Mental Health Services, A. (2017). *Confidentiality of Substance Use Disorder Patient Records: 42 CFR Part 2.* Retrieved from Washington, DC. https://www.ecfr.gov/current/title-42/chapter-I/subchapter-A/part-2

Jordan, M. I., & Mitchell, T. M. (2015). Machine learning: Trends, perspectives, and prospects. *Science, 349*(6245), 255–260. https://doi.org/10.1126/science.aaa8415

Kotseva, K., Wood, D., Bacquer, D. D., Backer, G. D., Rydén, L., Jennings, C., Gyberg, V., Amouyel, P., Bruthans, J., Castro Conde, A., Cífková, R., & Vulić, D. (2015). EUROASPIRE IV: A European Society of Cardiology Survey on the lifestyle, risk factor and therapeutic Management of Coronary Patients from 24 European countries. *European Journal of Preventive Cardiology, 23*(6), 636–648. https://doi.org/10.1177/2047487315569401

Laney, D. (2001). 3D data management: Controlling data volume, velocity and variety. *META group research note, 6*(70), 1.

Lee, J. C., Lee, B. J., Park, C., Song, H., Ock, C. Y., Sung, H., Woo, S., Youn, Y., Jung, K., Jung, J. H., & Ahn, J. (2023). Efficacy improvement in searching MEDLINE database using a novel PubMed visual analytic system: EEEvis. *PLoS One, 18*(2), e0281422. https://doi.org/10.1371/journal.pone.0281422

Lee, S. R., Prasad, A., Choi, Y. S., Xing, C., Clopton, P., Witztum, J. L., & Tsimikas, S. (2017). *LPA* gene, ethnicity, and cardiovascular events. *Circulation, 135*(3), 251–263. https://doi.org/10.1161/circulationaha.116.024611

Lin, H., Karusala, N., Okolo, C. T., D'Ignazio, C., & Gajos, K. Z. (2024). " come to us first": Centering community organizations in artificial intelligence for social good partnerships. *Proceedings of the ACM on Human-Computer Interaction, 8*(CSCW2), 1–28. https://doi.org/10.1145/3687009

Liu, S., & Guo, L. (2024). Data ownership in the AI-powered integrative health care landscape. *JMIR Medical Informatics, 12*, e57754. https://doi.org/10.2196/57754

Mahmood, R., Lucas, J., Acuna, D., Li, D., Philion, J., Alvarez, J. M., Yu, Z., Fidler, Law, M. T. (2022). *How much more data do I need? Estimating requirements for downstream tasks.* Paper presented at the arXiv preprint / CVPR 2022. https://doi.org/10.48550/arXiv.2207.01725

McKinsey, Company. (2023). What is Gen Z? Retrieved from https://www.mckinsey.com/featured-insights/mckinsey-explainers/what-is-gen-z

Prensky, M. (2001). Digital natives, digital immigrants part 1. *On the Horizon, 9*(5), 1–6. https://doi.org/10.1108/10748120110424816

Privé, F., Luu, K., Blum, M. G. B., McGrath, J. J., & Vilhjálmsson, B. J. (2020). Efficient toolkit implementing best practices for principal component analysis of population genetic data. *Bioinformatics, 36*(16), 4449–4457. https://doi.org/10.1093/bioinformatics/btaa520

Raffel, C., et al. (2020). Exploring the limits of transfer learning with a unified text-to-text transformer. *Journal of Machine Learning Research, 21*(140), 1–67. https://www.jmlr.org/papers/volume21/20-074/20-074.pdf

Shokri, R., Stronati, M., Song, C., & Shmatikov, V. (2017). Membership Inference Attacks Against Machine Learning Models. 3–18. https://doi.org/10.1109/sp.2017.41

van Engelen, J. E., & Hoos, H. H. (2020). A survey on semi-supervised learning. *Machine Learning, 109*(2), 373–440. https://doi.org/10.1007/s10994-019-05855-6

World Health Organization. (2021). Global strategy on digital health 2020–2025. In *Global strategy on digital health 2020–2025.* https://www.who.int/publications/i/item/9789240020924

Wortsman, M., Ilharco, G., Gadre, S.Y., Roelofs, R., Gontijo-Lopes, R., Morcos, A.S., Namkoong, H., Farhadi, A., Carmon, Y., Kornblith, S., & Schmidt, L. (2022). Model soups: averaging weights of multiple fine-tuned models improves accuracy without increasing inference time. *Proceedings of the 39th International Conference on Machine Learning.* https://proceedings.mlr.press/v162/wortsman22a.html

Zhu, X., & Goldberg, A. B. (2009). Introduction to semi-supervised learning. *Synthesis Lectures on Artificial Intelligence and Machine Learning, 3*(1), 1–130. https://doi.org/10.2200/S00196ED1V01Y200906AIM006

Chapter 6
Public Health Domain Data for AI

6.1 Introduction for Public Health AI Data

6.1.1 AI Pipeline Perspective

Let's introduce some concepts from the artificial intelligence (AI) pipeline perspective. *Static data* in public health, such as clinical records, administrative data, survey data, environmental risk data, and historical registries, can be updated yearly. *Self-reported data* in public health, such as HRQoL surveys, mental health self-reports, and chronic symptom tracking, are updated monthly. *Streaming data* in public health, such as wearable and mobile health, bio-surveillance data, social media and web signals, and environmental sensors, is updated daily or in real-time. *Initial training* is where you build the first version of the AI model. You train a model using *static data* to learn general patterns. *Continuous retraining* is when the model adapts to *streaming data* over time to remain accurate and relevant. The *user feedback loop* incorporates human input (*self-reported data*) to improve relevance and accuracy.

Like cooking a dish, initial training is needed to develop the recipe. Static data is the ingredients you gathered. You test combinations of ingredients, cooking time, and methods to discover what works. After a few iterations, you settle on a reliable base recipe that most people enjoy. In AI terms, you use static data to train a base model that captures general patterns. Continuous retraining is to adjust the recipe over time. Fresh ingredients that come in daily are streaming data. You refine the recipe regularly to keep it relevant and delicious. In AI terms, the model is updated as new data comes in, ensuring predictions stay accurate in real-world settings. The user feedback loop is to listen to your eaters. They give feedback after every meal. Over time, your dish is not just better but tailored to each eater. In AI terms, self-reported data helps fine-tune the model based on real-world human preferences and needs.

M. Wu, *Artificial Intelligence in Public Health*,
https://doi.org/10.1007/978-3-032-15872-7_6

EMR and EHR

EMR (electronic medical record) is a digital patient chart in a single clinic or healthcare organization. EHR (electronic health record) includes everything in an EMR plus medical history across clinics and hospitals, immunizations, allergies, radiology images, social determinants, referrals, and insurance data. EHR is designed to be shared across providers, labs, specialists, and patients.

Data Interoperability

AI models depend on diverse, high-quality, and harmonized data in public health, such as EMRs, lab reports, social determinants of health, environmental sensors, syndromic surveillance, mobile and wearable data, and policy interventions. Suppose these data cannot "talk to each other." In that case, AI models will struggle to generalize, miss context-specific patterns, propagate bias or fragmentation, and cannot be validated across populations. Data interoperability is one of public health informatics' most significant and persistent challenges.

There are some solutions or research directions for data interoperability. For example, federated learning is AI training across siloed data without sharing raw data. Data harmonization pipelines are AI-assisted data cleaning and structure mapping. Data interoperability can be partially improved using AI. AI can assist in overcoming technical and semantic mismatches across systems, formats, and vocabularies. However, AI alone *cannot s*olve governance and standards, legal and ethical barriers (e.g., consent management requires policy, not algorithms), and contextual knowledge (need human oversight for public health).

6.1.2 EMR and Meaningful Uses (MU)

Let's review some history of EMR and Meaningful Uses (MU). A chain reaction is shown in Fig. 6.1. "Every cloud has a silver lining." It means that even in dire situations, there's potential for something positive to emerge. The US faced the collapse of major financial institutions in 2008. In response, the US passed the American Recovery and Reinvestment Act (ARRA) in February 2009, a $787 billion stimulus package. HITECH Act(Health Information Technology for Economic and Clinical Health Act) is a part of ARRA and got $35 billion for digital medical records. The US government reimburses EMR costs for healthcare providers and improves EMR adoption. It lays the groundwork for public health surveillance and data exchange. Creating Meaningful Uses (MU) standards ensures EMRs are used effectively (Slight et al., 2015). MU was rolled out in 3 stages between 2011 and 2018, each with stricter requirements for data capture and sharing (e.g., e-prescribing, demographics, lab results), advanced clinical processes (e.g., secure messaging, CDS tools), and improved outcomes (e.g., population health, public health reporting), as shown in Table 6.1. MU requirements for EMR enabled data pipelines for surveillance, made large-scale public health research and predictive modeling possible, and created standardized, structured data for AI innovations today.

In the early stages, the MU requirement was that hospitals and providers had to report public health data electronically to agencies. But many public health agencies weren't ready. They lacked the infrastructure to receive and process the data. Their systems were not interoperable with hospital EHRs. There were funding and staffing limitations. Data standards weren't uniformly implemented. Over a decade after the launch of MU, many public health agencies in the US are better prepared than in the early 2010s.

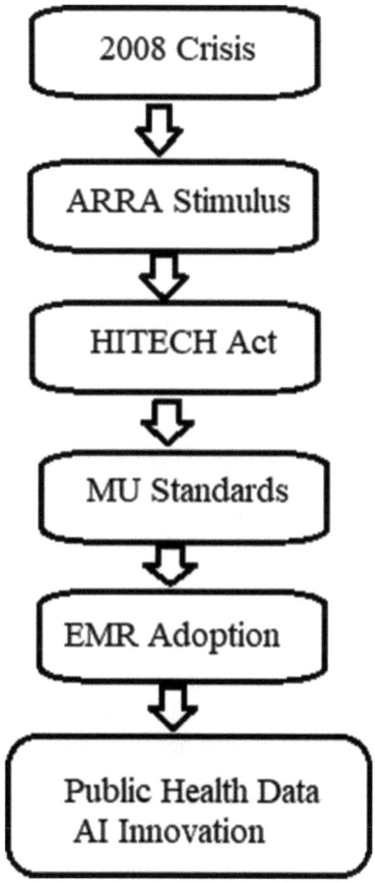

Fig. 6.1 Chain reaction for meaningful uses of EMRs

Table 6.1 Core objectives of MU for public health

Objectives	Description
Electronic reporting to immunization registries	EMRs must be able to send electronic immunization data to public health agencies Supports real-time vaccine tracking and outbreak response
Syndromic surveillance reporting	Sharing anonymized data on patient symptoms (before diagnosis) to detect outbreaks or bioterrorism threats Helps in early detection of disease trends in communities
Reportable lab results	Automatically report certain lab results (like infectious disease tests) to public health agencies Increase timeliness and accuracy in disease tracking
Electronic case reporting (eCR)	Automatically generate and transmit case reports (e.g., COVID-19, STDs [Sexually Transmitted Diseases]) from EMRs to public health Reduces manual reporting burden and improves consistency
Cancer registries and specialized registries reporting	Submit data to state or national cancer registries and other specialty registries (e.g., birth defects) Facilitates longitudinal tracking and research

6.2 Domain Data for Systemic-Factor Public Health AI[1]

6.2.1 Domain Data for Disease Monitoring

Let's look at some diseases for monitoring, such as communicable diseases (respiratory diseases, vector-borne diseases, vaccine-preventable diseases, gastrointestinal and waterborne diseases, sexually transmitted infections (STIs), and antimicrobial-resistant infections), non-communicable conditions (drug overdose, substance use disorders, mental health crises, and environmental health-linked conditions).

Sentinel

In public health, a sentinel refers to a system, site, or provider as an early warning indicator of disease trends or health events. It's like a lookout post to monitor key

[1] Suppose you focus on the impact of AI on public health. In this case, systemic-factor public health AI has a greater potential for population-level impact. Systemic factors AI can affect and improve health for millions, rather than digitally connected people. In short, systemic-factor AI has more transformative potential. Our public health informatics students should learn how to design public health systemic-factor AI applications.

signs to detect problems early before they spread widely. Sentinel is useful when full population-level surveillance isn't feasible.

Data Types Related to Disease Monitoring

Let's group some data types related to disease monitoring in Table 6.2. It'll help you to use them at the different stages of diseases, such as early signs of illness or confirmed case reporting. For example, social media can be used to detect diseases early.

Data for Disease Monitoring from AI Pipeline Perspectives

There are many disease monitoring systems and applications such as ESSENCE (Electronic Surveillance System for the Early Notification of Community-based Epidemics) (Centers for Disease Control and Prevention, 2025a), National Syndromic Surveillance Program (NSSP) (Centers for Disease Control and Prevention, 2022), ILINet (Influenza-like Illness Network) (Centers for Disease Control and Prevention, 2023b), "Flu Near You"/"Outbreaks Near Me", Wastewater Surveillance for SARS-CoV-2 (Centers for Disease Control and Prevention, 2024), ProMED-Mail (International Society for Infectious, 2025), and "HealthMap" (HealthMap, 2025). AI doesn't replace systems, but it powers them. AI models will use those platforms' data, enabling smarter, faster, and more adaptive predictions. In Chapter 7, we will apply our design models to AI applications for disease monitoring. In this section, let's focus on the domain data for disease monitoring from AI pipeline perspectives, as shown in Table 6.3. This is a conceptual analysis of data issues for disease monitoring. AI models heavily depend on domain data for continuous training.

Table 6.2 Data types related to disease monitoring

Categories	Examples of data types
Syndromic surveillance data (focuses on detecting early signs of illness before confirmed diagnosis, often in real-time)	Chief complaints (from ER or clinic visits) Self-reported symptoms Syndromic data (ER [Emergency Room] visits, ICD [International Classification of Diseases] codes) Reports from sentinel healthcare providers Search engine trends Social media signals
Informal or alternative signals (Non-traditional, less structured data sources for early warning or public sentiment)	News reports Social media Search engine trends Self-reported symptoms (if collected outside formal health systems)
Diagnostic and clinical data (Structured clinical data, often used for confirmed case reporting)	Discharge diagnoses Lab test reports EHRs (Electronic Health Records) Medication purchases

Table 6.3 Domain data for disease monitoring from AI perspective

Training use	Data type	Examples	Pipeline role
Initial training	EHRs	Hospital records (HIPAA-regulated)	Static data
Continuous retraining	Syndromic data (ER visits, ICD codes)	ESSENCE BioSense Hospital feeds	Stream data
	Lab test reports	COVID-19 test results Flu test results	Stream data
	Social media signals	Twitter (early signal) Reddit (early signal)	Stream data
	Search engine trends	Google Trends (e.g., "fever near me")	Stream data
	Self-report symptom data	Flu Near You Zoe Health Study	Self-report data

6.2.2 *Domain Data for Epidemiological Forecasting*

What Do We Forecast in Epidemiology?

The short answer is to forecast future disease trends. The long answer is to predict disease incidence or case counts, disease spread and transmission patterns, hospitalizations and mortality, vaccine impact, emergence of variants or mutations, public behavior and intervention effects, and environmental and vector-borne risks.

SEIR Model

The SEIR (Susceptible, Exposed, Infectious, Recovered) model is a mathematical model used in epidemiology to describe how a disease spreads through a population. It divides the population into four groups: susceptible people (S), exposed people (E), infectious people (I), and recovered people (R) (Hethcote, 2000). This relies on some assumptions to make disease dynamics mathematically tractable, as shown in Table 6.4.

SEIR is a rule-based system, and these rules are derived from epidemiological theory. AI systems (like machine learning models) are data-driven and learn patterns from data rather than being explicitly programmed with fixed rules. *Why do you still need to know some rule-based models, such as SEIR?* The short answer is that rule-based models help you understand the structure of epidemiological input data and interpret the output of AI models. The long answer is that the rule-based models provide foundational domain knowledge (principles of infectious disease transmission), help AI generate synthetic training data based on rule-based models, act as baselines, and provide transparency (for policymakers).

Table 6.4 Assumptions of the SEIR model

Category	Assumptions
Population structure assumptions	Homogeneous mixing: every individual is equally likely to interact with every other individual Fixed population size: no births, non-disease deaths, immigration, or emigration Closed system: no external introductions of infection unless modeled explicitly
Disease progression assumptions	Fixed transition rates: infection rate, incubation rate, recovery rate Instantaneous compartment transitions: movement between S, E, I, R follows exponential waiting times No asymptomatic transmission: only infectious individuals transmit disease (basic model)
Pathogen and immunity assumptions	No reinfection: recovered individuals are immune for life Pathogen does not mutate: virus characteristics (transmissibility, incubation time, etc.) are stable

Assumptions in Epidemiological Forecasting

Let's explore the assumptions of epidemiological forecasting in Table 6.5. You should be aware of what data is needed to support those assumptions. Vaccine effectiveness depends on "pathogen properties stay the same" and "population behavior is stable".

Data Types Related to Epidemiological Forecasting

Let's group some data types related to epidemiological forecasting in Table 6.6. It'll help you to use them for different forecasting tasks. For example, forecasting disease spreads and transmission patterns need mobility and movement data, population data, modeling parameters, epidemiological surveillance data, and behavioral and public sentiment data.

Table 6.5 Assumptions in epidemiological forecasting

Category	Assumptions
Modeling assumptions	Disease transmission follows predictable patterns Model parameters are estimated correctly
Data-related assumptions	Data is accurate and timely
Behavioral and policy assumptions	Population behavior is stable Public health interventions remain constant or are predictable
Biological assumptions	Pathogen properties stay the same
Environmental assumptions	Environmental conditions are stable or modeled

Table 6.6 Data types related to epidemiological forecasting

Category	Examples of data types
Epidemiological surveillance data	Case reports (lab test, testing) Confirmed cases (testing data) Daily case reports (testing data) Historical case counts (history flu trends) Hospitalization data Deaths (outbreak alerts) National reporting Official health data
Population data	Population demographics (age, sex, socio-economic indicators) Population density (urban/rural classification, geographic clustering)
Mobility and movement data	Mobility patterns (commuting data, geolocation data) Population movement (air traffic, airline ticketing data)
Environmental and climate data	Weather and climate data (temperature, humidity, rainfall, wind speed, UV (Ultraviolet) index, etc.)
Immunization and health protection data	Vaccination coverage (vaccination rates by age, location, vaccine type, time period)
Clinical and health records	Electronic Health Records (EHRs) (ICD codes, syndromic surveillance, symptom surveys) Claim data (ICD codes)
Genomic and pathogen data	Genomic data (pathogen mutations [spike protein variants, antiviral resistance mutations, lineage tracking])
Behavioral and public sentiment data	Self-reported data (survey) Search engine trends (Google search queries) Social media (Twitter, Facebook, Reddit)
Media and informal reporting sources	News reports Official reports (government alerts, health ministry updates)
Modeling parameters and assumptions	SEIR model assumptions (disease incubation rate, transmission rate, recovery period)

Data for Epidemiological Forecasting from AI Pipeline Perspectives

There are many epidemiological forecasting systems and applications such as "FluSight" (CDC) (Centers for Disease Control and Prevention, 2025b), "HealthMap" (HealthMap, 2025), "BlueDot" (BlueDot, 2025), "Gleamviz/GLEAM" (Van den Broeck et al., 2011), Google COVID-19 Mobility Reports, "DELPHI (CMU)" (Delphi Research, 2025), and COVID-19 Forecast Hub (Cramer et al., 2022). AI doesn't replace systems, but AI models empower them using the platform's data. Let's regroup those data types for epidemiological forecasting from

AI pipeline perspectives, as shown in Table 6.7. This is a conceptual analysis of data issues for epidemiological forecasting.

Table 6.7 Data for epidemiological forecasting from AI perspectives

Training use	Data type	Examples	Pipeline role
Initial training	Population data	Census data, Demographic surveys (age, sex, SES), UN population projections	Static
	Modeling parameters and assumptions	SEIR assumptions (incubation/transmission rates, recovery period estimates)	Static
Initial training and continuous retraining	Epidemiological surveillance data	CDC (Centers for Disease Control and Prevention)/WHO (World Health Organization) weekly reports, daily case counts ILI data FluView EuroFlu	Static and streaming
	Environmental and climate data	NOAA weather data, temperature/humidity trends, rainfall patterns	Static and streaming
	Immunization and protection data	Vaccination coverage (CDC, WHO) Immunization rates	Static and streaming
Continuous retraining	Mobility and movement data	Google mobility reports Airline ticketing Geolocation data Air traffic	Streaming
	Clinical and health records	EHRs ICD codes Syndromic surveillance Hospital admission data	Streaming
	Genomic and pathogen data	Pathogen sequencing (e.g., GISAID [Global Initiative on Sharing All Influenza Data], NCBI [National Center for Biotechnology Information]) Mutation reports	Streaming
Feedback loop	Behavioral and sentimental data	Symptom trackers (e.g., Flu Near You) Social media Google trends	Self-report and streaming
	Media and informal reports	News reports Government alerts Outbreak news on Twitter	Streaming

6.2.3 Emergency and Disaster Response

In public health, there are natural disasters, biological disasters, and man-made disasters. Natural disasters include floods, hurricanes/typhoons, earthquakes, wildfires, heat waves/cold waves, droughts, tsunamis, landslides, and volcanic eruptions. Biological disasters include pandemics and vector-borne outbreaks. Man-made disasters include chemical spills/exposures, radiological/nuclear incidents, infrastructure failures, mass casualty events, wars, refugee crises, food insecurity, etc.

All disasters will cause public health issues; we should have disaster recovery plans and systems to respond to them. For example, satellite communication should be available to key public health personnel in disaster-prone or communications-vulnerable settings. Many disasters (e.g., hurricanes, earthquakes, wildfires, blackouts, etc.) can destroy cellular networks. A smartphone with satellite communication capabilities (like those enabled for text, voice, or SOS without relying on cellular networks) is extremely valuable in disaster response.

In public health, there are many disaster response systems and applications such as ESSENCE (Centers for Disease Control and Prevention, 2025a), National Syndromic Surveillance Program (NSSP) (Centers for Disease Control and Prevention, 2022), HealthMap (HealthMap, 2025), WebEOC/EMResource/HICS (Hospital Incident Command System) (Juvare, 2025), State/regional HIE platforms, NOAA/NWS Alerts, Global Disaster Alert and Coordination System (GDACS) (Global Disaster, 2025), PulsePoint (real-time emergency alerts) (PulsePoint, 2025), Epi Info (CDC) (Centers for Disease Control and Prevention, 2025c). AI doesn't replace those disaster systems, but AI models empower them using the platform's data.

Let's look at flooding as an example of a disaster and explore AI data pipelines to respond to flooding. Why choose flooding? Flooding is one of the most common and frequent natural disasters globally (Jonkman et al., 2024).

Data for Flooding Responses from AI Pipeline Perspectives

Before flooding, based on the static data, we can conduct initial training for AI models for flooding response. We need streaming and self-report data to continuously retrain the AI models during and after flooding. The data for flooding responses from AI pipeline perspectives are shown in Table 6.8. This is a conceptual analysis of data issues for flooding.

6.2.4 Population Health Analytics

Evaluation of a Community's Health

Evaluating a community's health is like checking the pulse of an entire city, not just whether people are sick but how safe, supported, and thriving they are across all aspects of life. Why is it complex? It includes health outcomes (e.g., mortality, morbidity), behaviors (e.g., diet, exercise, smoking), environmental exposures (e.g.,

Table 6.8 Data for flooding response from AI pipeline perspectives

Training use	Data type	Examples	Pipeline roles
Initial training	Flood zones	FEMA (the Federal Emergency Management Agency) flood maps, historical inundation	Static
	Transportation routes	Highway flood susceptibility	Static
	Location of health facilities	Hospitals in flood-prone areas	Static
	Population density	High-risk urban areas	Static
	Travel patterns	Commuter flows near rivers	Static
	Electronic Health Records (EHRs)	Diagnoses, flood-related injuries	Static (historical)
	Lab results	Waterborne disease tests (e.g., cholera)	Static/Streaming
	School/work absenteeism	Sudden drops in attendance post-flood	Static/Streaming
Continuous retraining	Real-time incident locations	Live flood sensors, road closures	Streaming
	Satellite imagery	Post-flood damage assessment	Streaming
	Weather/climate forecasts	Rainfall predictions, storm tracks	Streaming
	Air/water quality data	Contaminant levels post-flood	Streaming
	911 call logs	"Water rising in basement" reports	Streaming
	Social media trends	Twitter hashtags (Flood Alert)	Streaming
	Mobility data (from phones)	Evacuation route patterns	Streaming
	Resource availability	Shelter bed shortages	Streaming
	Mutual aid requests	Mutual aid requests	Streaming
	Emergency department complaints	"Difficulty breathing" (flood mold)	Streaming
	Over-the-counter medication sales	Anti-diarrheal meds spike	Streaming
Feedback loop	Crowdsourced reports	Flood damage submissions	Self-report

(continued)

Table 6.8 (continued)

Training use	Data type	Examples	Pipeline roles
	Geo-tagged photos/ videos	Citizen flood documentation	Self-report
	Incident reports	NGO (Non-Governmental Organizations) flood response logs	Streaming/Self-report

air, water quality), social determinants (e.g., income, housing, education), and access to care and trust in systems. We know AI and "citizen science" are transformative in the AI era. Is it possible to make community health assessments faster and more accurate? Data-driven AI models depend on data. Let's explore data issues for those components one by one.

What is "Citizen Sciences?"

Citizen science refers to data collection or participation by the public, often using digital tools (e.g., mobile apps, web platforms, wearable devices) to contribute to surveillance. It augments traditional datasets for broader or more equitable surveillance. Key benefits are collecting real-time and hyperlocal data and cost-effective extension of surveillance networks.

Priorities (Root Causes)

There are some priorities among many components. Suppose a community's health is like a tree's health. The tree's soil is like the "social determinants of health (SDOH)" of the community. Income, education, housing, and neighborhood conditions strongly predict life expectancy and disease burden. It is often the root cause of poor health. The water for a tree is like "health behaviors" in a community. Behaviors like smoking, diet, physical activity, and substance use are major, modifiable risk factors. The sunshine for a tree is like "access to care" for a community. It determines timely prevention, diagnosis, and treatment. Access gaps often widen inequities, especially for underserved populations. The air for a tree is like "environmental exposure" for a community. It is usually invisible but critical. It includes air/water quality, pollution, lead, and climate risks. Long-term exposures influence chronic disease and child development. One more thing is "trust in systems." It affects compliance, vaccine uptake, health-seeking behavior, and data sharing. It is increasingly important in the era of misinformation and AI. The soil, water, sunshine, and air for a tree are available, and the tree will naturally grow, which is a "health outcome." It is a result, not a cause. SDOH is the top priority for a community's health. The whole session must be dedicated to exploring SDOH in the next session. Let's explore health behaviors in this session, which contribute to a large portion of premature deaths.

Substance Use (One of Health Behaviors)

Let's focus on substance use (one of health behaviors) as a case scenario. Chapter 5 explored data privacy and security issues for "substance use and addiction." You can review them to see the whole picture. There are some systems for substance use below. BRFSS is a "behavioral risk factor surveillance system," an annual survey of adults via phone interviews (Centers for Disease Control and Prevention, 2023a). YRBSS is a "youth risk behavior surveillance system," a school-based survey of U.S. high school students (Centers for Disease Control and Prevention, 2023c). NHANES is a "national health and nutrition examination survey" with gold-standard biomarker datasets for substance use and health risks (National Center for Health Statistics, 2023). WHO STEPS is a WHO's global risk factor framework (World Health, 2023). We treat the data as "static data" if it is updated annually.

Let's explore data issues from AI pipeline perspectives in Table 6.9. This is a conceptual analysis of domain data related to substance use.

6.2.5 Social Determinants of Health (SDOH)

Social Determinants of Health (SDOH) Analysis

SDOH is often the root cause of poor health in a community. SDOH includes income, education, employment, housing, food security, discrimination, transportation, and community safety. The elephant in the room is "income," a foundational determinant. It affects access to housing, food, education, and healthcare and strongly predicts morbidity, mortality, and life expectancy. In the AI era, income inequality may initially worsen, driven by job displacement and automation, before potential policy responses such as AI taxation or universal basic income (UBI) mitigate the impact. It is a long-term challenge for us, and more researchers should investigate "income inequality" and find solutions. For example, how do we redirect AI gains locally, such as community-based AI applications in public health based on local community data?

Education

As a case scenario, let's discuss the second priority of SDOH, education, which is a strong predictor of long-term health outcomes, employment, and health literacy. It affects income and health behaviors. In the AI era, education for "upskilling" is a part of the solution for SDOH (see Chapter 10). Many education systems and tools are part of SDOH. For early childhood literacy, programs like "Reach Out and Read" address literacy before school begins, a major predictor of long-term health (Reach et al., 2025). For k-12 students (e.g., attendance and engagement monitoring), Ed-Fi and Panorama help flag students who may be at risk due to unstable housing, food insecurity, or stress (Ed-Fi, 2023). There are initiatives for community schools to act as comprehensive SDOH hubs (healthcare, food, education) in low-income areas. For continuous education in the AI era, many AI-powered apps (e.g., Khan Academy,

Table 6.9 Data for substance use from AI pipeline perspectives

Training use	Examples of data types	Example data	Pipeline roles
Initial training	Self-reported surveys (cross-sectional)	BRFSS phone survey (e.g., smoking frequency)	Static, self-reported
	Demographics and lifestyle data	WHO STEPS Step 1 (sociodemographic and behavior data)	Static, self-reported
	Biomarkers and physical exams	NHANES urine nicotine test WHO STEPS Step 2 and 3 (BP, blood/ urine tests)	Static, sensor-generated
	School-based youth surveys	YRBSS teen alcohol and tobacco use reports	Static, self-reported
	Historical EHRs	Historical ICD-10 codes for substance use	Static
Continuous retraining	EHR updates	New ICD-10 code for substance use Treatment adherence logs	Periodic, clinical
	Longitudinal surveys	NHANES follow-up: change in e-cigarette use WHO STEPS repeated measures	Dynamic (with temporal aspect)
	Clinician feedback	Provider: "intervention success" flag Manual correction of AI prediction	Human-in-the-loop, outcome labeling
	Sensor and wearable data	Fitbit: sleep disturbance after substance use Apple Health: elevated heart rate	Streaming, passive collection
	Mobile app logs	MyFitnessPal: logged alcohol calories Recovery app: daily check-ins	Streaming, user-initiated
	Location data	Geotagged check-ins near liquor stores GPS data from recovery apps	Streaming, contextual data

(continued)

Table 6.9 (continued)

Training use	Examples of data types	Example data	Pipeline roles
	Social media content	Tweets: "relapse," "overdose" posts Reddit: substance use forums	Streaming, public user-generated
	Daily mood and craving logs	App log: "craving level today" User: "felt triggered at party"	Self-report, real-time, user-initiated
	Citizen science inputs	Narratives of local use hot spots	User-initiated, participatory, continuous
	App survey updates	Monthly in-app relapse self-checks Weekly stress scale updates	Self-report, recurring
User feedback loops	Follow-up surveys	Monthly user survey: "how many drinks this week?" Post-intervention outcome survey	Self-report, longitudinal, reflective
	User corrections	Sensor was wrong Wrong number of drinks	Real-time correction, human-in-the-loop
	Behavior changes	App detects reduced relapse frequency after alerts Decrease in craving logs after coping suggestion	Dynamic behavioral feedback, reinforcement learning signal

Duolingo, Zearn, DreamBox) can scale tutoring, personalized learning, and life-skill development in under-resourced regions. There are equity dashboard systems (e.g., Opportunity Atlas) that help communities visualize where educational investments are most needed.

Table 6.10 provides domain data for education from AI pipeline perspectives. This is a conceptual analysis of data issues for education in a community.

Table 6.10 Data for education from AI pipeline perspectives

Training use	Examples of data types	Examples of data	AI pipeline roles
Initial training	K–12 administrative data	Attendance, test scores, GPA (Grade Point Average)	Static data
	State accountability metrics	Test scores, subgroup performance, English learner progress	Static data
	Cradle-to-career metrics (StriveTogether, 2023)	High school graduation/dropout rates	Static data
	Longitudinal socioeconomic outcomes	Adult income based on childhood census tract	Static data
Continuous retraining	Literacy screening	Number of books read	Self-reported data
	Social-emotional learning (SEL) surveys	"I feel safe at school"	Self-reported data
	Longitudinal academic and social outcomes	Long-term program performance metrics	Longitudinal data
	Student-conducted research (e.g., YPAR)	Peer surveys or interviews	Periodic data
	Learning activity logs (AI-powered)	DreamBox mastery levels	Streaming data
	Language learning metrics (AI-powered)	Duolingo language logs	Streaming data
	Math learning metrics (AI-powered)	Skill proficiency (Zearn logs)	Streaming data
	Opportunity Atlas metrics	Income mobility by education level	Periodic, longitudinal
User feedback loop	Community voice and advocacy data	Student videos, youth-led policy suggestions	Self-reported data
	YPAR action outcomes	Policy audits by youth	Self-reported data

6.2.6 Resource Management

Resource Allocation Optimization

The limited resources in public health include funding, personnel, equipment, vaccines, etc. Some urgent challenges are ICU (Intensive Care Unit) bed allocation and vaccine distribution. AI can help with resource allocation optimization. In this session, let's explore vaccine resource allocation optimization (Zhou et al., 2021). The vaccine demonstrates how public health prevents diseases through organized societies' efforts (Wouters et al., 2021). The key components related to vaccine

Table 6.11 Data for vaccine equity from AI pipeline perspectives

Training use	Public health strategy	Example data
Initial training	Risk stratification (train models to prioritize based on clinical risk)	Age-related risk (e.g., older adults) Medical risk (e.g., people with chronic diseases, immunocompromised individuals) Occupational risk (e.g., frontline healthcare workers) Historical severity data (e.g., populations with higher past rates of hospitalization) Congregate setting risk (e.g., residents of nursing homes, shelters, or correctional facilities)
	Equity adjustment (including systemic disparities in the baseline model)	Social vulnerability index (SVI) Insurance status, rural access, language data
Continuous retraining	Gap monitoring (detection) (detect and adapt to real-time failures or inequities)	Live coverage by ZIP code and demographic Missed appointments, no-show trends ZIP codes with low vaccination despite high vulnerability Missed second doses Low uptake in minority or rural communities
User feedback loop	Reprioritize based on findings (improve equity and coverage during rollout)	Low-uptake alerts Community sentiment Outbreaks in underserved areas

resource optimization include "when and where vaccine needed," "who get vaccines," "how to distribute and store vaccines" and "maintain vaccines safety and trust."

Let us look at the data issues of one of the vaccine distribution processes, such as how to handle vaccine equity. Suppose that you will train an AI model to decide who gets vaccines. Table 6.11 lists key data elements from AI pipeline perspectives.

6.2.7 *Policy Optimization*

Public health policy modeling is a core skill and a foundational lens in public health education. Table 6.12 lists some examples of public health policy modeling.

Policy Modeling

To demonstrate how to conduct public health policy modeling, let's choose a case scenario to explore: early warning systems for heatwaves. The policy goal is to reduce

Table 6.12 Examples of public health policy modeling

Category	Examples of subcategory	Examples of policy modeling
Infectious disease control	Vaccination	COVID-19 vaccine allocation (e.g., herd immunity, logistics, equity)
	Travel restrictions	Airport screening during outbreaks (e.g., delay vs. containment trade-offs)
Chronic disease prevention	Sugar tax	20% soda tax (e.g., obesity, diabetes reduction)
	Nutrition labeling	Traffic-light food labeling (e.g., consumer behavior, weight trends)
Environmental and occupational health	Air quality	Emission limits near schools (e.g., Asthma rates in children)
	Heatwaves	Early warning systems (e.g., mortality reduction in vulnerable populations)
Maternal and child health	Paid maternity leave	National paid leave program (e.g., breastfeeding rates, child development)
	Prenatal care access	Rural telemedicine for prenatal care (e.g., birth outcomes, equity)
Health equity and access	Medicaid Expansion	State-level ACA (Affordable Care Act) policy (e.g., uninsured rates, preventable deaths)
	Telehealth Incentives	Rural telehealth subsidies (e.g., service access, digital divide)
Behavioral and mental health	Suicide prevention	School-based mental health programs (e.g., suicide rates, early identification)
	Alcohol sales limits	Ban on late-night sales (e.g., injury, violence, DUIs [Driving Under the Influence])
Emergency preparedness	PPE (Personal Protective Equipment) stockpiling	Federal mask reserves (e.g., resilience under demand surges)
Health financing and cost control	Value-based payment	Pay-for-performance programs (e.g., cost-effectiveness, quality improvement)

mortality and morbidity among vulnerable populations (e.g., elderly, low-income, chronically ill) during extreme heat events.

First, you should define the structure of the system. It includes actors (public health agencies, emergency services, media, residents), components (weather data systems, alert infrastructure, local services, hospitals), scope (city or regional level, over summer months), and interactions (heat alerts trigger responses like hydration centers, outreach to seniors). Second, it should include relevant variables, such as temperature thresholds, humidity, population age and comorbidities, access to air conditioning, emergency response capacity, and timing and coverage of alerts. Third, you should establish relationships between variables. For example, the key relationships include heat index for hospitalization risk, heat alerts for behavior change (e.g., visiting cooling centers), and AC (Air Conditioner) access for mortality risk reduction. Finally, you will design the rules and behaviors of the system. For example, vulnerable people visit cooling centers if a heatwave alert is issued. The risk increases with every degree if there is no AC and no alert. The system has resource constraints, such as limited transportation or staffing for outreach.

As public health officials or practitioners, you realize that public health policy modeling is a reasoning problem. They involve cause-effect thinking, trade-offs, and system dynamics, which require reasoning across multiple levels. Policy models require assumptions about population behavior, system capacity, funding, compliance, and politics. Policy modeling is context-specific. What works in one region may not apply elsewhere. Political, economic, and cultural factors all matter. There are often conflicting priorities (e.g., privacy vs. surveillance of pandemics).

In the AI era, AI will help use reasoning with agent-based modeling (ABM) or reinforcement learning (RL), which are needed to simulate policy dynamics properly.

Agent-Based Model (ABM) Data Needed

Agent-based modeling is a bottom-up reasoning (Karsai et al., 2016). It simulates individual agents (e.g., residents, responders, hospitals) and their interactions under heatwave scenarios. Table 6.13 lists the example data for ABM (early warning systems for heatwaves).

Reinforcement Learning (RL) Data Needed

Reinforcement learning is a "goal-oriented" adaptive reasoning (Liu et al., 2015) (You can review the RL concept in Chapter 2). It simulates dynamic decision-making over time to optimize actions like when to issue alerts, allocate ambulances, or open shelters. Table 6.14 lists the example data for RL (early warning systems for heatwaves).

Table 6.13 Example data for "agent-based" policy modeling

ABM data types	Examples of data
Agent characteristics	Demographics (e.g., age, gender, income, housing type, social isolation) Health status (e.g., chronic diseases, disability, mobility limitations) Behavioral traits (e.g., response to alerts, trust in government messages, likelihood of using cooling centers)
Environmental data	Geospatial data (e.g., neighborhoods, zip codes, distances to cooling centers or hospitals) Urban heat zones (e.g., microclimate variations, tree cover, building density) Infrastructure (e.g., AC availability, transportation access, health facility distribution)
Interaction rules and triggers	Social networks (e.g., who checks on whom, info-sharing patterns) Alert triggers (e.g., what threshold activates behavioral response) Policy rules (e.g., when outreach begins, who gets prioritized)

Table 6.14 Example data for "reinforcement learning" policy modeling

RL data types	Examples of data
State space (what the AI sees at each decision point)	Temperature, humidity forecasts AC access by neighborhood Current hospitalization counts Resource availability (staff, shelters, transport)
Actions	Issue warning alert (Yes/No) Open cooling centers (location/time) Allocate outreach teams to districts Adjust alert thresholds dynamically
Rewards	Reduction in heat-related ER visits or deaths Equity improvement (e.g., reduced disparities) Cost-efficiency (e.g., avoid unnecessary alerts)
Transition dynamics	How people respond to alerts How fast resources can be mobilized Effect of previous actions on outcomes

6.3 Domain Data for Personal-Responsibility Public Health AI[2]

6.3.1 Concept Maps for Personal Health Data

The domain data for personal responsibility in public health is relatively minor compared to systemic factors in public health. However, they are still rich and complex. This session will explore the various data types and usages of domain data for personal responsibility in public health. A concept map is drawn and shown in Fig. 6.2. They are involved in many concepts such as personal health records, individual profiles, medical snapshots, objective signals (e.g., wearable and biosensor data), subjective data (e.g., self-reported data), contextual data, interaction logs, etc.

Personal Health Records (PHR) (Roehrs et al., 2017)

Both medical records (MR) and personal health records are about your life's story related to your health. Medical records are chapters written by your medical doctors (health care providers). MRs are structured and formal, but only from clinical encounters. While personal health records are your complete autobiography, they include doctors' chapters, plus your journal entries, fitness logs, feelings, goals, and photos.

If every citizen maintains a PHR, even before becoming a "patient" (MR), the PHR becomes a universal health intelligence tool for public health. It can capture everyday health behaviors (sleep, nutrition, physical activity), environmental exposures (location, air quality, stressors), preventive care (vaccination history, screening status), self-reported symptoms and mental health states, as well as social determinants (housing, employment, access to food). Public health will benefit from PHR. They will enable community-level health trend monitoring, risk prediction and early intervention, personalized preventive recommendations, faster emergency response planning, and inclusive public health policymaking.

One of the key reasons for the historically low adoption of PHRs has been the knowledge gap in health between citizens and healthcare professionals. Most people haven't used PHRs because they don't understand the data, are overwhelmed by medical jargon, and don't know what to do with it. PHRs are passive or isolated (like a dusty filing cabinet). In the past, a PHR was like a notebook where you had to write everything and hope a doctor would read it later.

---

[2] Public health AI for personal responsibility has seen more consumer-facing applications recently because those AI applications are highly personalized, data-rich, and relatively easier to deploy at scale in commercial markets. In this session, let's focus on personal responsibility AI applications in public health. Every person has 100% health concerns for themselves, and people will invest in it if the benefit is clear and accessible. Payers and employers want a short-term return on investment (ROI). Behavior-focused AI applications give them measurable returns (lower absenteeism, fewer claims). In the AI era, AI made personalization affordable and scaled to millions. Finally, humans have an unprecedented opportunity to improve health literacy and reduce the knowledge gap between the public and healthcare providers. AI democratizes access to health information.

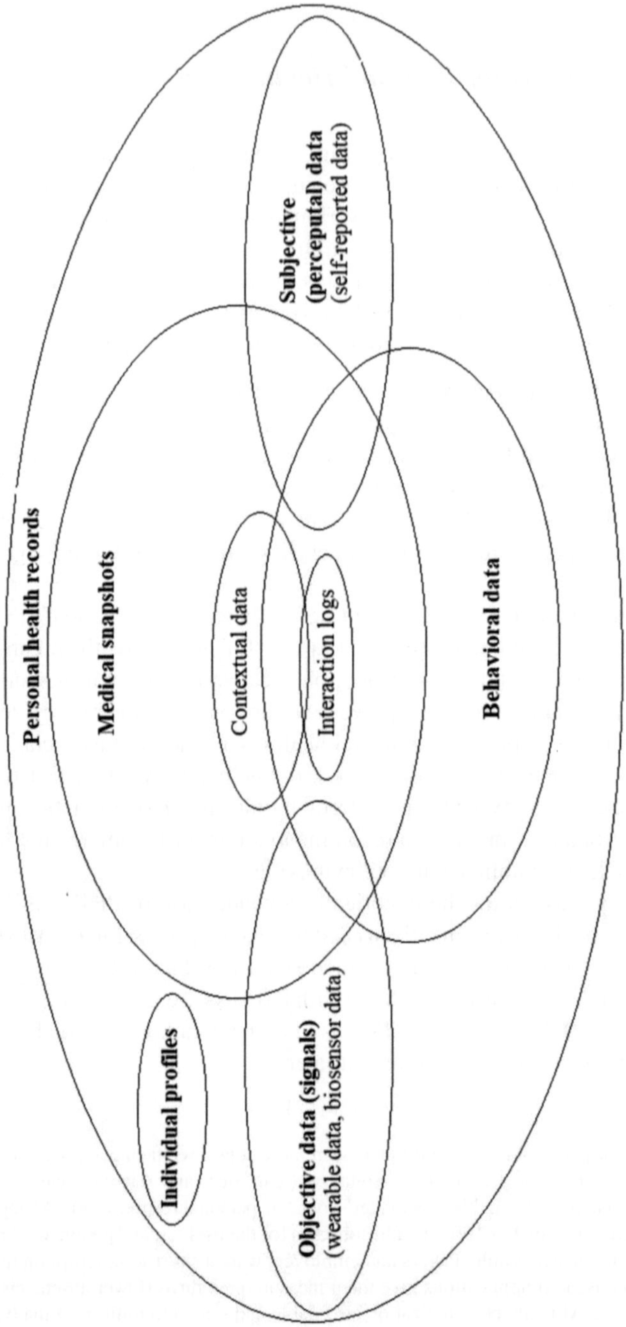

Fig. 6.2 A concept map for domain data type for PHR

Now, in the AI era, a PHR has the potential to become a smart journal that reads what you write, understands its meaning, and gently helps you make better choices every day. Firstly, AI is your health literacy companion, translating complex health data into clear, meaningful information. For example, "HbA1c = 7.8%" means "Your blood sugar is a little high. This means you may be at risk for type 2 diabetes. Let's look at small steps to help." Secondly, based on the PHR, AI copilot for self-care guides citizens on what symptoms to track, when to seek care, and how lifestyle choices affect health. It becomes a "digital health coach," tailored to you. PHRs can become real-time behavioral tools, offering reminders for vaccines or checkups, encouragement to meet health goals, and warnings when a trend looks concerning.

What is N-of-1 Learning?

Public health targets the population, and the larger the sample size in public health research, the more effective it is. While personal health records are targeting one person. N-of-1 learning is a personalized, continuous feedback process where an individual becomes their own "case study," learning from their own data over time to optimize health decisions. It comes from N-of-1 trials in medicine, where "N" (the sample size) is one person, and the goal is to *test what works for you, not just the population.*

Medical Snapshots

A medical snapshot is a concise, structured summary of a person's health status at a specific point in time. It is often used in PHRs to give users or AI systems a readable, timely view of key clinical information. Medical snapshots are not the same as medical records. They are simplified views of selected health information, designed for understanding, monitoring, and action. Medical snapshots are short and naturally improve patient understanding and health literacy.

How do you decide the "relevance" of a short data set (snapshot) to filter from complete medical records? They are many ways, such as, purpose/use-case (what matters for this user/action/context), recency (what's recent enough to affect today), problem-linkage (what's directly tied to current conditions), risk/impact (what's urgent, unusual, or changing), personalization (what's practical or understandable to the reader) and narrative simplicity (what builds a coherent, actionable picture). You can find more metadata ideas in the following sessions.

Individual Profiles

The individual profile is a component of the PHR. It's a foundational layer that defines who the person is. It includes static or slowly changing characteristics, such as demographics (age, sex, race, language), social determinants (education, income, housing), health literacy, access to technology, care preferences, genetic risk factors, or family history.

Contextual Data

Contextual data is the environmental and situational layer in PHR. It can be location, time, weather, calendar, and work shifts. It will support the interpretation of behavior (e.g., missed steps due to rain), wearable data (e.g., sleep interrupted by travel), and interaction logs (when and why a user skipped or responded).

Objective Data/Signals

Objective signals or data refer to measurable and quantifiable information. For example, wearable data are collected from wearables (e.g., heart rate, steps). Biosensor data are physiological measurements (e.g., glucose levels, ECG [Electrocardiogram]).

Subjective (Perceptual) Data

Subjective (perceptual) data can be self-reported data (e.g., pain levels, mood, stress, energy). It contrasts with objective signals, which are measured. It is frequently paired with objective data for reasoning. It is often used to enrich behavioral and interaction logs.

Interaction Logs

In the digital age, users frequently interact with digital devices, including apps, chatbots, and wearables. Interaction logs record how, when, and why a user interacts with a system (e.g., a mobile app, wearable device, chatbot, or PHR platform). They are records of digital interactions. They overlap with behavioral data (actions), subjective data (user reports), and contextual data (such as timing and triggers). Interaction logs are extremely valuable for AI learning about habits, preferences, and health literacy. They feed the AI model training and is a goldmine for AI-powered PHR.

Behavioral Data

Before the advent of AI, PHR adoption was limited. At that time, PHRs were a moral duty or an ethical ideal. PHRs will become real in the AI era. Behavioral data captures how people live, act, and engage with their health in everyday life. It is becoming a core pillar of PHRs and goes far beyond clinical notes and lab results. Behavioral data are actions and patterns, such as steps, meals, sleep, screen time, and medication adherence. They are records of habits (e.g., exercise, diet, sleep).

AI-powered PHRs will have a real and transformative impact on individuals in the coming years. For example, you can help your family members manage their pre-diabetes. AI-powered PHRs can track behavioral data, such as steps per day, food photos, skipped meals, sugar intake, and sleep patterns.

6.3.2 Metadata for Personal Health Records

Metadata is data about data, such as indexes. In traditional medical records (MRs), the indexes (metadata) primarily revolve around time, location, and the problem list. In the AI era, AI-powered PHRs called for a richer, multidimensional metadata architecture. For example, encounter time in MRs will become continuous behavioral and contextual timelines in PHRs. Locations in MRs will be environmental and social setting metadata in PHRs. Problem lists in MRs are multimodal symptom-behavior-intervention-outcome chains. Let's explore the metadata for AI-powered personal health records in this session. Table 6.15 lists the key metadata examples used in PHRs for public health AI applications, shown in Fig. 6.3.

The conceptual framing is crucial for leveraging AI as a thinking partner. In short, as a public health informatics student, you should understand concept maps and key metadata for PHRs. Metadata literacy is a core skill for AI-driven public health. These metadata will support many public health AI applications for personal responsibilities, such as continuous, multimodal data streams, contextual reasoning and personalization, causal inference and predictive modeling, and real-time feedback and explainability.

6.4 Discussion Questions

Question 6.1. How should public health practitioners choose between static, streaming, or self-reported data sources when developing AI models for disease surveillance? What are the tradeoffs in terms of accuracy, timeliness, and implementation complexity for each data type?

Question 6.2. What are the most significant barriers to extracting meaningful insights from Electronic Medical Records (EMR) for public health AI? How can these be addressed while maintaining patient privacy and data integrity?

Question 6.3. Why is continuous retraining significant for AI models in disease surveillance compared to other public health applications? What challenges arise when maintaining an AI pipeline that relies on real-time streaming data versus periodic static updates?

Question 6.4. Compare the data characteristics (e.g., granularity, frequency, sources) required for population-level surveillance AI versus personalized health AI.

Question 6.5. How should personal health record metadata be structured and standardized to maximize its utility for AI applications while protecting individual privacy? What tradeoffs exist in this design process?

Table 6.15 Metadata for AI-powered personal health records

Metadata examples	Example data	Use examples in AI-powered PHRs
Temporal metadata	Timestamps (exact time of data entry, capture, or event) Duration (of symptoms, behaviors, interventions) Sequencing (temporal order of events) Recurrence patterns (e.g., cyclical migraines, monthly mood dips) Lag time (between trigger and outcome)	Sequencing, event tracking, pattern discovery, anomaly detection, causal modeling (causality)
Contextual metadata	Location (home, work, clinic, outdoor) Environment (weather, pollution, pollen, noise) Time of day/day of week Social context (alone, caregiving, at a party) Life events/stressors (job loss, school exams)	Situation-aware reasoning, predicting triggers, understanding situational variance
Behavioral feature vectors	Daily metrics across multiple dimensions (sleep hours, steps, meals, hydration; stress/mood ratings; screen time, alcohol, medication adherence, etc.) Optionally tagged with confidence or quality score (manual vs. auto-sensed)	Daily prediction, habit modeling, AI-driven risk scoring, adaptive coaching, forecasting health dips
Health events and intervention tags	Clinical events: symptoms, diagnoses, treatments Self-care actions: meditation, exercise, diet changes Triggers: pain onset, social conflict, missed dose Outcomes: "Pain decreased," "mood improved," "BP normalized"	Feedback loops, N-of-1 learning, intervention tracking, response modeling
Personal knowledge graph metadata	Nodes (Symptoms, diagnoses, drugs, meals, goals, questions, apps used) Edges/links (Causal, temporal, semantic) Attributes (frequency, importance, relevance score)	Structured relationships for explainability (explainable AI), query-based summaries, personal reasoning chains

(continued)

Table 6.15 (continued)

Metadata examples	Example data	Use examples in AI-powered PHRs
Psychosocial and readiness indicators	Motivation level (low/moderate/high) Health literacy score or style (visual/verbal, metric/narrative) Behavior stage (pre-contemplation → maintenance) Barriers (cost, fear, forgetfulness, tech) Engagement history (app opens, message replies, symptom tracking frequency)	Tailored education and nudging, micro-segmentation, chatbot personalization, equity-aware nudges
Provenance metadata	Data source (device, app, clinician, self-report) Confidence score (wearable sensor reliability, user consistency) Authorship (AI-generated summary, user log, clinician note) Timestamp of processing (when AI last updated or interpreted the data)	Data trust, model validation, auditability (audit trail)
Goals and preference metadata	Short- and long-term health goals Preferred terminology or conditions of concern Risk tolerance or alert thresholds Communication preferences (tone, timing, channel)	AI personalization, ethics, engagement, user-controlled care plans

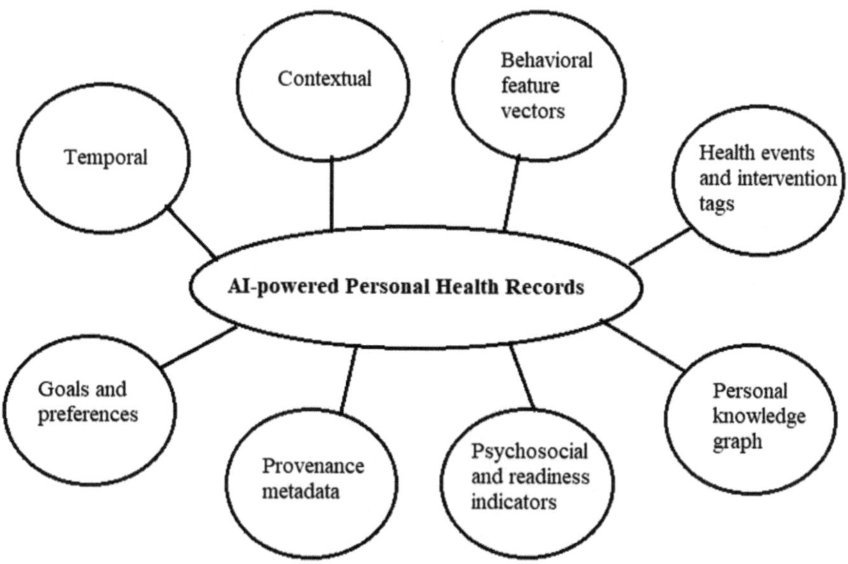

Fig. 6.3 Metadata for AI-powered personal health records

References

BlueDot, I. (2025). BlueDot: Outbreak Intelligence. Retrieved November 30, 2025, from https://bluedot.global/

Centers for Disease Control and Prevention. (2022). *National Syndromic Surveillance Program (NSSP)*. https://www.cdc.gov/nssp/index.html

Centers for Disease Control and Prevention. (2023a). *Behavioral Risk Factor Surveillance System (BRFSS)*. https://www.cdc.gov/brfss/

Centers for Disease Control and Prevention. (2023b). *U.S. Outpatient Influenza-like Illness Surveillance Network (ILINet)*. https://wwwn.cdc.gov/ILINet/

Centers for Disease Control and Prevention. (2023c). *Youth Risk Behavior Surveillance System (YRBSS)*. https://www.cdc.gov/yrbs/

Centers for Disease Control and Prevention. (2024). *National Wastewater Surveillance System (NWSS)*. https://www.cdc.gov/nwss/wastewater-surveillance.html

Centers for Disease Control and Prevention. (2025a). *ESSENCE|National Syndromic Surveillance Program (NSSP)*. https://www.cdc.gov/nssp/php/onboarding-toolkits/essence.html

Centers for Disease Control and Prevention. (2025b). *FluSight: Influenza Forecasting*. https://www.cdc.gov/flu/weekly/flusight/index.html

Centers for Disease Control and Prevention. (2025c). *Epi Info™*. https://www.cdc.gov/epiinfo/index.html

Cramer, E. Y., Huang, Y., Wang, Y., Ray, E. L., Cornell, M., Bracher, J., et al. (2022). The United States COVID-19 Forecast Hub Dataset. *Scientific Data, 9*, 462. https://doi.org/10.1038/s41597-022-01517-w

Delphi Research, G., & Carnegie Mellon, U. (2025). *Delphi: Epidemic Forecasting*. Retrieved November 30, 2025, from https://delphi.cmu.edu/

Ed-Fi, A. (2023). *Ed-Fi Data Standard and Technology Suite*. Retrieved November 30, 2025, from https://www.ed-fi.org/

Global Disaster, A., Coordination, S., United Nations Office for the Coordination of Humanitarian, A., & European, C. (2025). *GDACS: Global Disaster Alert and Coordination System*. Retrieved November 30, 2025, from https://gdacs.org/

HealthMap, & Boston Children's, H. (2025). *HealthMap: Global Disease Alert Map*. Retrieved November 30, 2025, from https://www.healthmap.org/en/

Hethcote, H. W. (2000). The Mathematics of Infectious Diseases. *SIAM Review, 42*(4), 599–653. https://doi.org/10.1137/S0036144500371907

International Society for Infectious, D. (2025). *ProMED-Mail: Program for Monitoring Emerging Diseases*. https://promedmail.org/

Jonkman, S. N., Curran, A., & Bouwer, L. M. (2024). Floods Have Become Less Deadly: An Analysis of Global Flood Fatalities 1975–2022. *Natural Hazards, 120*(7), 6327–6342. https://doi.org/10.1007/s11069-024-06444-0

Juvare. (2025). *WebEOC: Emergency Operations Center Crisis Management Platform*. https://www.juvare.com/webeoc/

Karsai, I., Montano, E., & Schmickl, T. (2016). Bottom-Up Ecology: An Agent-Based Model on the Interactions Between Competition and Predation. *Letters in Biomathematics, 3*(1). https://doi.org/10.30707/lib3.1karsai

Liu, D., Li, H., & Wang, D. (2015). Feature Selection and Feature Learning for High-Dimensional Batch Reinforcement Learning: A Survey. *International Journal of Automation and Computing, 12*(3), 229–242. https://doi.org/10.1007/s11633-015-0893-y

National Center for Health Statistics, Centers for Disease Control and Prevention. (2023). *National Health and Nutrition Examination Survey (NHANES)*. https://www.cdc.gov/nchs/nhanes/

PulsePoint, F. (2025). *PulsePoint: Real-Time Emergency Alerts*. Retrieved November 30, 2025, from https://www.pulsepoint.org/

Reach, O., & Read National, C. (2025). *Reach Out and Read: National Literacy Program*. Retrieved November 30, 2025, from https://reachoutandread.org/

Roehrs, A., da Costa, C. A., Righi, R. d. R., & da Silva, A. F. (2017). Personal Health Records: A Systematic Literature Review. *Journal of Medical Internet Research, 19*(1), e13. https://doi.org/10.2196/jmir.5876

Slight, S. P., Berner, E. S., Galanter, W., Huff, S., Lambert, B. L., Lannon, C., & Bates, D. W. (2015). Meaningful Use of Electronic Health Records: Experiences From the Field and Future Opportunities. *JMIR Medical Informatics, 3*(3), e30. https://doi.org/10.2196/medinform.4457

StriveTogether. (2023). *Cradle-to-Career Metrics Framework*. Retrieved November 30, 2025, from https://www.strivetogether.org/cradle-to-career-network/

Van den Broeck, W., Gioannini, C., Gonçalves, B., Quaggiotto, M., Colizza, V., & Vespignani, A. (2011). The GLEaMviz Computational Tool, a Publicly Available Software to Explore Realistic Epidemic Spreading Scenarios at the Global Scale. *BMC Infectious Diseases, 11*, 37. https://doi.org/10.1186/1471-2334-11-37

World Health, O. (2023). *WHO STEPwise Approach to NCD Risk Factor Surveillance (STEPS)*. https://www.who.int/teams/noncommunicable-diseases/surveillance/systems-tools/steps

Wouters, O. J., Shadlen, K. C., Salcher-Konrad, M., Pollard, A. J., Larson, H. J., Teerawattananon, Y., & Jit, M. (2021). Challenges in Ensuring Global Access to COVID-19 Vaccines: Production, Affordability, Allocation, and Deployment. *The Lancet, 397*(10278), 1023–1034. https://doi.org/10.1016/s0140-6736(21)00306-8

Zhou, S., Zhou, S., Zheng, Z., & Lu, J. (2021). Optimizing Spatial Allocation of COVID-19 Vaccine by Agent-Based Spatiotemporal Simulations. *Geohealth, 5*(6). https://doi.org/10.1029/2021gh000427

Part IV
Cases Studies of AI Applications for Public Health

Chapter 7
AI Applications for Public Health Systemic Factors

7.1 Design Process of AI Applications in Public Health

Suppose you are interested in "disease monitoring," an essential public health task. In this case, let me introduce you to a simplified design process for artificial intelligence (AI) applications for disease monitoring. Data issues and public health domain data have been covered in Chapters 5 and 6. We will focus on selecting AI models and techniques to address the core public health tasks in this chapter and Chapter 8. Let me design a series of case scenarios in public health as unmet needs and demonstrate how to implement AI as a part of the solutions. A simplified design process for AI applications in public health is shown in Fig. 7.1.

Stakeholders Profiling

Disease represents an emergent or irregular demand for healthcare services and products. The suppliers include healthcare providers (e.g., hospitals and clinics) and health product manufacturers (e.g., pharmaceutical and diagnostics companies). Stakeholders include the public (as patients and taxpayers) and public health agencies/governments (as both funders and regulators). In this framework, disease monitoring functions as a form of market intelligence to collect and analyze data to understand disease burden, anticipate needs, and inform supply-side responses such as service delivery, medical product distribution, and public health policy. Unlike

---

There is a dilemma for the author: on the one hand, many clear and compelling public health problems are waiting to be explored; on the other, there is limited time to write this book. As a result, the first edition of the textbook includes only a limited number of case scenarios with step-by-step AI solutions. There are eight case scenarios in this chapter and Chapter 8. For most public health tasks, this textbook explores integrating AI into current public health solution frameworks and identifying AI strengths or weaknesses in those public health issues. Hopefully, this textbook will have a second edition, and the author can cover more popular case scenarios based on your feedback and interest.

M. Wu, *Artificial Intelligence in Public Health*,
https://doi.org/10.1007/978-3-032-15872-7_7

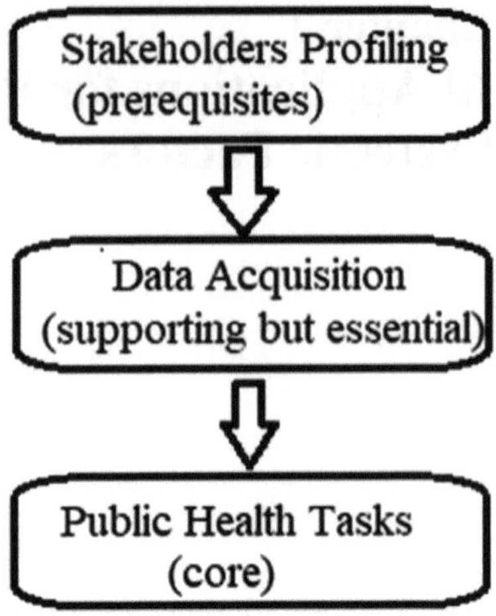

Fig. 7.1 A simplified design process of AI applications in public health

traditional markets, healthcare is heavily regulated, equity-focused, and frequently requires government intervention to address gaps or market failures.

The prerequisite of designing and developing AI applications for disease monitoring is stakeholder profiling for strategic and design input. It helps determine "What diseases to monitor (based on risk or policy priorities)?" "Which data to collect (based on stakeholder needs)?" and "How to communicate results (to different audiences)?"

Data Acquisition

Data acquisition plays a supporting role bu6t essential for data-driven AI application development. You can review traditional data collection for disease monitoring in Table 6.2 in Chapter. These tasks provide the raw inputs and context for effective monitoring. The new data collection approach is "citizen science" (see Chapter 6).

Public Health Tasks Design

The core of AI applications for public health is to handle public health tasks. In this case, the task is to identify the emergence and spread of disease early. There are clear and focused public health problems, such as surveillance and early detection, case tracking and mapping, genomic surveillance, and environmental and vector monitoring. You should select appropriate AI models for your AI systems.

This simplified design process for AI applications is like building a custom house. The stakeholder profiling is to meet the homeowners. Data acquisition is to gather construction materials. The core public health task design is to design the floor plan. In AI, this means defining what tasks the AI should perform? What outputs should be delivered to whom, and how? How does the model integrate with workflows, respect ethics, and protect privacy?

7.2 Surveillance and Forecasting

7.2.1 *Disease Monitoring*

Number of Diseases

Before discussing disease monitoring, let's answer the question: "How many human diseases are out there?" The short answer is that there are at least 10,000 to 30,000 distinct human diseases, depending on the classification system (World Health Organization, 2025). We do not know exactly the number. It's a significant number of diseases, and it is a challenging task for a medical student studying all of them. AI doctors are needed to help physicians remember all the details of human diseases. The good news for public health is that we only need to monitor a relatively small number. Currently, most countries monitor 50–150 priority diseases through formal public health surveillance systems (CDC, 2025), and global systems track 200–300+ diseases depending on the scope and region (World Health Organization, 2025). As a public health informatics student, you should know this number can be larger. Let's quickly mention the assumptions of current choices in Table 7.1. Suppose one of the assumptions changes in the future. In that case, you should be aware that the number of disease monitoring needs to be changed accordingly.

Surveillance and Early Detection

Public health domain data have been covered in Chapter 6. We will focus on selecting AI models and techniques to address the core public health tasks in this chapter. Let me propose Case Scenario 7a in disease monitoring and demonstrate how to implement AI as a part of the solutions.

Table 7.1 Assumptions of choices of diseases to monitor

Category	Assumptions
Resource and feasibility constraints	Countries do not have the capacity to monitor thousands of diseases
Public health impact is unevenly distributed	A small subset of diseases accounts for most of the illness, death, and economic cost (e.g., respiratory infections, TB, HIV, malaria, chronic diseases)
Surveillance systems are designed for actionable insights	Surveillance is meant for timely, population-level response
Epidemiological prioritization	Countries follow WHO (World Health Organization) guidelines, International Health Regulations (IHR), and regional health priorities
Formal surveillance is just one layer	Other diseases are monitored through different systems (e.g., hospital records, academic studies, or ad hoc outbreak investigations)

Case Scenario 7a. Respiratory disease monitoring: The emergence of a potential new respiratory disease outbreak in a large urban area. It is essential to detect it early before hospitals are overwhelmed. Suppose we design an AI system to address it.

Some literature about respiratory disease outbreaks in cities for disease monitoring (Abbas et al., 2021; McMichael et al., 2020) will provide background information for you to identify the key steps (tasks) in this scenario. This is a conceptual analysis of disease monitoring.

1. ***Signal Refinement and Noise Filtering***

Input data can be EHRs (Electronic Health Records) (e.g., rise in non-specific flu-like symptoms at urgent care clinics), over-the-counter pharmacy sales (e.g., a spike in cough and fever medications), and Google trends (e.g., increased searches for "chest tightness," "difficulty breathing."). You can find more input data types for disease monitoring in Table 6.2 and Table 6.3, which classified them as chief complaints (from ER [Emergency Room] or clinic visits), self-reported symptoms, syndromic data (ER visits, ICD [International Classification of Diseases] codes), and reports from sentinel healthcare providers, search engine trends, and social media signals. More data can come from *Citizen Sciences* approach in the future.

Before acting on any data, we need an AI system to clean it. This filters out false signals, misreported cases, and background noise (e.g., weekend effects). The AI system can select "*feature selection*" models (e.g., mutual information, recursive feature elimination) to refine signals. Hopefully, the output of this machine learning (ML) model is clean, smooth, and trustworthy signals.

2. ***Spike Detection***

With clean data, we can now identify statistical anomalies, which are sudden rises that deviate from historical norms. The AI system can select other machine learning models. For example, *clustering* (e.g., k-means [Jain et al., 1999], DBSCAN [Ester et al., 1996]) or *anomaly detection* (Chandola et al., 2009) (e.g., Isolation Forest, One-Class SVM) models to detect the spikes. Both models are unsupervised learning. Unsupervised learning is when the algorithm is given data without labeled outcomes. It doesn't know the "correct answer" in advance. Instead, it learns to identify patterns, structures, or relationships within the data. The output at this stage is flagged spikes or unusual trends. For example, the anomaly detection algorithm flags a larger than 2.5 standard deviation spike in respiratory complaints. "2.5 standard deviations" means something is way off from the usual. For example, a senior boy in high school who is 6′4″ tall is 2.5 standard deviations taller than the average (5′9″). That is rare, noticeable, and maybe even a red flag.

3. ***Early Outbreak Signal***

Spike does not equal an outbreak. This step interprets whether a spike across multiple sources or locations could indicate early outbreak potential. For example, there is a spike in ER visits, but some anomalies may be noise in one source. Let's confirm it across other sources, such as school absenteeism and social media chatter. This methodological approach in AI is called "multi-source fusion." Integrating data from multiple heterogeneous sources forms a more complete, reliable, and informative input. After you use multi-source data to validate whether detected spikes are meaningful. The output will be probable early warnings.

4. ***Hotspot Identification***

Once early outbreak signals are suspected, you must assess whether spikes occur in close time and space, indicating possible spread. For this task, the AI system can select spatiotemporal models (e.g., ST-GNN [Spatio-Temporal Graph Neural Network] [Li et al., 2018], LSTM [Long Short-Term Memory] with geospatial features [Shi et al., 2015]). Spatiotemporal models learn disease dynamics in space and time, making them highly suitable for outbreak hotspot detection. Spatial and temporal analysis helps identify where the disease may be spreading fastest. The output of this step is prioritized geographic areas (hotspots).

5. ***Context-Aware Forecasting***

We want to forecast short-term trends using past trends, geography, behavior, weather, etc., to anticipate what will happen in those hotspots.

Context-aware forecasting is where AI shows significant advantages over human capabilities. There are dozens to hundreds of contextual factors (e.g., past case trends, mobility, weather, social media chatter, vaccination rates). AI can simultaneously analyze all factors, while humans can only handle a few variables. AI (e.g., spatial–temporal models) can detect subtle space–time interactions beyond our human reasoning. Computers can process big data in seconds. AI is more logical and consistent than humans, while human forecasts are vulnerable to bias, fatigue, and inconsistency. Data-driven AI models (not static rules-based systems) can adapt to changing data (e.g., new variants or behavioral shifts). Human domain knowledge is crucial to correctly frame the models and select the right ones for tasks.

For this task, the AI system can select context-aware models (e.g., attention-based forecasting with location/time embeddings). In this scenario, time embedding is day-of-week, and location embedding is urban or region ID. The output of this step is short-term trend predictions by region (e.g., case counts forecasts, trend direction, hotspot risk scores, temporal risk alerts).

6. ***Uncertainty Modeling***

Forecasts are rarely precise. Like weather forecasting, the meteorologists come with a cone of uncertainty, showing where the storm is likely to go and how confidence decreases the further out in time or space you look. This step adds confidence intervals to estimates of cases, transmission rates, or future spread. It provides scenario bounds (e.g., best-case to worst-case outbreak sizes). It quantifies how sure or unsure we are for communications, depending on data quality, missing information, or model assumptions; it will help users understand what we don't know. For this task, the AI system can select one of the probabilistic and generative models, such as Bayesian models (e.g., Bayesian time-series models). The output will be disease forecasts with ranges and probabilities.

7. ***Scenario Simulation***

This is used for "what if" analysis. For example, when planning a road trip with GPS apps, you use Google Maps to check different routes ("What if I take the highway vs. local roads?") and see estimated arrival times based on traffic or construction. There are many "what-if" scenarios in a road trip, such as "What if it rains?" or "What if I stop for lunch?" Your brain can simulate how a road trip might change under those conditions. What if vaccination increases or a new variant arrives for disease monitoring? We need to simulate how a disease might behave under different conditions. This step helps decision-makers evaluate actions and help policy planning.

In this case, we need to handle the random nature of respiratory disease transmission (stochastic variability), which includes transmission dynamics (e.g., random interactions, super-spreading events, and environmental factors), population heterogeneity (e.g., behavioral difference, age, and health status), incubation and latency, testing and reporting delays, and intervention effectiveness.

For this task, the AI system can select one of the probabilistic and generative models, such as simulation-based models (e.g., agent-based models) (Schelling, 1971). The model can simulate detailed outbreak scenarios (e.g., how people interact, spread the disease, and respond to policies). It can model stochastic variability of respiratory diseases with unpredictable spread. The output is forecasts of "what might happen" under different conditions. They are policy-relevant futures based on simulated conditions.

7.2.2 Epidemiological Forecasting

Epidemiological forecasting is like "weather forecasting for diseases." It predicts future disease outbreaks, estimates how many people might get sick, and guides public health decisions.

Humans have been familiar with infectious diseases (e.g., measles, whooping cough, tick-borne disease, foodborne illness) for many years and have successfully developed models and systems for epidemiological forecasting based on historical or real-time data.

Antimicrobial resistance (AMR)-related infections are rising and becoming public health concerns (Walsh et al., 2023). AMR is a category of infections caused by microorganisms (bacteria, fungi, viruses, parasites) that have developed resistance to antimicrobial treatments like antibiotics, antivirals, or antifungals. AMR increases the severity, duration, and mortality of infections. Even infections with low R_0 (reproduction number) can become a significant threat if resistant strains spread unchecked, especially in healthcare settings (Walsh et al., 2023). AMR is one of the top ten public health problems. Table 3.3 in Chapter 3 summarizes the systemic factors for AMR, such as overuse and misuse of antibiotics in healthcare (e.g., excessive antibiotic prescriptions).

Let's look at a case scenario for AMR-related infections and explore how to design an AI application for AMR-related infections. Carbapenem-resistant enterobacterales (CRE) bloodstream infections (BI) are a critical antimicrobial resistance (AMR)-related infection, classified as an "urgent threat" by the CDC (Centers for Disease Control and Prevention) and WHO due to high mortality rates and limited treatment options.

Some literature about CRE bloodstream infections forecasting (Aslan et al., 2024; Liang et al., 2024; Zheng et al., 2024; Onorato et al., 2022) will provide background information for you to identify the key steps (tasks) in this scenario.

Case Scenario 7b. AMR-related epidemiological investigations: During the epidemiological investigation for CRE-BI, there are many tasks such as case definition and case finding, descriptive epidemiology (e.g., patient characteristics), source identification and transmission pathways, microbiological and genomic characterization, trend and pattern analysis, etc. One urgent and labor-intensive daily task is to find CRE-BI cases.

AI-Powered Case Finding

Based on the concept-based design model (see Chapter 3), AI can mimic human cognitive functions and empower those tasks above. Let's explore how AI can empower us to identify confirmed and probable CRE-BI cases. This is a conceptual analysis.

Step 1. Extract Raw Signals

It is a labor-intensive process for humans to review documents (e.g., EHR, progress notes, discharge summaries) and extract raw signals for CRE-BI cases. For example, public health workers need to identify keywords like "CRE-positive," "Klebsiella pneumonia," "carbapenem-resistant," or "sepsis of unknown origin." They must parse microbiology reports for culture results indicating *Enterobacteriaceae* growth and antibiotic susceptibility profiles (e.g., resistant to imipenem, meropenem). Fortunately, AI (NLP) can do data mining on EHR and unstructured data (e.g., clinical notes). This step aims to extract symptoms, diagnoses, or case indicators from free text related to CRE-BI cases.

Step 2. Standardization

To run AI or rule-based algorithms reliably for identifying CRE-BI cases, we need to standardize the input data and prepare consistent data for AI. For example, mapping text like "Klebsiella pneumoniae in blood" to a structured pathogen code ensures the AI treats it like "CRE in the bloodstream." This step aims to match symptoms, pathogens, and lab findings to structured concepts (e.g., SNOMED CT [Systematized Nomenclature of Medicine—Clinical Terms], ICD-10, LOINC [Logical Observation

Identifiers Names and Codes]). The AI system can select "named entity recognition" (NER) and ontology mapping tools for this standardization step.

Step 3. Initial Classification

If clear, well-defined rules exist, such as clinical guidelines (based on best practices), the rule-based systems are still used in many applications. In this case, the classification of CRE-BI cases has clear rules. CDC's NHSN (National Healthcare Safety Network) provides definitions for bloodstream infections, as shown below:

> Confirmed case = positive blood culture for CRE + signs of systemic infection (Centers for Disease Control and Prevention, 2024)

Surveillance needs to be broader to catch early or community-acquired cases. There are rules for "probable case" as shown below:

> Probable case = recent hospitalization + risk factors + mention of CRE in other sites (e.g., urine, wound) (Weiner et al., 2016)

The rule-based AI system can classify patients as confirmed, probable, or excluded cases. Rule-based systems are only as good as the rules they are built on. If those rules are too many and too complex to manage. Any changes require manually updating rules, so running a rule-based system on a large-scale level in real time is impractical.

We can use supervised machine learning classifiers (Hastie et al., 2009) (e.g., decision trees, random forest, logistic regression) to classify patients. ML models are trained on labeled cases from historical infection control data. Features may include lab values (e.g., WBC [White Blood Cell] count, CRP [C-Reactive Protein]), vitals (fever, blood pressure), microbiology results, and time series of antibiotic prescriptions (e.g., carbapenem use before culture) (Taylor et al., 2016). Machine learning models are flexible: they adapt better to complex patterns, but they can amplify bias, fail on rare events, or underperform in data-scarce environments. Machine learning is limited by its data.

Step 4. Use LLMs (Large Language Models) to Find Missed Probable Cases

Machine learning classifiers work best with structured data (lab values, coded diagnoses, vital signs). ML alone might miss a case if the lab test isn't entered or the diagnosis isn't coded yet. Besides structured data, there are unstructured clinical text (narrative notes) in the EHR where doctors, nurses, and other staff document patient information in their own words, such as progress notes, microbiology interpretation notes, discharge summaries, and consult notes. LLMs (large language models) can help. Transformer-based LLMs can be GPT-4. First, LLMs can convert free text into usable features (structured data), which can be added to the ML model. Secondly, LLMs read clinical notes to catch missed clues. LLMs can combine weak signals across notes and give a probability score, like: *"Based on those notes, there's an 80% chance this is CRE-BI."*

Step 5. Real-Time Surveillance and Ongoing Epidemiological Investigation

Suppose you successfully find confirmed cases or probable cases. In this case, what should you do next? Firstly, you must maintain real-time surveillance on those cases by updating data (e.g., new lab results). Secondly, you may prepare cases for the following stages of the ongoing epidemiological investigation, such as descriptive epidemiology (e.g., patient characteristics) and microbiological and genomic characterization. This step can pull information from different sources together and flag cases that need human attention (e.g., data is unclear or evolving). Source identification and transmission pathways are essential in this ongoing epidemiological investigation, so this step can prepare cases for tracking the patient's journey over time. Patients might move between units or hospitals (e.g., ER → ICU (Intensive Care Unit) → regular floor → discharge).

ML in Step 3 (data-driven pattern recognition) and LLMs in Step 4 (text understanding) are middle levels of reasoning. Dynamic task integration (e.g., human-like multi-step thinking) in Step 5 is the highest-level reasoning. It's challenging for AI to mimic complex human cognitive functions (e.g., task management, multi-step planning). Cognitive architectures are like the "operating system of the mind," providing structure for how an intelligent system should think, reason, and solve problems over time (Anderson et al., 2007). For example, ACT-R (Adaptive Control of Thought-Rational) was created by John R. Anderson at Carnegie Mellon University, and it aims to simulate human cognitive processes like memory, attention, and learning (Anderson et al., 2007). Soar was developed by John Laird and colleagues at the University of Michigan, and it targets general problem-solving and multi-task reasoning (Laird, 2012). There are many new cognitive architectures and frameworks in AI, such as SOFAI (Selection Of Framework for AI) (Fabiano et al., 2023), ToT (Tree of Thoughts) framework (Yao et al., 2023), OlaGPT (The Holistic GPT) (Xie et al., 2023), CoALA (Conceptual Abstraction and Logical Architecture) (Sumers et al., 2023), latent reasoning in AI, and ARC-AGI-2 Benchmark (Chollet et al., 2025).

Case Scenario 7c. AMR-related infection forecasting: Several hospitals in a major city have reported increasing CRE bloodstream infections in ICU patients over the past 3 months. Hospitals and public health officials want to forecast the spread so that they can respond effectively.

AI-Powered CRE-BI Forecasting Modeling

CRE-BI has complex nonlinear dynamics involving patient behavior (e.g., patient movement, adherence), microbial evolution (e.g., resistance mechanisms), healthcare practices (e.g., antibiotic prescribing), and policy shifts (e.g., infection control). There is no forecasting model specific to AMR. Fortunately, AI can help provide "black box models" if you have enough data on CRE-BI to train AI models. About the "black box" concept, you can review the neural network section in Chapter 2. AMR is rising, and we will have more data on it. We may be ready to train data-driven AI models for modeling complex CRE-BI forecasting. Let's explore an AI pipeline for creating "black box" AI models for CRE-BI forecasting. This is a conceptual analysis.

Stage 1: Before Initial Training (Data Preparation and System Setup)

The first step is to collect and organize data from EHRs, labs, patient movement, whole genome sequences, and infection control logs. Before we can use data in an AI model, we must prepare it. This step is called data cleaning and pre-processing (see Chapter 5). Sometimes, data is incomplete (e.g., a patient's age or test result is missing). Instead of throwing away that data, AI can fill in intelligent guesses using patterns from the rest of the dataset. Hospitals report cases at different periods (e.g., weekly or daily). AI helps line up the timelines so we can compare everything fairly. Other sources may use different scales. One hospital records temperature in Celsius, another in Fahrenheit. AI can help us to put everything in the same format or scale. AI helps "harmonize" data from various sources. This process is called intelligent data integration. Currently, you need to know which static data (monthly or yearly updated), define streaming data (daily or real-time updated) pipelines for this task, and validate self-reported data for user feedback for the AI system. We should partition datasets into training, validation, and test splits (by time/facility).

The next step is to set up the system. It includes building key variables, such as weekly case counts, resistance frequencies, transfer rates, hygiene scores, etc. AI functions are feature engineering or temporal feature alignment. We must label targeting variables for supervised models to define outcome labels (e.g., new CRE-BI case in a week in a location).

Stage 2: Initial Training (Modeling and Simulation)

This stage focuses on training foundational models using historical static data. Firstly, we can simplify the case scenario and treat it as a linear situation in a short time (e.g., weekly). The AI system can train time-series models (e.g., LSTM [Hochreiter et al., 1997], Prophet [Taylor et al., 2018]) on weekly CRE-BI counts per ward. The AI system can have trend learning from historical data. Secondly, we should include more factors (biology, patient behavior, and policy shift) and treat it as a non-linear complex situation for a long time by adding mechanistic models. Using population, movement, and resistance data, the system will simulate ward/facility transmission dynamics and fit mechanistic models (e.g., SEIR [Susceptible, Exposed, Infectious, Recovered] [Hethcote, 2000], agent-based). It can become a complex multimodal learning, and the system will train hybrid models that combine statistical, mechanistic, and genomic inputs.

When we build an AI model, we need to ensure it works, not just on the data we trained it with but also on new data it hasn't seen before. We save some of the data for testing, which is called "held-out data" or the test set. Using held-out data shows how well the model works on new, unseen cases. Models have "settings" called hyperparameters (like the number of layers in a neural network or how fast it learns). We can tune these settings to get better performance.

We do not know which is the best AI model for CRE-BI complex situations. You must try multiple models with different settings. You prepare a small portion of the data as a validation set. You use them to see which model performs best and select that model for this case scenario.

When the model is out of the lab, plug it into a real system, like a hospital epidemiological investigation tool for CRE-BI forecasting. The goal is to make the predictions usable by public health officials in hospitals and integrate them into their daily workflow. For example, it can be linked to the hospital's infection control dashboard for public health officers who want to forecast the CRE-BI trends.

Stage 3: Continuous Retraining and Adaptive Forecasting

This stage keeps the models responsive to evolving microbial, behavioral, and hospital system dynamics. For short-time trend forecasting, we depend on the time-series AI models. Firstly, we need dynamic data integration and ingest real-time/weekly streaming data from EHRs, labs, and logs. Then, we can retrain time-series models periodically. A rolling window is used when working with time series data (like weekly case counts of CRE-BI). For example, you use a 4-week rolling window to predict Week 5. In the next window, you will use Weeks 2–5 data to predict Week 6. This helps you train models on recent patterns, which can be more relevant for dynamic trends like hospital infections. LSTM fine-tuning is another continuous retraining method. You start with a pre-trained LSTM model (trained on general data) in Stage 2. Then, you train it more on your specific data (e.g., your hospital's CRE-BI data) in Stage 3. This helps the model adapt better to your unique situation.

For long-term forecasting, we need complex models, such as agent-based simulations. We can update agent-based simulations based on new patient movement, resistance patterns, and feedback from evolving system states. If there are health policy shifts, we can run updated simulations to test policies (e.g., hand hygiene boost, antibiotic restriction). AI will be helpful in scenario testing and policy optimization. You can retrain mechanistic models and generate real-time forecasts and alerts, such as ward-level risk, strain replacement, and resistance trajectory. This will be a continuous learning and retraining process.

The interventions and outcomes should be logged and will feed back into the next round of model retraining. It is a closed-loop learning. The AI predicts that a specific unit is at high risk. The infection control team acts, such as cleaning or patient screening. Later, you see what happened. That real outcome gets fed back into the model. The AI updates itself and learns to make better predictions next time.

7.3 Emergency and Disaster Response

After many years of fighting disasters, humans have developed structured thinking frameworks, such as Incident Command Systems (ICS), to respond to disasters (Barbera et al., 2011). ICS is the most established structured framework for emergency response. It was initially developed for wildfires but is now used globally for disasters of all types. Key features include modular hierarchy, unified command, standardized communication, and five Cs of command (Command, Control, Communications, Coordination, and Cooperation).

The role of AI in emergencies and disaster response is transformative. For example, AI processes satellite/UAV (Unmanned Aerial Vehicle or drone) imagery much faster than humans to map disaster zones (e.g., wildfires, floods). AI models (e.g., Google's Flood Hub) predict floods seven days in advance with 90% accuracy, outperforming traditional forecasts (Nearing et al., 2024). AI-driven logistics platforms optimize evacuation routes and supply chains during crises. AI-powered sensors detect gas leaks/structural faults post-earthquakes without human fatigue.

Integration of AI into Emergency and Disaster Response Frameworks

AI can be integrated into emergency and disaster response frameworks (e.g., ICS, systems thinking approaches, SoS (System of systems), Senge's five disciplines) and has unique strengths and weaknesses, as shown in Table 7.2. This is a conceptual analysis.

Table 7.2 AI strengths and weaknesses for disaster response

Structured frameworks	AI strengths	Human edges
Incident command system	Real-time data integration: AI processes satellite imagery, sensor data, and social media feeds faster than humans to map disasters Resource allocation: optimizes deployment of personnel and supplies using predictive analytics Automated reporting: generates ICS-compliant reports	Leadership: ICS requires human commanders to make ethical decisions Adaptability: humans adjust protocols for novel scenarios
Systems thinking approaches (e.g., causal loop diagrams, complex adaptive systems)	Pattern recognition: identifies feedback loops in disaster systems Dynamic modeling: simulates Complex Adaptive System (CAS) behaviors	Contextual nuance: humans interpret socio-political factors
System of systems (SoS) (Bajwa et al., 2025)	Interoperability: AI integrates disparate systems Anomaly detection: flags vulnerabilities in critical infrastructure	Holistic oversight: humans manage trade-offs
Senge's five disciplines (McNulty et al., 2025)	Shared vision: AI aggregates stakeholder inputs for consensus Mental models: challenges biases in risk assessments	Team learning: humans foster trust and collaboration

Next-Generation Public Health Practitioners Treating AI as a Thinking Partner

Emergency and disaster situations are high-pressure and can affect many people's health and safety. Public health officials must consider the whole system, not just one part. This is called systems thinking. It means understanding how different parts of a situation (like hospitals, supplies, weather, transportation, and communities) are connected and using that big-picture view to make smart, fast decisions that help most people.

In an emergency or disaster, things can get complex fast. There's a lot of data from hospitals, weather reports, social media, emergency calls, and more. It's hard for one person to process all that alone. That's where AI as a thinking partner comes in. It doesn't replace the public health officials, but it helps them. AI can quickly analyze data, spot patterns, and suggest possible actions. When used this way, AI supports systems thinking, assisting officials to see how different parts of the crisis connect so they can make better, faster decisions to protect public health.

Just like you practice public speaking or writing, you must also practice thinking with AI to get good at it. That's where "meta-AI homework" comes in (see Appendix A). It's a new assignment for you to build AI-guided reasoning skills. That means you learn how to work with AI as a competent helper so you can make better decisions in complex public health situations like during emergencies or when analyzing health data.

7.4 Population Health Management

Population Risk Stratification

With limited resources in public health, we focus our efforts on those citizens who are most in need, without ignoring anyone. Population risk stratification in public health is like sorting passengers (e.g., low-risk, medium-risk, or high-risk travelers) at an airport security checkpoint based on their likelihood of posing a risk. In public health, there are numerous population risk stratification systems with various focuses, including community vulnerability (see Table 7.3) and health event prediction (see Table 7.4).

Traditional risk stratification is like handing out umbrellas to people before a storm based solely on a few fixed factors, such as age, income, and medical history. But there are many problems with this system. For example, some people who are already indoors, others who are outside, far from shelter, or in flood-prone areas get missed entirely; no one checks if they can *use* the umbrella or even reach it in time. In the AI era, we should design better risk stratification systems, such as equity-aware risk stratification models (see next session).

Table 7.3 Population risk stratification for community vulnerability

Model/System	Stratification bases	Key uses
CDC social vulnerability index (SVI) (Centers for Disease Control and Prevention, 2024)	Socioeconomic status, minority status, housing, transportation	Disaster preparedness, response, resource allocation, equity planning
Area deprivation index (ADI) (University of Wisconsin–Madison, 2023)	Income, education, employment, housing quality	Targeting interventions, resource allocation, understanding geographic health disparities
Healthy places index (HPI) (California) (Public Health Alliance of Southern California, 2024)	25+ social determinants: education, housing, healthcare access	Guide public health funding, planning, and equity-focused programs
Environmental justice index (EJI) (Centers for Disease Control and Prevention, 2022)	Environmental burden and social vulnerability	Identify communities overburdened by pollution and risk
CDC BRFSS (behavioral risk factor surveillance system) (Centers for Disease Control and Prevention, 2023)	Self-reported behavioral and demographic data	Monitoring population-level health risks and informing public health policy

Table 7.4 Population risk stratification for health event prediction

Model/System	Stratification bases	Key uses
CMS-HCC (Medicare risk adjustment)	Diagnoses, demographics, healthcare utilization	Adjust Medicare payments, forecast health costs
Johns Hopkins ACG system (Johns Hopkins, 2024)	Diagnoses, pharmacy data, utilization history	Predict healthcare needs, manage population health
QRisk (UK) (ClinRisk Ltd., and University of Nottingham, 2024)	Age, BP, cholesterol, smoking, ethnicity, comorbidities	Predict 10-year cardiovascular disease (CVD) risk
LACE index (Mdcalc, 2024)	Length of stay, acuity, comorbidities, ED (Emergency Department) visits	Predict 30-day hospital readmission or death

7.5 Health Equity-Aware Risk Stratifications

Equity-Aware Risk Stratification

The design principle (in Chapter 3) for AI applications in public health is "encoding justice", and we should apply health equity and social determinant analysis into public health practices. Only in the AI era are AI-empowered equity-aware public health applications possible and actionable. Let me propose an equity-aware risk stratification model (***EquiRisk***) first and design an AI application using the EquiRisk model for diabetes patients in food deserts (***EquiRisk-DF-AI***).

EquiRisk model in the AI Era is like using smart umbrellas that know where the storm is hitting hardest in real time; adapt who gets help, based on not just health status but location, housing, social support, transit access; deliver umbrellas where and when they're needed, and make sure people can reach them; and learn from each storm to get better every time.

Core Assumptions

In the AI era, the EquiRisk model broke away from rigid, one-size-fits-all rules and instead thrives on real-world, real-time complexity. Below are key assumptions that underpin this new generation of models. First, risk is dynamic, not static. People's risk levels change in real-time based on environment, context, and access to opportunities. Secondly, equity requires contextual awareness. Fairness depends on recognizing local and historical disadvantages (e.g., redlining, digital divide, systemic barriers). Thirdly, stratification must be linked to opportunity. It's unethical to label someone high-risk without ensuring actionable support is available. Fourthly, feedback loops are required. Equity-aware systems must learn from their own outcomes and user engagement (or lack thereof). Finally, transparency must be built in. Stakeholders (clinicians, communities, policymakers) must understand how risk scores are produced and used. Let's design the *EuitRisk* model based on those assumptions above.

Equity

Equity is not just about being fair. It's about being functional as a species. Without equity, our systems will break politically, socially, ecologically, and medically. In the AI era, this becomes urgent: If we don't encode justice into AI, it will encode something else (e.g., efficiency, control, profit, or power), and that can be dangerous. To guide superintelligent systems safely, equity must be a foundational design principle. In this textbook on AI in public health, we emphasize that "Encoding Justice" is a design principle, as discussed in Chapter 3.

EquiRisk Model

"Equity-aware risk stratification" is to combine risk with context. Moving from individual-level risk to community-level context is at the heart of being "equity-aware." It's not just how sick you are, but how well your environment can support you. The equity-aware risk stratification (EquiRisk) model comprises three components, as illustrated in Fig. 7.2.

Let's explore the functions in each component in Table 7.5. You can review population risk stratification in the last session.

Imagine two drivers driving cars on different roads. Traditional models measure the vehicle alone, while the EquiRisk model measures the road as well.

Why is the AI Era Crucial for Equity-Aware Risk Stratification?

Equity-aware models require combining diverse data sources (e.g., health event risk prediction and community vulnerability) in real time. AI excels at ingesting, cleaning, and fusing these heterogeneous datasets dynamically. Traditional statistical models

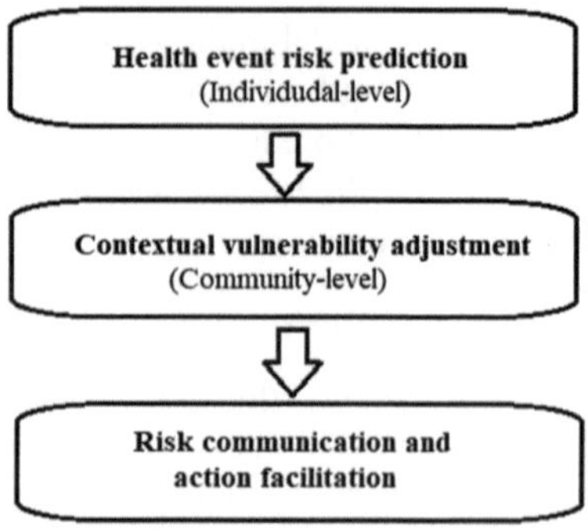

Fig. 7.2 Equity-aware risk stratification model (EquiRisk)

Table 7.5 Functions of equity-aware risk stratification model (EquiRisk)

No	Stage name	Function summary
1	Health event risk prediction	Uses health data (e.g., diagnosis, utilization, age, etc.) to predict likelihood of events (e.g., hospitalization, complications). Draws from models like CMS-HCC (Centers for Medicare and Medicaid Services—Hierarchical Condition Categories), ACG (Adjusted Clinical Groups), LACE (Length of stay, Acuity of admission, Comorbidities, Emergency department visits), QRisk
2	Contextual vulnerability adjustment	Adjust risk based on local vulnerability indicators (e.g., SVI, ADI, redlining history, digital divide), correcting for systemic disadvantage. recalculating risk tiers and refining who is at greatest need
3	Risk communication and action facilitation	Delivering tailored risk reports, prioritization lists, outreach plans, and intervention recommendations in understandable, actionable formats

often use fixed factors and linear assumptions. AI/ML enables the capture of complex, nonlinear interactions between individual risk and contextual vulnerabilities (e.g., how living in a food desert affects diabetes outcomes over time). AI systems can continuously learn from new health data, engagement patterns, and intervention outcomes, adjusting risk predictions and equity weights as populations and environments change. AI-powered natural language generation, user profiling, and channel selection enable the delivery of culturally sensitive and accessible messages on a large scale.

EquiRisk on Diabetes Within Food Deserts

While the EquiRisk model is designed as a generalizable framework for equity-aware risk stratification across multiple public health domains, this project focuses on ***diabetes within food deserts*** to test its feasibility and effectiveness. We plan to design an AI application for diabetes within food deserts using our EquiRisk model (***EquiRisk-DF-AI***). This ***focused*** application allows validation with well-defined clinical and social data, providing a robust proof of concept. Future work will explore expansion to other conditions and vulnerability factors. This application is feasible because there is clear data availability, strong existing public health programs targeting food access and chronic disease, and a broad consensus on addressing social determinants of health. This topic is relatively more straightforward to engage community organizations and clinics.

In the past, food deserts were often treated as background noise. In the EquiRisk model, they become central equity modifiers that reshape our understanding of risk at both the individual and community levels. There are three stages in the conceptual design of the EquiRisk-DF-AI application.

Case Scenario 7d. EquiRisk on diabetes within food deserts: In a small city with several food desert neighborhoods, adults with type 2 diabetes have limited access to nutritious food. Currently, patients' clinical data (HbA1c, blood pressure, comorbidities) are not connected with social determinants (e.g., food access). Suppose we design an AI system to address this, such as generating an equity-aware risk score and using this score to stratify patients. This AI system will guide current intervention programs to better serve diabetes patients in this city.

Stage 1. Health Event Risk Prediction (Diabetes Focus)

The first stage is to estimate the probability and severity of specific adverse health events in people with diabetes who live in food deserts. Its focus is on near-term and medium-term health risks (weeks to months), not general prevalence.

The input data includes clinical indicators (e.g., A1C, fasting glucose, blood pressure, cholesterol levels, weight/BMI trends), medical history and events (e.g., past ER visits/hospitalizations for hypo/hyperglycemia, history of diabetic complications), medication and treatment data (e.g., insulin or oral medication regimen), and recent clinical encounters (e.g., visit frequency, most recent lab results, and provider notes).

At this stage, AI models can assist with feature engineering and data fusion. For example, AI integrates longitudinal clinical data with continuous glucose monitor streams and handles missing data through imputation strategies. The primary AI models in this stage are predictive modeling, which operates as a predictive analytics engine. For example, survival analysis models (e.g., Cox [Therneau et al., 2000], deep survival networks [Ranganath et al., 2016]) can estimate time-to-event for hospitalizations or complications. Gradient boosting (Friedman, 2001)/random forest models (Breiman et al., 2001) can be used for binary or multi-class event risk prediction. Recurrent neural networks (RNNs/LSTMs) (Hochreiter et al., 1997) can be utilized to identify temporal patterns in laboratory results, vital signs, and medication usage.

The output of this stage is risk profiles for everyone. They can be probability scores for key diabetes-related adverse events (e.g., ER visit for hypoglycemia or hyperglycemia, cardiovascular event, hospitalization within 3 months) or risk trajectories to project trends over the next 3–6 months.

Stage 2. Contextual Vulnerability Adjustment (Food Desert Focus)

The goal of Stage 2 is to adjust health event risk predictions to reflect the systemic disadvantage caused by food deserts. This stage consists of identifying individuals whose health risks are likely to be exacerbated by restricted access to healthy food and developing refined risk tiers for targeting limited public health resources.

The input data for Stage 2 consists of two categories: one is the output from Stage 1, and the other is contextual vulnerability data. In this focused application, the contextual vulnerability are food desert indicators, such as geographic identifiers (ZIP code, census tract, GPS coordinates), USDA (U.S. Department of Agriculture) or local government food desert maps, distance to nearest grocery store or fresh produce vendor, food environment quality indices (e.g., % of healthy vs. unhealthy food outlets), and public transportation access to food sources.

The first AI models used in this stage are geospatial linking and feature mapping. They can geocode patient addresses and overlay them on food desert maps and create vulnerability scores from food environment indices. The main equity-aware risk adjustment models include Bayesian hierarchical models to adjust base risk estimates based on contextual vulnerability scores, reweighting algorithms to correct for systemic underestimation of risk in disadvantaged geographies, and causal inference frameworks to estimate the *incremental risk* attributable to living in a food desert. Ultimately, AI systems require recalibration of risk tiers. It will calibrate risk thresholds so individuals in high-vulnerability areas are more likely to be placed in higher alert categories when justified by context. At the same time, an AI system can use bias and fairness validation models to check that no subgroup is systematically downgraded inappropriately.

The outputs are context-adjusted individual risk profiles (e.g., updated probability scores and/or risk trajectories incorporating food desert disadvantage) and refined risk tiers (e.g., Low/Moderate/High/Critical) for prioritization.

Stage 3. Risk Communication and Action Facilitation

The goal of Stage 3 is to translate the adjusted risk profiles and tiers from Stage 2 into clear, actionable information for those who need to act, including patients, care teams, public health workers, and community organizations.

The basic input is output data from Stage 2, such as context-adjusted individual risk profiles and refined risk tiers. Depending on your goals for action facilitation, you should enable rapid coordination between healthcare and community support resources. Additional input data for Stage 3 may include action and intervention resource data, such as available local interventions (e.g., food delivery programs, diabetes education, transportation to clinics) or contact information for community health workers, dietitians, case managers, or program eligibility rules and capacity limits.

AI models for communication are "Tailored risk narrative generation". They are natural language generation (NLG) to produce individualized reports in patient-friendly terms. Current AI models have reading level and language adaptation for diverse literacy backgrounds. AI models for action facilitation are "Prioritization and outreach planning". The optimization algorithms or routing algorithms can efficiently assign community health workers.

The outputs are intervention recommendations or reports. AI systems can provide audience-specific formatting such as patient-facing summaries (e.g., tailored risk reports), clinician-facing dashboards (e.g., clinical flags or tailored risk reports), or public health/community organization reports (e.g., aggregated risk maps, priority lists, or outreach plans). The AI recommendation systems in Stage 3 can suggest the most relevant interventions for each patient based on risk tier, needs, and available resources.

Uniqueness of EquiRisk-DF-AI

Community vulnerability indexes (e.g., SVI and ADI) are typically applied in broad population health planning. Still, they are rarely combined with individual clinical risk to guide personalized interventions. Regarding the food deserts issue, the USDA is typically used independently of clinical risk models. The proposed "EquiRisk-DF-AI" framework is unique. First, this conceptual AI framework combines real-time clinical risk prediction with detailed local equity adjustments for food desert metrics. Secondly, this AI framework can establish a link to opportunity and intervention. It moves beyond risk stratification by embedding a communication and action facilitation stage that personalizes outreach and connects individuals to context-specific resources (e.g., food box programs, transportation support).

7.6 Discussion Questions

Question 7.1. How do systemic public health challenges differ from individual-level challenges, and why might AI be especially valuable for addressing them?
Question 7.2. In what ways could case scenarios and step-by-step frameworks help practitioners bridge the gap between conceptual AI models and practical implementation?
Question 7.3. How does the choice of input data shape both the strengths and limitations of AI applications in public health case scenarios?
Question 7.4. What criteria should guide the selection of AI models (e.g., predictive, generative, classification) for different types of public health challenges?
Question 7.5. How can the outputs of AI frameworks be designed to ensure they are actionable, understandable, and equitable for both policymakers and individuals?
Question 7.6. How might equity-aware risk stratification help ensure that systemic AI solutions do not reinforce existing health disparities?

Question 7.7. How can public health agencies strike a balance between the need for rapid AI deployment in crises (such as disasters or pandemics) and the need for transparency and accountability?

References

Abbas, M., Nunes, T. R., Cori, A., Cordey, S., Laubscher, F., Baggio, S., & Harbarth, S. (2021). Explosive Nosocomial Outbreak of SARS-CoV-2 in a Rehabilitation Clinic: The Limits of Genomics for Outbreak Reconstruction. *Journal of Hospital Infection, 117*, 124–134. https://doi.org/10.1016/j.jhin.2021.07.013

Anderson, J. R. (2007). *How Can the Human Mind Occur in the Physical Universe?* New York, Oxford University Press.

Aslan, A. T., Ezure, Y., Harris, P. N. A., Paterson, D. L. (2024). Scoping Review of Risk-Scoring Tools for Early Prediction of Carbapenem-Resistant Enterobacterales Bloodstream Infections. *Journal of Antimicrobial Chemotherapy, 6*(1), dlae032. https://doi.org/10.1093/jacamr/dlae032

Barbera, J. and K. Stambler (2011). "Engineering the Incident Command and Multiagency Coordination Systems." *Journal of Homeland Security and Emergency Management 8*(1): 1–27.

Bajwa, A. (2025). AI-based emergency response systems: a systematic literature review on smart infrastructure safety Am. J. Adv. *Technol. Eng. Solution, 1* (1) , pp. 174–200, https://doi.org/10.63125/xcxwpv34

Breiman, L. (2001). Random Forests. *Machine Learning, 45*(1), 5–32. https://doi.org/10.1023/A:1010933404324

Centers for Disease Control and Prevention. (2023). *Behavioral Risk Factor Surveillance System (BRFSS).* https://www.cdc.gov/brfss/

Centers for Disease Control and Prevention. (2024). *National Healthcare Safety Network (NHSN) Patient Safety Component Manual: Chapter 4—Bloodstream Infection (BSI) Event.* https://www.cdc.gov/nhsn/pdfs/pscmanual/4psc_clabscurrent.pdf

Centers for Disease Control and Prevention, & Agency for Toxic Substances and Disease Registry. (2024). Substance priority list. Retrieved November 30, 2025, from https://www.atsdr.cdc.gov/

Centers for Disease Control and Prevention. (2025). *New Home for NNDSS Weekly and Annual Tables.* https://www.cdc.gov/nndss/infectious-disease/weekly-and-annual-disease-data-tables.html

Centers for Disease Control and Prevention, Agency for Toxic Substances and Disease Registry. (2022). *Environmental Justice Index (EJI).* https://www.atsdr.cdc.gov/place-health/php/eji/index.html

Centers for Disease Control and Prevention, Agency for Toxic Substances and Disease Registry. (2024). *CDC/ATSDR Social Vulnerability Index.* https://www.atsdr.cdc.gov/place-health/php/svi/index.html

Chandola, V., Banerjee, A., & Kumar, V. (2009). Anomaly Detection: A Survey. *ACM Computing Surveys, 41*(3), 1–58. https://dl.acm.org/doi/10.1145/1541880.1541882

Chollet, F., Knoop, M., Kamradt, G., Landers, B., & Pinkard, H. (2025). ARC-AGI-2: A New Challenge for Frontier AI Reasoning Systems. *arXiv preprint* arXiv:2505.11831. https://doi.org/10.48550/arXiv.2505.11831

ClinRisk Ltd., & University of Nottingham. (2024). *QRisk®*. Retrieved November 30, 2025, from https://qrisk.org/

Ester, M., Kriegel, H. P., Sander, J., & Xu, X. (1996). A Density-Based Algorithm for Discovering Clusters in Large Spatial Databases with Noise. *Proceedings of the 2nd International Conference on Knowledge Discovery and Data Mining (KDD-96)*, 226–231. https://www.aaai.org/Papers/KDD/1996/KDD96-037.pdf

Fabiano, F., Pallagani, V., Ganapini, M. B., Horesh, L., Loreggia, A., Murugesan, K., & Srivastava, B. (2023). Fast and Slow Planning. *arXiv preprint* arXiv:2303.04283. https://arxiv.org/abs/2303.04283

Friedman, J. H. (2001). Greedy Function Approximation: A Gradient Boosting Machine. *The Annals of Statistics, 29*(5). https://doi.org/10.1214/aos/1013203451

Hastie, T., Tibshirani, R., & Friedman, J. (2009). *The Elements of Statistical Learning: Data Mining, Inference, and Prediction.* https://doi.org/10.1007/978-0-387-84858-7

Hethcote, H. W. (2000). The Mathematics of Infectious Diseases. *SIAM Review, 42*(4), 599–653. https://doi.org/10.1137/S0036144500371907

Hochreiter, S., & Schmidhuber, J. (1997). Long Short-Term Memory. *Neural Computation, 9*(8), 1735–1780. https://doi.org/10.1162/neco.1997.9.8.1735

Jain, A. K., Murty, M. N., & Flynn, P. J. (1999). Data Clustering: A Review. *ACM Computing Surveys, 31*(3), 264–323. https://dl.acm.org/doi/10.1145/331499.331504

Johns Hopkins, U. (2024). *The Johns Hopkins ACG® System.* https://www.hopkinsacg.org/

Laird, J. E. (2012). *The Soar Cognitive Architecture.* MIT Press. https://doi.org/10.7551/mitpress/7688.001.0001

Li, Y., Yu, R., Shahabi, C., & Liu, Y. (2018). *Diffusion Convolutional Recurrent Neural Network: Data-Driven Traffic Forecasting.* Paper presented at the International Conference on Learning Representations (ICLR). https://arxiv.org/abs/1707.01926

Liang, Q., Ding, S., Chen, J., Chen, X., Xu, Y., Xu, Z. (2024). Prediction of Carbapenem-Resistant Gram-Negative Bacterial Bloodstream Infection in Intensive Care Unit Based on Machine Learning. *BMC Medical Informatics and Decision Making, 24*, 123. https://doi.org/10.1186/s12911-024-02504-4

McMichael, T. M., Currie, D. W., Clark, S., Pogosjans, S., Kay, M., Schwartz, N. G., & Duchin, J. S. (2020). Epidemiology of Covid-19 in a Long-Term Care Facility in King County, Washington. *New England Journal of Medicine, 382*(21), 2005–2011. https://doi.org/10.1056/nejmoa2005412

McNulty, E. J., Spisak, B. R., & Marcus, L. J. (2025). AI-Augmented Learning Organizations in Crisis Management: Applying Senge's Five Disciplines. *Journal of Emergency Management, 23*(3), 112–130. https://doi.org/10.5055/jem.0836

Mdcalc. (2024). *LACE Index for 30-Day Readmission.* https://www.mdcalc.com/calc/3805/lace-index-readmission

Nearing, G., Cohen, D., & Matias, Y. (2024). Global Prediction of Extreme Floods in Ungauged Watersheds Using AI. *Nature, 627*, 559–563. https://doi.org/10.1038/s41586-024-07145-1

Onorato, L., Sarnelli, B., D'Agostino, F., Signoriello, G., Trama, U., D'Argenzio, A., Montemurro, M. V., Coppola, N. (2022). Epidemiological, Clinical and Microbiological Characteristics of Patients with Bloodstream Infections Due to Carbapenem-Resistant *K. Pneumoniae* in Southern Italy. *Antibiotics, 11*(5), 633. https://doi.org/10.3390/antibiotics11050633

Public Health Alliance of Southern California. (2024). *Healthy Places Index (HPI).* Retrieved November 30, 2025, from https://www.healthyplacesindex.org/

Ranganath, R., Perotte, A., Elhadad, N., & Blei, D. (2016). Deep Survival Analysis. *Proceedings of the 1st Machine Learning for Healthcare Conference, 56*, 101–114. https://proceedings.mlr.press/v56/Ranganath16.html

Schelling, T. C. (1971). Dynamic Models of Segregation. *The Journal of Mathematical Sociology, 1*(2), 143–186. https://doi.org/10.1080/0022250X.1971.9989794

Shi, X., Chen, Z., Wang, H., Yeung, D.-Y., Wong, W.-K., & Woo, W.-C. (2015). *Convolutional LSTM Network: A Machine Learning Approach for Precipitation Nowcasting.* Paper presented at the Advances in Neural Information Processing Systems. https://proceedings.neurips.cc/paper/2015/hash/07563a3fe3bbe7e3ba84431ad9d055af-Abstract.html

Sumers, T. R., Yao, S., Narasimhan, K., & Griffiths, T. L. (2023). Cognitive Architectures for Language Agents. *arXiv preprint* arXiv:2309.02427. https://arxiv.org/abs/2309.02427

Taylor, R. A., Pare, J. R., Venkatesh, A. K., Mowafi, H., Melnick, E. R., Fleischman, W., & Hall, M. K. (2016). Prediction of In-hospital Mortality in Emergency Department Patients With Sepsis:

A Local Big Data–Driven, Machine Learning Approach. *Academic Emergency Medicine, 23*(3), 269–278. https://doi.org/10.1111/acem.12876

Taylor, S. J., & Letham, B. (2018). Forecasting at Scale. *The American Statistician, 72*(1), 37–45. https://doi.org/10.1080/00031305.2017.1380080

Therneau, T. M., & Grambsch, P. M. (2000). *Modeling Survival Data: Extending the Cox Model.* Springer. https://doi.org/10.1007/978-1-4757-3294-8

University of Wisconsin–Madison. (2023). *Neighborhood Atlas—Area Deprivation Index.* Retrieved November 30, 2025, from https://www.neighborhoodatlas.medicine.wisc.edu/

Walsh, T. R., Gales, A. C., Laxminarayan, R., & Dodd, P. C. (2023). Antimicrobial Resistance: Addressing a Global Threat to Humanity. *PLoS Medicine, 20*(7), Article e1004264. https://doi.org/10.1371/journal.pmed.1004264

Weiner, L. M., Webb, B. J., Limbago, B., et al. (2016). Antimicrobial-Resistant Pathogens Associated With Healthcare-Associated Infections: Summary of Data Reported to the National Healthcare Safety Network at the CDC, 2015–2017. *Infection Control & Hospital Epidemiology, 37*(11), 1288–1301. https://doi.org/10.1017/ice.2016.174

World Health Organization. (2025). *World health statistics 2025.* Retrieved November 30, 2025, from https://www.who.int/data/gho/publications/world-health-statistics

Xie, Y., Xie, T., Lin, M., Wei, W. T., Li, C., Kong, B., Chen, L., Zhuo, C., Hu, B., Li, Z. (2023). OlaGPT: Empowering LLMs With Human-like Problem-Solving Abilities. *arXiv preprint* arXiv:2305.16334. https://arxiv.org/abs/2305.16334

Yao, S., Yu, D., Zhao, J., Shafran, I., Griffiths, T. L., Cao, Y., & Narasimhan, K. (2023). Tree of Thoughts: Deliberate Problem Solving with Large Language Models. *arXiv preprint* arXiv: 2305.10601. https://arxiv.org/abs/2305.10601

Zheng, G., Cai, J., Deng, H., Yang, H., Xiong, W., Chen, E., Bai, H., He, J. (2024). Development of a Risk Prediction Model for Subsequent Infection After Colonization with Carbapenem-Resistant Enterobacterales. *Antimicrobial Resistance & Infection Control, 13*, 46. https://doi.org/10.1186/s13756-024-01394-5

Chapter 8
AI Applications for Public Health Personal Responsibilities

8.1 New Concepts for Public Health Personal Responsibility

Shift in Public Health Philosophy

In the past, public health often used blame (e.g., "You're unhealthy because you made bad choices") or encouragement alone (e.g., "Try harder! Eat better! Exercise more!") as behavior change strategies. Personal responsibility becomes a kind of "moral burden" for individuals, such as "you should eat healthier," "you need to exercise more," "you should know your health risks," and "it's your responsibility to get vaccinated." However, research and practice have shown that they are ineffective. Blame rarely leads to lasting change. Encouragement without capacity-building can be hollow, especially when people face structural barriers (e.g., poverty, time, stress, and lack of access).

The COM-B model (Capability, Opportunity, Motivation-Behavior) is a widely used framework for understanding and designing behavior change interventions. It was developed by Susan Michie and colleagues as part of the *Behaviour Change Wheel (BCW)* framework (Michie et al., 2011). The COM-B model is often applied

Systemic public health AI has a high potential and can improve millions of outcomes (e.g., optimizing Medicaid, detect outbreaks, reduce structural inequities). However, the value of those AI applications is societal, not directly monetizable. In the AI era, humans have an unprecedented opportunity to improve health literacy and reduce the knowledge gap between the public and healthcare providers. AI democratizes access to health information. This chapter will cover personal responsibility AI applications related to health literacy, behavior change, lifestyle, and chronic disease prevention. Public health AI for personal responsibility has seen more consumer-facing applications recently. Every person has 100% health concerns for themselves, and people will invest in it if the benefit is clear and accessible. The short-term return on investment (ROI) may be larger than one. Users are willing to pay. Employers see productivity gains, and health insurers can save. For example, behavior-focused AI applications give them measurable returns (lower absenteeism, fewer claims).

M. Wu, *Artificial Intelligence in Public Health*,
https://doi.org/10.1007/978-3-032-15872-7_8

in public health to design interventions that target the most influential determinants of behavior. In the era of artificial intelligence (AI), a critical shift occurred in the public health sector. The key change for personal health behaviors is from "motivation-only" to "AI-powered personalized motivation, capability, and opportunity". Let me define a public health behavior framework in the AI era (PMCO-AI) as an extension of the COM-B model by adding AI-powered personalization into it as follows:

> **PMCO-AI** (Personalized Motivation, Capability, and Opportunity, empowered by AI) is a framework for behavior change in the AI era that integrates individualized drivers, practical skill-building, and context-aware access.

Why do we need this PMCO-AI concept? First, AI makes personalization realistic at scale in public health. For example, with smart devices, apps, and wearables, we can now observe, learn, and adapt in real time. Secondly, this concept could bridge the gap between responsibility and reality. This PMCO-AI could be timely and meaningful in the context of AI-powered public health. Older public health models often asked people to "take responsibility" without providing them with the necessary skills (capability), access (opportunity), or tailored encouragement (motivation). This PMCO-AI potentially could help build a human-AI partnership model for behavior change. Human-AI partnership models will study motivations (which are personally resonant), capabilities (which align with individual strengths-building), and opportunities (which are contextually relevant and accessible) in public health topics. Table 8.1 provides examples of personalized motivations, capabilities, and opportunities in public health.

Personalization: AI-Powered Real-Time Pattern Recognition

AI's strength in real-time pattern recognition can significantly empower personal responsibility in public health, mainly by providing individualized, timely, and actionable insights. Pattern recognition is the core data-driven strength of AI, not reasoning. Several examples of AI applications with real-time pattern recognition for public health personal responsibility are provided in Table 8.2. The PMCO-AI concept is applied in Table 8.2 to categorize those personalized AI applications. In the PMCO-AI concept, "personalized motivation" refers to encouragement and emotional readiness to act, "personalized capability" encompasses health knowledge, guidance, or skill support, and "personalized opportunity" pertains to a timely context where action is possible or impactful.

Realistic expectations

Another application of the PMCO-AI model is to assess what realistically shapes a citizen's ability to take personal responsibility in public health. Suppose you are interested in "heatwaves," an urgent public health issue every summer due to climate change. In this case, let me explain the ranking of PMCO-AI components based on realistic expectations regarding heatwave issues (Fig. 8.1).

Table 8.1 Examples of PMCO-AI

Category	Examples of AI-powered actions	Examples of cases
Personalized motivation	AI can adjust tone, timing, and content to intrinsic drivers	"Walk with your daughter to the park to boost her mood and yours." (Walk for 30 min)
	AI uses convenience framing for workplace wellness, digital ergonomics, and stress management	"You've got 6 min before your next Zoom meeting. Do you want to stretch now to relieve that shoulder pain?"
Personalized capability	Teaching health literacy, cooking, and digital skills at the user's level	AI tutor explains food labels at a 6th-grade reading level in Spanish
	An AI voice assistant reminds an elderly user when and how to take medications	Use simple spoken instructions
Personalized opportunity	AI systems can integrate with local maps, hours, and services	"Where can you get a healthy meal within 1 mile and $7?"
	AI-powered mental health resource linker	A student feels depressed at midnight. The AI doesn't suggest therapy (closed at that hour) but connects them to a 24/7 crisis text line or peer-support discord server

First, personalized opportunities are the most fundamental. A worker with no AC, no cooling center nearby, and extended outdoor shifts cannot protect himself from the heat even if he wants to. AI can notify this worker: "Nearest cooling shelter 0.5 miles, open now." Opportunity sets the real-world limit. Secondly, personalized capability is the second most important. If someone doesn't know what to do (e.g., a person doesn't understand the signs of heatstroke or how to rehydrate safely), they can't take the correct action even with access. In the AI era, AI can help improve health literacy and decision-making skills. Finally, personalized motivation is essential. Someone may choose not to act due to denial, fear, or misinformation. In a heatwave, a teen ignores heat alerts because "I'm young and healthy", and it is a poor risk perception. AI can provide social norm cues for this young kid: "All other kids in your neighborhood are staying indoors today."

Table 8.2 Real-time pattern recognition in personal AI applications

PMCO-AI components	Examples of AI applications	Descriptions (personal level)	Examples of data and AI models
Personalized motivation	Activity nudging via smartwatch	Smartwatches notice you're inactive for 90+ minutes and nudge you to stretch or walk based on your prior routine	Accelerometer, heart rate, user schedule; activity recognition, habit modeling
Personalized capability	Smart nutrition coaching	AI-powered nutrition app sees how certain foods spike your sugar and suggests healthier alternatives in real time	Food logs, continuous glucose monitors, time-series eating patterns; models for glycemic response prediction
	Cough/ speech health monitors	Phone detects early signs of a respiratory illness from your cough and suggests testing or early care	Voice recordings, audio patterns (frequency, tone); CNN (Convolutional Neural Network)/ RNN (Recurrent Neural Network) models trained on illness acoustic features (Laguarta et al., 2020)
Personalized opportunity	Air quality alerts for respiratory risk	Before going for a walk, your AI warns that outdoor air is hazardous for your asthma today and suggests indoor alternatives	Real-time AQI (Air Quality Index), GPS (Global Positioning System), medical profile (e.g., asthma); pattern matching with environmental health thresholds
	Flu tracker and clinic locator	If you're feeling feverish, your app finds a flu testing clinic nearby that has walk-in slots within the next hour	Local outbreak maps, self-reported symptoms, GPS; real-time illness heatmaps and recommendation systems

(continued)

Table 8.2 (continued)

PMCO-AI components	Examples of AI applications	Descriptions (personal level)	Examples of data and AI models
	Infection risk alerts	Phone alerts you when you're near high-risk flu/COVID areas or recently exposed, so you can test, mask, or avoid crowds	GPS, proximity, health surveillance data; spatial–temporal clustering and predictive heatmaps
Personalized motivation and capability	Mental health AI check-ins	AI chatbot detects stress or sadness from your journal or voice and guides you to calming activities or professional support	Text input, speech tone, typing patterns, circadian rhythm; NLP (Natural Language Processing) mood classification models (e.g., BERT (Bidirectional Encoder), LSTM (Long Short-Term Memory))
	Sleep quality advisor	AI tracks your sleep and offers better nighttime habits like turning off screens early or doing breathing exercises	Wearable sleep stages (HRV (Heart Rate Variability), motion), digital behaviors (screen use); unsupervised pattern models for sleep disruption
	AI journaling for teen mental health	AI reflects subtle signs of mood decline in your journaling and helps you recognize when to seek help early	Typed/voice journal tone, emotional trajectory over days/weeks; NLP sentiment/emotion tracking
Personalized motivation and opportunity	Smart medication reminders	AI assistant predicts when you're likely to forget meds and reminds you in a friendly tone, at your ideal time	App usage, wearable timing, historical adherence trends; temporal behavior prediction models

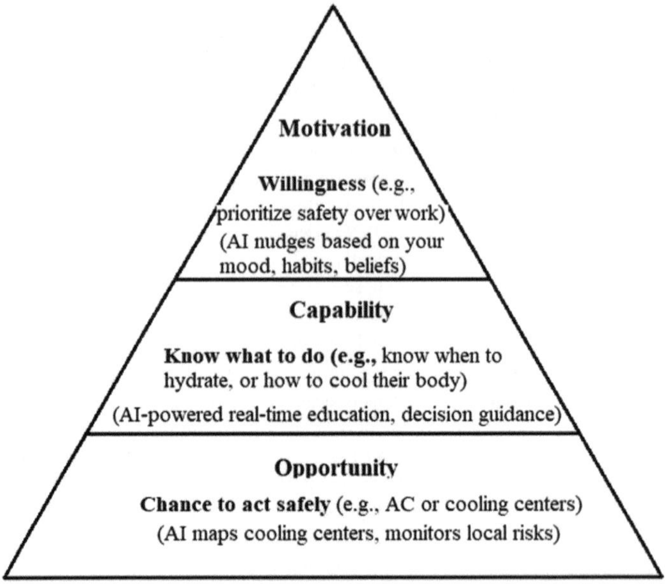

Fig. 8.1 Ranking of PMCO-AI components based on realistic expectations

8.2 PMCO-AI Model with AI Engines

To pilot or develop real AI applications (products), we need to revise the PMCO-AI behavior framework by adding AI engines. The AI application has a user-friendly front, connected to intelligent engines (brains), that answer specific questions (through APIs). API stands for Application Programming Interface. Table 8.3 explores clarity, insight, and companion engines.

Table 8.3 Explorations of clarity, insight, and companion engines

AI Engines	Example use cases	Key API modules
Clarity engine	Explain lab results in patient portals Translate discharge instructions Localize vaccine risk explanations	/explain-lab /simplify-term /translate-cultural /generate-metaphor
Insight engine	Provide feedback on symptom logs Reflect on diet and activity patterns Guide public health behavior change	/analyze-pattern, /summarize-journal, /correlate-behaviors, /generate-insight
Companion engine	Conversational health check-ins Coach for chronic disease Long-term guidance in underserved areas	/ask-question, /track-goal, /check-in, /conversational-learning

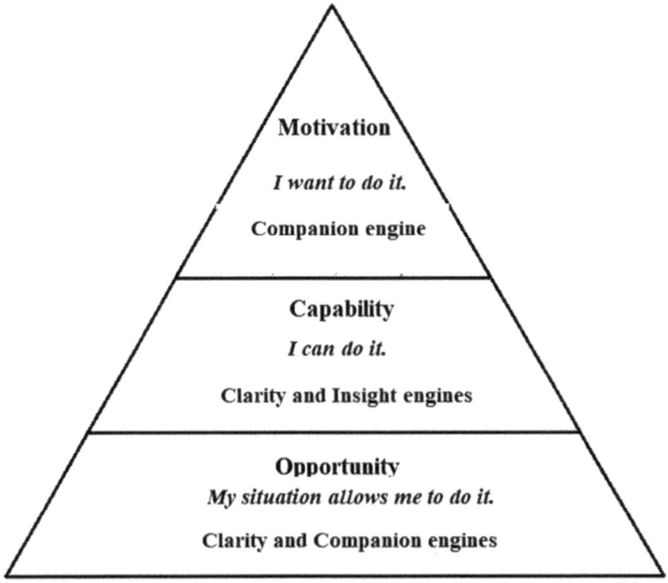

Fig. 8.2 PMCO-AI-Engine: Behaviour change pyramid with AI engines

Let's revise the PMCO-AI model as a realistic behavior change pyramid and embed the three engines (Clarity, Insight, and Companion) accordingly (see Fig. 8.2). This session will propose a PMCO-AI-Engine concept framework that is both behaviorally accurate and technically actionable.

8.3 Personalized Opportunity Empowered by AI

Personal AI Empowerment Tools

Knowing what you're entitled to is a precondition for "Opportunity." No opportunity feels real or actionable if it's unknown or unclear. A personal AI empowerment tool is crucial in helping people understand their health rights, protections, and system-level access. Table 8.4 lists some key functions of AI empowerment tools. Building awareness of what you're entitled to is foundational for public health personal responsibility.

Personal AI Navigation Tools

Personalized opportunities are fundamental because they define what is realistically possible and actionable for a person *right now*. Opportunity is time-bound and context-dependent. It's the "when and where" of action. Without an AI guide, they miss real-world opportunities due to a lack of navigation in complex situations. Modern health care systems are highly complex, and that complexity is a significant

Table 8.4 Key functions of AI empowerment tools

Key function	Description	Examples
Health coverage and care entitlement guidance	Explains what healthcare services or programs a person is eligible for, based on insurance, location, or identity	AI those answers "Am I eligible for Medicaid?" Tools that break down Medicare coverage State-by-state benefit explainer bots
Privacy and data rights support	Clarifies legal rights around medical data (access, sharing, consent) and alerts users to potential violations	HIPAA chatbot that explains data rights in plain English Tools that analyze which apps share your health data AI that walks users through consent forms
Insurance benefit optimization	Help users interpret and use their health insurance efficiently: understanding what's covered, what costs apply, and how to get the most out of their plan	AI that decodes EOBs (Explanation of Benefits) and coverage summaries Personalized deductible/co-pay calculators GPT (Generative Pre-trained Transformer) that explains out-of-network vs. in-network rules
Appeals and grievance assistance	Guides users through challenging denied claims or unfair treatment: offering clear, actionable steps to file and follow through on complaints	Tools that generate appeal letters for denied procedures Chatbots that file grievances with insurers step-by-step Templates for medical billing disputes

barrier to people recognizing and acting on real opportunities. A navigation tool is needed to help users discover and access personalized, actionable health opportunities. This tool enables you to act on your options and navigate choices. It should highlight guidance, wayfinding, and customized recommendations. Table 8.5 lists some key functions of AI navigation tools.

8.4 Personalized Risk Management and Prediction

Personalized risk management or prediction is a critical first step in fostering personal responsibility in public health. Your health is a journey, and risk prediction is the GPS.

Let's look at a case scenario for personalized risk management and explore how to design an AI application for this topic. Some literature about personalized health risk prediction will provide background information for you to identify the key steps

Table 8.5 Key functions of AI navigation tools

Key function	Description	Opportunity types	Examples
Preventive service matching	Identifies free or low-cost health screenings and preventive services (based on age, risk factors, or location)	Time-bound (events, age milestones, seasonal eligibility) Context-dependent (risk level, insurance coverage, location	AI alerts for free mammogram events near you Personalized screening schedules based on risk profile Medicaid-eligible flu shot reminders
Social support program finder	Help users discover eligibility and enrollment options for non-medical programs that affect health, like food assistance, housing, fitness, or caregiving support	Context-dependent (income, family size, ZIP code) Time-bound (application windows, program cycles)	AI tools that screen for SNAP, WIC, or housing vouchers Local fitness or walking group finder based on ZIP code Tools that match caregivers to respite programs
Local care access and logistics help	Finds nearby clinics, pharmacies, urgent care, and community health centers — and supports logistical needs like transportation or hours	Time-bound (operating hours, appointment availability) Context-dependent (geographic location, income eligibility)	Maps of open walk-in clinics or mobile health units AI tools that find providers who accept sliding scale Ride-share coordination for doctor appointments
Research and innovation matching	Matches users to clinical trials, pilot programs, or digital health innovations they qualify for, based on condition, demographics, or geography	Time-bound (trial enrollment periods, pilot windows) Context-dependent (health condition, demographics, location)	AI tools that match cancer patients to clinical trials Notifications for local wearable tech studies Apps that recruit underserved populations for digital health pilots
Personalized digital wellness tools	Recommends apps or services for mental health, sleep, fitness, or self-care based on the user's specific needs, goals, or conditions	Context-dependent (psychological state, user goals, behavior patterns) Less time-bound, but may include dynamic timing (e.g., reminders, daily routines)	Depression screening → recommends a CBT-based app Sleep disruption → matches with mindfulness or circadian rhythm tools AI-curated wellness plans for chronic stress or anxiety

(tasks) in this scenario (Alaa et al., 2019; Choudri et al., 2020; Desye, 2024; Zhang & Pan, 2022).

Case Scenario 8a: Personalized health risk management. A 50–55-year-old male office-based professional is beginning to experience health concerns, including being slightly overweight (BMI 27), elevated cholesterol, and a history of migraines triggered by stress, bright light, and sleep loss. He also reports mild cognitive issues, such as forgetting daily tasks. The concerns are amplified by a family history of heart disease, poor sleep quality, and a high-stress work environment. Motivated to take proactive steps, he is particularly interested in monitoring his cardiovascular health, migraine risk, and his brain health, with a focus on memory and attention. Suppose we design a personal AI application to address it.

Step 1. Digital Consent and Transparency

The first task for personal AI applications is to establish privacy, trust, and user control. For example, AI allows the user to see and selectively approve data sources used for risk prediction and memory health tracking. In this case, the user data could be self-reported symptoms (e.g., memory slips, brain fog logs), wearable data (e.g., heart rate, sleep), medical records (e.g., cholesterol, medications), and screen time, etc. The AI application can help you review and understand consent terms by utilizing a consent recommendation engine or NLP summarization. Data visualization may be helpful in deciding which input is needed for risk prediction.

Step 2. Personalized Risk Awareness Alerts

The aim of this step is to deliver real-time or daily alerts about acute health risks based on fused personal and environmental data. First, let's look at the input, which are real-time physiological and contextual signals. In this scenario, wearable data includes sleeping duration, HRV, and body temperature. The self-report can be related to memory lapses or headaches. The environmental data includes the heating index and air quality. The medical records will consist of medication (e.g., statins for migraine treatment).

Second, you need to select AI models for this step. LSTM (Long Short-Term Memory) (Hochreiter & Schmidhuber, 1997) can predict short-term worsening trends like migraine recurrence or cognitive dips based on recent patterns. GRU (Gated Recurrent Unit) can efficiently track variables like sleep disruption or stress variability for triggering daily alerts (Melvin et al., 2019). Bayesian network (McLachlan et al., 2020) calculates the probability of migraine or memory issues based on fused signals (even if some data is missing). The rule-based logic layer ensures alerts make sense to users. Personalized-threshold model prevents alert fatigue by only providing alerts when the risk is significant for that user. A decision tree for interpretability presents easy-to-understand logic.

The output of this step is personalized risk awareness alerts, specifically for cardiac, migraine, or brain fog. For example, "You are at high risk today for both migraines and mental fog." Contributors are "3.8 h of sleep", "92°F heat index", "7.2 h of screen time", or "Statin-related fatigue sensitivity".

Step 3. Risk Calculators and Scenario Simulations

The goal of this step is to help users understand long-term risk trends (CVD, migraine frequency, memory clarity) and how behavior changes can affect them. The data input includes EMRs (e.g., cholesterol history, medication), self-reports (e.g., exercise, diet, headache frequency, memory logs), wearables (e.g., HR trends, sleep quality), and other inputs (e.g., screen time, alcohol/caffeine use, stress perception).

The AI models for cardiovascular risk can be a logistic regression (Hosmer & Lemeshow, 2000) (e.g., ASCVD (Atherosclerotic Cardiovascular Disease)), which predicts the chance (risk) that someone will have a heart problem (like a heart attack or stroke) in the next 10 years. The AI models for migraine recurrence can be a Gradient Boosting Machine (GBM) (Friedman, 2001), which predicts how likely you are to get a migraine in the next few days, based on many daily habits or triggers. The AI models for cognitive trend scoring can be time series regression or LSTM models, which track your mental clarity and memory over time and help you see patterns or declines. AI can provide scenario simulations, allowing you to test different lifestyle changes and see how they could improve your health risks. For example, you can run simulations like "What if you go to bed 30 min earlier?" "What if you drink less coffee?" "What if you walk 15 min every day?".

This is a strong personalization through lifestyle and biometric modeling. The output in this step could be some suggestions. For example, "Your 10-year heart disease risk is 20%. With 30 min of walking 5x/week, risk drops to 14%.", "Your migraine frequency is 3 times per month. Better sleep (avg 7 h/night) may reduce this to one time per month." "Your memory slips are twice per week. Improved hydration and focus breaks may cut this by 50%."

Step 4. Community Risk Alerts Tailored to User Profile

The aim of this step is to blend population-level health and environmental risks with the user's personal profile to adjust alerts for contextual decision-making. The local risk will be integrated with the user profile and symptom history. The data input could include local flu/virus prevalence, heat waves, air quality index (PM2.5, AQI), and user-specific risk factors (e.g., migraines, cholesterol, sleep deprivation).

You need to select the AI models for this task. Geospatial clustering (e.g., DBSCAN (Density-Based Spatial Clustering of Applications with Noise) (Ester et al., 1996)) finds community-level risk events (e.g., flu outbreak in a ZIP code, spike in migraines reported nearby). Environmental data APIs and NLP feed location-specific events (e.g., pollen spike, poor air quality alert) into the risk prediction pipeline. Bayesian updating adjusts user-specific risk scores as new local information comes in. Federated learning helps models learn from distributed data (e.g., symptom trends) while preserving privacy. Personalized filtering rules send only relevant alerts (e.g., pollen alert only if users have migraines triggered by allergies).

The output of this step will be community-aware risk alerts. For example, "Air quality in your ZIP code is unhealthy (AQI 138)." "Because of your migraine and memory sensitivity history, you may experience fatigue and fog today." "Use an air purifier indoors. Delay high-focus tasks until air improves."

Your City's Climate Risk Profile

Unfortunately, the window to prevent catastrophic climate change is closing fast. Still, political systems move slowly and cannot avoid the damage related to climate change (e.g., heatwaves related to Arctic warming patterns). Some cities in the world may become functionally unlivable in the summer (e.g., more than 3 weeks with temperatures above 38 °C or 100°F). AI tools could map your current city's climate risk profile (such as heat, water, and health). Your ZIP code can matter as much as your genetic code when it comes to long-term wellness.

8.5 Personalized Health Education

Your health is a journey, and risk prediction is the GPS. Personalized health education is your driver's intelligence. It's not enough to have a GPS (risk model). You need to know what it means when the GPS says, "sharp turn ahead". Health literacy teaches what signs to look for (recognizing early warning symptoms, lab changes, or health trends), how to handle a sudden detour (responding to unexpected events: illness, side effects, stress triggers, environmental risks), when to pull over and get help (understanding when symptoms are urgent or need professional attention), understanding road maps and dashboard alerts (interpreting test results, medication instructions, or wearable data), why it's worth staying on course (connecting health goals with daily decisions and building long-term commitment).

Let's look at a case scenario for personalized health education and explore how to design an AI application for this topic. Some literature about personalized health education will provide background information for you to identify the key steps (tasks) in this scenario (Barello et al., 2016; Hibbard et al., 2004; Ryan & Deci, 2000).

Case Scenario 8b: Personalized health education. A 52-year-old male construction project manager with a business background, no health training. He avoids checkups, lives a high-stress lifestyle with a poor diet, and little exercise. After experiencing chest tightness, the ER reveals several warning signs: high blood pressure, high LDL (Low-Density Lipoprotein), prediabetes, and overweight (BMI (Body Mass Index) 28). He wants to take better control of his health but feels overwhelmed and uninformed. Suppose we design a personal AI application to address it to improve health literacy.

Stage 1. Activation

The triggers for users to activate personal health education can be an ER (Emergency Room) visit or a diagnosis shock. This is a timely awareness of the need for health education. The goal of the AI tool is to help users immediately understand new health information and reduce anxiety. The tool can be a "lab result translator", which can translate raw clinical data into easy-to-understand language tailored to the user's condition and context. We aim to prevent hallucinations or errors when interpreting health-sensitive data. Because lab results follow clinical rules (e.g., "normal," "borderline," "high") and apply clinical thresholds (e.g., "A1c > 6.5% = diabetes"), the first selection of the AI model in this case can be "rule-based NLP (Natural Language Processing)". It's fast, safe, and predictable. This is like a highly structured dictionary that knows how to match lab values with basic explanations. For example, "Your A1c is 6.2%, which means you're in the prediabetes range." Another AI model is RAG (Retrieval-Augmented Generation) (Gao et al., 2023; Izacard et al., 2022). It adds a brain that can "look things up" before answering and then explain the lab result in a more personal, context-aware way. It avoids overwhelming the user by presenting only the necessary information. For example, "This shows your average blood sugar is higher than normal. The good news: lifestyle changes at this stage can often reverse the trend." The outcome of this stage of education is that the user feels informed and calm and begins to engage meaningfully with their health.

Stage 2. Reflection

The second stage of education will be reflection, a daily self-awareness. The triggers can be new medication or experiencing daily symptoms like dizziness. The goal of the AI tool is to recognize symptom patterns and understand personal responses to treatment. The tools can be a "conversational symptom coach" and a "medication experience simulator". Symptoms are not one-time events; they follow specific timelines. While human memory is imperfect, AI can track small changes more accurately. We can select LSTM (Long Short-Term Memory) or time-aware models to help detect subtle, personal health rhythms. LSTM is a type of neural network that remembers patterns across time. For example, AI can detect migraine every third day or find that sleep quality worsens after a dose increases. Medications can be complex, but users often want clarity. AI can select "knowledge graphs" to explain known medication effects in user-friendly language. For example, "Many people feel dizzy the first 3 days of this medication. If it continues, you may need a dose adjustment." The education outcome of this stage is that the user becomes more aware of body signals, medication effects, and when to seek help.

Stage 3. Skill-Oriented Learning

The next stage of education is skills-oriented learning, such as health reasoning and critical thinking. This can be triggered by encountering confusing or false health claims. People are vulnerable to overhyped "natural cures", miracle quick-fix claims, distrust in medicine, and social media misinformation. For example, "You can reverse diabetes in ten days with this detox smoothie plan." Prediabetes can improve with lifestyle, but not overnight. Extreme detoxes can be unsafe. AI tools can serve as a "misinformation explainer bot" or a "critical thinking prompter." The goal of these educational tools is to develop reasoning skills and foster trust in evidence-based decision-making. The AI models can use LLM (large language models) with RAG

(Retrieval-Augmented Generation). Generative AI can perform fact-checking and draw from clinical guidelines and systematic reviews. High-quality domain data sources include the CDC, WHO, Cochrane (Cochrane, 2024), UpToDate (Wolters, 2024), and PubMed. The AI tool can select AI models, such as "Socratic Dialogue Trees" or "Logic-Based Prompting", for building reasoning skills. These use structured question chains to simulate a critical-thinking coach without giving direct answers too soon. AI can promote "guided reasoning", not just information consumption. For example, AI: "What evidence supports this claim about reversing diabetes in ten days?" "Is that anecdote the same as scientific evidence? What would a good study look like?" The educational outcome of these tools is that users can intelligently question health content, resist misinformation, and become more confident decision-makers.

Stage 4. Knowledge Growth and Motivation

This stage of education is knowledge growth and motivation. The goal of AI tools is to reinforce engagement, support deeper learning, and motivate progress. The AI tool can serve as a "learning dashboard and health timeline" (displaying progress). It can track what a user has learned or struggled with over time and build a personal profile of knowledge gaps and progress. AI can select "knowledge tracing models" such as deep knowledge tracing (DKT) (Yeung & Yeung, 2018) or Bayesian knowledge tracing (Corbett & Anderson, 1995). Temporal data modeling, also known as time-series AI, can enable the timeline to be interactive and predictive, rather than just static. For example, timelines for health metrics of BP, glucose, and weight. Visualizing timelines can detect patterns, improvements, or stagnation for user learning. The educational outcomes are that the user sees progress, stays motivated, and continues building health knowledge and behaviors.

8.6 Behavioral Nudging and Coaching

Behavioral nudging and coaching closely align with the personalized motivation component of the PMCO-AI model (see Session 8.1). Behavioral nudging is a "motivation engine" that triggers intrinsic drive and leverages external cues. Medication adherence is a prime example of behavioral nudging in both personal and public health. Health is a journey. Medication adherence is like remembering to fuel your car regularly. It may not feel urgent on a day-to-day basis, but without it, the engine slowly breaks down.

Let's examine a case scenario for "medication adherence support" and explore how to design an AI application for this purpose. Some literature on this topic will provide background information to help you identify the key steps (tasks) in this scenario (Arno & Thomas, 2016; Conn & Ruppar, 2017; Munro et al., 2007; Patel et al., 2015).

Case Scenario 8c: Medication adherence support. A middle-aged male was recently diagnosed with hypertension and prediabetes. He's been prescribed statins and metformin but struggles to take them consistently due to his hectic, irregular schedule. Often forgetting doses. He also feels unsure whether the medications are truly helping, which adds to his skepticism and sense of being overwhelmed. The goal is to support the user in building a consistent habit of taking his daily medications to better manage his health. Suppose we design a personal AI application, "Medication Adherence Tool (MAT)", to address it.

Stage 1. Clarify the Why

The first stage of the medication adherence tool (MAT) involves building personal motivation by connecting medication to values, beliefs, and goals. This process is powered by an AI clarity engine. It synthesizes patient input and health data, infers motivation-relevant themes, produces clear, coherent, and emotionally resonant output, and it can loop with the user iteratively for better alignment. The related AI models include conversational LLMs (Large Language Models) for motivational interviewing, value alignment models, risk modeling, and narrative generation models (such as storytelling). For example, "What matters most to you, such as your energy at work, time with family, or reducing stroke risk?" "Take this medication to stay active for your grandchildren." "Without meds, your 10-year heart attack risk is 22%. With them, it's 12%."

Stage 2. Support the How

This stage of MAT supports users with well-timed, emotionally intelligent, and context-aware nudges and habit-building scaffolds, enabling medication-taking to become automatic and sustainable. The first task is to sense user's real-world context (location, time, activity). The AI models are "mobile context detection modeling" to detect daily patterns and suggest optimal contexts for medication prompts: home vs work, active vs sedentary, busy vs idle. For example, "You're usually at home at 9 pm in the kitchen. Shall I set a gentle reminder for that window?" The next task of MAT is to choose optimal timing/channel for reminder. The selected AI model can utilize reinforcement learning (RL) for smart reminder timing, allowing it to learn and adapt to the user's routine and identify when and how reminders are most likely to lead to success. Feedback loop allows the system to learn what works best for user. AI needs to generate tone-matched messages. The selected AI models can be emotion-aware LLMs to tailor messages in tone and framing to match the emotional state or preference, such as supportive, funny, serious, urgent, gentle, etc. For example, "You're doing great! Just one tiny step left today: your BP med". The goal of MAT is to provide habit-building scaffolds that support user's learning. The selected AI models can be habit modeling engines (knowledge graphs or probabilistic graphical models of behavior routines) that reinforce the cue-action-reward loop and update the scaffold. For example, "After brushing teeth? That's a good anchor."

Stage 3. Discover What's Working

This stage for MAT is to discover what is working. AI can help users reflect on progress, understand their own behavior, adjust routines, and learn personalized strategies that are sustainable. First, AI can detect adherence trends and shifts in context. Time-series analysis models (e.g., LSTM networks (Hochreiter & Schmidhuber, 1997), Hidden Markov Models (HMMs) (Rabiner, 1989), or Temporal Convolutional Networks (TCNs) (Lea et al., 2017)) can be used for pattern detection. The selected AI models can identify adherence patterns over time (e.g., weekday vs. weekend drops, monthly cycles, or contextual shifts). For example, "You consistently miss your meds on weekends after 10 am." Secondly, MAT can prompt users to reflect on progress or obstacles. The AI models can be self-reflection prompting with Socratic LLMs. Socratic dialogue is a method of discussion where you ask thoughtful questions to help individuals clarify their own thoughts and feelings. It guides users in reflecting on their routines, beliefs, obstacles, and successes, gently eliciting self-insight and fostering learning. For example, "What made Saturday harder, and what might you change next time?" Then, MAT can generate interpretable feedback about "what works", using explainable AI (XAI) (Gilpin et al., 2018; Guidotti et al., 2018). XAI will convert behavioral data and prediction model outputs into clear, understandable insights for the user. For example, "Your reminders work best when you're at home and have low calendar activity." Finally, MAT will suggest tailored strategies based on behavioral twins, by using behavior clustering for personalized strategy suggestions. Unsupervised learning models (e.g., K-means (Jain et al., 1999), DBSCAN (Ester et al., 1996), t-SNE (van der Maaten & Hinton, 2008) and clustering) can be applied to multi-dimensional behavioral features. It will identify user archetypes (e.g., "morning-focused self-trackers," "evening routine stackers," "emotional responders") and tailor strategy recommendations accordingly. For example, "Try linking to lunch or using pill pack?".

Stage 4. Sustain with Others

Another feature of MAT is to "sustain with others," which adds social reinforcement, peer norms, system-level support, and fosters long-term habits. Before we explore the AI models for this stage. Let's see some specific real-world cases showing why the "sustain with others" feature in MAT becomes especially important, depending on age group, health condition, or life context (see Table 8.6).

This stage aims to help users stay on track over time, supported by peers, family, clinicians, and systems, leveraging AI-driven social intelligence and connected data. First, the selected AI models can be AI recommender systems for social norms and peer modeling. For example, "People with your schedule tend to take meds just before breakfast." Second, AI gamification engines can learn when users need extra encouragement or challenge. For example, "You and five peers earned a five-day badge this week. Great teamwork!" Gamification is especially impactful for children with chronic conditions because it turns routine, often frustrating, self-management tasks into playful, empowering experiences. Then, social comparison AI (with privacy-safe, personalized benchmarking) can show how the user compares

Table 8.6 Real-world cases for the need of "sustain with others."

Examples of real-world cases	The needs of "sustain with others"
Children with chronic conditions (e.g., Asthma, Epilepsy)	Children depend on caregivers to manage medication Forgetfulness or misunderstanding dosage is common Schools and daycares may play a role
Older adults with memory decline or low digital literacy	May forget doses or confuse medications Reluctant to use tech independently Risk increases with isolation and polypharmacy
Pregnant women with new supplement or medication routines	Pregnancy often includes new medications (e.g., iron, prenatal vitamins) Emotional and physical changes make consistency harder Peer advice is influential and comforting
College students managing ADHD or mental health meds	High independence but chaotic schedules Peer norms, stigma, and forgetfulness are key barriers Students may not tell family or clinicians when they struggle
People managing stigma-associated conditions (e.g., HIV, depression)	Isolation, shame, or cultural barriers may block routine care Support from people "who get it" can be lifesaving
Workers with unpredictable schedules (e.g., gig workers, shift-based roles)	Irregular shifts, unstable routines, high risk of missed doses May lacks health insurance or consistent care

to an anonymized group, in an encouraging, non-shaming way. For example, "Most people in your age group also struggle with weekends but see a big improvement by adding a morning alarm." Finally, you need integration APIs (e.g., pharmacy, health portals, smart devices) to pull external data for real-time reinforcement and system-level feedback. For example, "Your smart pillbox shows consistency. Time to celebrate your 30-day streak!".

8.7 Policy-Aware Personalized Opportunity (PAPO) Model

Personalized Opportunity

Opportunities represent the intersection between systemic factors (such as policy implementation) and personal responsibility in public health (see Fig. 8.3). Without accessible, tailored opportunities, even well-designed policies cannot translate into population-level behavior change. The policy-aware personalized opportunity (PAPO) model is like a "smart translator" between public policy and individual

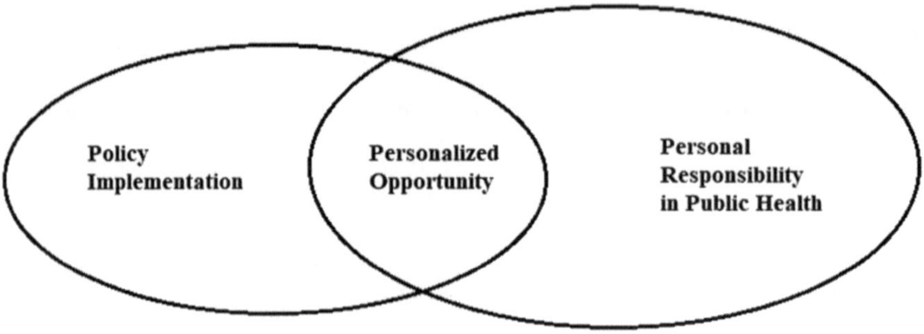

Fig. 8.3 Personalized opportunities in public health

lives. Only in the AI era was PAPO actionable. It requires AI to speak in millions of personalized voices and adjust messages based on context, language, access, and values.

In this session, a policy-aware personalized opportunity (PAPO) model is proposed, and an AI application for heatwaves using PAPO is designed. The core assumptions of the PAPO models or the PAPO-heatwave AI application is that opportunities are the most immediate and actionable link between policy implementation and personal responsibility in public health.

8.7.1 PAPO Model

Uniqueness

Most public health personalization is citizen-first: "Who is at risk? What do they need?" The proposed model is policy-first: "What public resources now exist? Who can benefit from this?" AI applications will make public policies actionable at the individual level in real time, for real people.

Instead of creating generic policy alerts or long-term programs, this model allows on-demand matching of time-bound interventions (e.g., 4-h bus schedule), location-bound resources (e.g., cooling shelters), and context-specific needs (e.g., elderly diabetic patients without AC (Air Conditioner)).

Model Design

PAPO has four components, as shown in Fig. 8.4.

1. ***Policy input layer***

The policy input layer defines system-wide interventions, including alerts, services, resource deployments, guidelines, and restrictions. It can capture real-time or updated public health policies and environmental alerts. In public health, system-level interventions, driven by policy, are core tools for protecting population health.

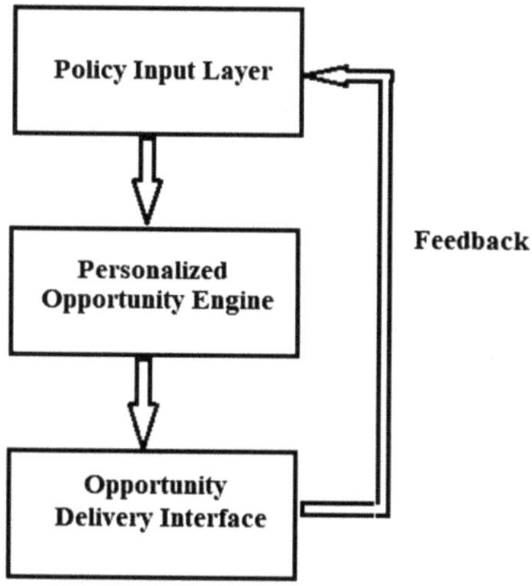

Fig. 8.4 The design of the policy-aware personalized opportunity model

Here are some examples of health policies, such as vaccination mandates in infectious disease control, smoking bans in public places in chronic disease prevention, air quality alerts in environmental health and safety, building codes for fall prevention in aging populations, shelter location and operation policies in disaster response, funding for school-based counselors in mental health, and food recall systems for nutrition.

2. ***Personalized opportunity engine***

The personalized opportunity engine translates policy data into individualized opportunities by combining policy context with personal factors (e.g., location, health status, access to resources) to generate actionable insights tailored for each person. It translates policies into *localized*, *timely*, and *person-specific* opportunities (micro-opportunities). For example, during a wildfire, the engine can output: "Air quality is hazardous in your ZIP code. N95 masks are available free at the nearest library—open until 6 PM today." For water contamination or boil alerts, the engine may output: "Boil water advisory in your area. A pickup station for clean drinking water is available at [school name], open now. Map?".

3. ***Opportunity delivery interface***

The user interface provides personalized, timely recommendations and notifications to individuals via apps, SMS, or other communication channels, encouraging protective behaviors. It will communicate opportunities to the person at the right time, in the correct format. For example, the interface can be voice alerts for elderly populations. The interface should provide a nudge action by reducing friction and increasing salience.

4. ***Feedback loop***

The feedback component collects behavioral data and contextual responses from individuals to inform policymakers and personalize algorithms, enabling continuous refinement of both policy strategies and personalized support. For example, for heatwaves, the feedback is "Cooling center X was underused." Those behavior and usage data can be gathered in anonymized or consented formats.

8.7.2 PAPO-Heatwave AI

To apply the PAPO model to an urgent public health issue, I first chose the heatwave issue. The name of the first AI application using the PAPO model is "PAPO-heatwave AI".

Why Choose Heatwaves?

Unlike hurricanes or earthquakes, heatwaves often kill people silently and invisibly, especially among vulnerable populations like older adults living alone, people with chronic conditions (e.g., heart disease, diabetes), low-income communities without air conditioning, outdoor or manual laborers, and the unhoused homeless. In the summer of 2025, record-breaking temperatures during heatwaves reached 50 °C in some regions and exceeded 40 °C across the U.S. and EU.

Deploying an AI application in public health is a complex project that requires the support of the community, professionals, and regulators. In heatwaves, regardless of one's socioeconomic status, people are feeling the heat. Even in politically polarized or economically unequal societies, heat doesn't discriminate. This creates a rare moment of shared vulnerability and shared motivation to act. Let's design a PAPO-heatwave AI for our cities that will be well-prepared for heatwaves in future summers due to climate change.

> **Case Scenario 8d: PAPO-heatwave AI.** In a small city, there are more frequent heatwaves due to climate change. The local government aims to optimize heatwave responses and reduce mortality rates in the upcoming summer. Suppose we design an AI system to address it, using the PAPO model. This system will analyze real-time weather data, population vulnerability (e.g., elderly residents), and policy constraints (e.g., budget limits) to generate tailored recommendations.

PAPO-Heatwave AI application[1]

[1] There is a trade-off for the author between the clarity of concept for public health readers and the technical depth for developers. Due to the urgency of climate change, I hope the PAPO-heatwave AI application design can be deployed in the real world as soon as possible to save lives. Therefore, I will integrate domain data analysis in Chapter 6 with AI model selections for the AI application in this session. The technical depth may increase, making it more actionable for developers. Let's quickly review some key concepts (see Chapter 6 for more details) about domain data. Rules are strategic or operational logic derived from policy (e.g., "prioritize elderly"). Data are used as input to

Pre-heatwave:

Before the heatwave, we need to have sufficient domain data (e.g., policy elements and personal information) for training AI systems. There are related AI models or tools to support the stages of "policy input layer" and "personalized opportunity engine" in pre-heatwave.

Stage 1 Policy Input Layer

Let's provide some examples of pure policy elements in pre-heatwaves in this stage (see Table 8.7).

AI can empower many tasks in policy input layer. For example, AI can perform document ingestion using an OCR (Optical Character Recognition) and NLP pipeline to extract text from PDFs, memos, and budgets. AI can parse those files for the logic layer and infer activation rules or budget logic from formal plans. The AI entity extraction can identify actors (e.g., "Office of Emergency Management"), targets, and dates. In this stage, AI can use geographic tagging to map ZIP code references to actual geographic data (GIS (Geographic Information System) layers).

Table 8.7 Examples of pure policy elements in pre-heatwaves

Policy element	AI role (data type)	Description and examples
Strategic intent	Rules (extracted from static text)	High-level goals (e.g., "reduce elderly heat mortality"); translated into logic or weights
Policy equity focus	Rules (extracted from static text)	Equity goals (set the ethical and strategic direction of the intervention; Thresholds for action (Rules that define eligibility or priority tiers; These define when and where to act.); Resource Allocation Rules (These guide operational priorities)
	Data (static)	SVI (Social Vulnerability Index) (Centers for Disease Control and Prevention, 2024); ADI (Area Deprivation Index) (University of Wisconsin-Madison, 2023); ZIP-level demographic and infrastructure data; Health outcome baselines
Preparedness architecture	Data (static)	SOPs (standard operation procedurals), roles (emergency command), response timing, agency responsibility (used to time/trigger recommendations)
Resource distribution	Data (static and GIS)	Budget allocations (e.g., cooling centers), location of services (inputs to spatial opportunity matching)
Institutional capacity	Data (static and inventory)	Staff numbers, assets (vans, shelters). Numbers of AC-equipped buses. Constraints for AI feasibility checks

algorithms or models. Static data is rarely changed, such as plans and infrastructure maps. Streaming data is updated frequently. Self-report data are collected from human feedback or community input.

Stage 2. Personalized Opportunity Engine

Let's provide some examples of personal information related to heatwaves in this stage (see Table 8.8).

AI can empower many tasks in the pre-heatwave stage of this personalized opportunity engine. Let's look at some examples. AI can prepare eligibility inference and proxy inference (e.g., detect likely AC insecurity status or flag households for cooling device programs). AI can generate vulnerability scoring and risk profiling (e.g., combining age, chronic disease, and housing status to assign a risk tier). During heat waves, AI can utilize scores to prioritize outreach and deliver tailored warnings. AI can create constraint modeling (e.g., identify transportation challenges or digitally disconnected populations).

During Heatwave:

During the heatwaves, environmental alerts are active, policies are implemented, public services are deployed, mobility support is adjusted, and community outreach is operationalized. There is a flow in this process, including triggers, logic, services, access, engagement, and feedback. Both domain data (e.g., more streaming data) and AI models during heatwaves will be explored in this session.

Stage 1. Policy Input Layer

Let's provide some examples of real-time policy elements related to heatwaves at this stage (see Table 8.9). During the heatwaves, the policy input layer includes new input elements, such as environmental alerts and community outreach.

Table 8.8 Examples of static personal data in pre-heatwaves

Examples of personal data element (pre-heatwave)	Data type	Sources
Location (home)	Static	Health records, public registries, housing programs
House type (e.g., AC access)	Static	Public housing data, utility subsidies, survey/enrollment forms
Demographics (e.g., age, income)	Static	Census-linked data, social service enrollment
Health risk factors	Static	Medicaid/Medicare, chronic disease registries, local health dept data
Access needs (mobility, disability, caregiver status)	Static	Transit access data, disability registry, human services records
Preferred contact method	Self-report	Community outreach, sign-up campaigns
Digital access	Self-report and static	Broadband data, prior survey responses

Table 8.9 Examples of policy elements during heatwaves

Policy element	Data type	Role	Example inputs
Environmental alerts	Streaming	Workflow trigger	Heat advisories, UV index, heat risk indices
Policy logic (active rules)	Static rules and real-time	Decision trigger conditions	SOPs (Standard Operating Procedures) with thresholds, event timelines
Public services availability	Streaming and static	Personalized opportunity source	Open cooling center status, capacity, geolocation
Mobility support	Streaming and static	Accessibility filter and routing support	Real-time bus feed, adjusted GTFS (General Transit Feed Specification) routes
Community outreach	Self-report and event-driven	Feedback and adaptive targeting	Volunteer check-ins, unmet need reports, wellness surveys

AI can power many tasks, such as detecting environmental alert levels and activating corresponding policies or workflows. AI can evaluate dynamic conditions against policy rules to determine subsequent actions. At that time, AI can match individuals with the nearest available services, prioritizing those with high-risk profiles. AI models can recalculate accessible routes to services in real-time and alert users. With community outreach data, AI learns where outreach is effective or ineffective, and adapts messages or deploys resources to underserved areas.

Stage 2. Personalized Opportunity Engine

Let's review some examples of real-time personal data during the heatwave for the personal opportunity engine (see Table 8.10). The target vulnerable population in heatwaves is also considered, including older adults living alone or individuals with chronic conditions.

Suppose policy elements and personal information (both static data before the heatwave and real-time data during the heatwave) are available. In this case, let's explore what key AI-powered tasks can be operated during a heatwave in "personalized opportunity engine" stage (see Table 8.11).

Stage 3. Opportunity Delivery Interfaces

Let's explore what key AI-powered tasks can be operated during a heatwave in "opportunity delivery interfaces" stage (see Table 8.12).

Stage 4. Feedback

Let's explore what key AI-powered tasks can be operated during a heatwave in feedback stage (see Table 8.13).

Table 8.10 Examples of real-time personal data during heatwaves

Examples of personal elements during the heatwaves	Data type	Data source	Target populations
Current location (mobile)	Streaming/ Real-time	Mobile apps, GPS, cell towers, wearables	• Outdoor/manual laborers • Homeless/unhoused • Older adults (if mobile)
Recent activity/ movement	Streaming	Transit logs, mobility apps, phone sensors	• Outdoor/manual laborers • Homeless/unhoused
Device connectivity status	Streaming/ Event-driven	App pings, SMS delivery receipts, IoT status	• All populations (especially older adults, low-income)
Check-in status	Event-driven/ Self-report	App/web forms, volunteer visits	• Older adults living alone • People with chronic conditions • Homeless
Cooling behavior feedback	Self-report	In-app surveys, text response, IVR	• Low-income residents without AC • Older adults
Symptoms or distress reports	Self-report/ Alert-triggered	Text/chat, hotlines, app forms	• People with chronic conditions • Older adults • Outdoor workers
Service utilization status	Streaming	Cooling center check-ins, transit card use	• Low-income families • Older adults • Homeless • Chronic illness group
Caregiver or neighbor alerts	Event-driven	Human networks, community health workers	• Older adults living alone • People with chronic conditions

Why is PAPO-Heatwave AI Unique?

Firstly, this PAPO-heatwave AI bridges *systemic policy* and *personal behavior* in real time. Most existing systems either broadcast heat alerts (generic, one-size-fits-all) or offer personal health tools with no live integration with public systems.

Secondly, "Opportunity" serves as the central unit in this design. This shift from *"awareness"* to *"opportunity"* is a significant innovation. Rather than just warnings or health advice, this system identifies concrete, real-world opportunities (e.g., a cooling center with a shuttle nearby) based on public policies and resources.

Thirdly, personalized delivery can be based on constraints. This makes the AI application design respectful, equity-aware, and practical. There are real possibilities to implement our design principle of *"encoding justice"*. It actively checks whether

Table 8.11 Key AI-powered tasks in personalized opportunity engine

AI-powered tasks	Description	Example AI models	Example data
Risk stratification in real time	Prioritize who needs help right now based on both static vulnerability and dynamic exposure	Ensemble risk scoring models (combine static and streaming data) Decision trees/gradient boosted trees (e.g., XGBoost (eXtreme Gradient Boosting) (Chen & Guestrin, 2016), LightGBM (Light Gradient Boosting Machine) (Natekin & Knoll, 2013)) Rule-based systems based on SOP thresholds (e.g., age > 75 + no. AC + no. recent check-in = high risk)	Static (age, AC access, chronic conditions) Real-time (location, check-in status, symptoms)
Personalized opportunity matching	Match individuals to actionable services (cooling centers, transit, hydration) based on their location, access needs, and service availability	Geospatial matching algorithms Constraint satisfaction (availability, distance, mobility filters) Recommender systems (e.g., top-N most accessible services)	Current location, mobility status, transportation options Service utilization status (real-time capacity, hours)

Table 8.12 Key AI-powered tasks in opportunity delivery interface

AI-powered tasks	Description	Example AI models	Example data
Multimodal communication	Matching opportunities must be delivered effectively via the right modality: SMS (Short Message Service), app, voice, caregivers, public display, etc	Contact preference model (email, SMS, call, visit) Communication success prediction (based on device connectivity)	Device Connectivity Real-time SMS/ app feedback Preferred contact method (from pre-heatwave data)
Outreach targeting	Uses delivery logic and community data to determine who should be reached via human outreach (CHWs (Community Health Workers), city workers). Social networks may help to identify informal caregivers, neighbors, or community groups that may act as secondary outreach agents	Decision rules: fallback pathways (e.g., escalate to in-person check) Social network-based models	Previous Outreach History Social support presence

Table 8.13 Key AI-powered tasks in feedback stage of PAPO model

AI-powered tasks	Description	Example AI models	Example data
Behavior monitoring and feedback loop	Detect when expected protective actions (e.g., going to a cooling center) are not happening, and trigger alerts or interventions	Time-series anomaly detection (e.g., expected check-in not received) Behavioral prediction models (e.g., who are likely to skip cooling resources) Event-driven rules (e.g., missing 2 check-ins = alert)	Cooling behavior feedback Service utilization Symptoms or check-in data
Resource reallocation support	Detect imbalances in service usage (e.g., one cooling center overwhelmed, another underused) and suggest redistribution	Dynamic Optimization/ Reinforcement Learning Demand Forecasting Models (e.g., short-term inflow to services) Equity-aware allocation algorithms	Real-time service utilization Neighborhood demand, transit access Heat maps of population movement and symptoms

an opportunity is usable by the person (considering mobility, time, location, and access). It chooses timing, wording, and channel based on each person's needs.

Finally, this design is a developer- and policy-maker-friendly architecture. The PAPO structure is *simple enough* to communicate clearly (especially to non-technical public health professionals), but *modular enough* for future integration with advanced AI (e.g., LLMs, geospatial systems, recommender engines). This makes it *implementable,* not just a theory.

Practical Considerations

The PAPO-AI system can work in a practical production setting only if policy data and services are digitized, personal risk and access data are collected ethically, and outreach and delivery logic are well-defined. Many cities experience heat waves in the summer, particularly those located near the equator. However, to pilot this PAPO-heatwave AI application ideally, we should choose a "data-ready" city. For example, this city already has well-documented emergency plans, digital maps of cooling centers and transit routes, open data APIs (Application Programming Interfaces), and policy-sharing agreements in place.

For cities that need PAPO-heatwave AI system but are not yet "data-ready", we can help them by providing related AI tools to get started, such as the "AI policy structuring advisor" or the "AI workflow reform assistant".

8.8 Discussion Questions

Question 8.1. How does the PMCO-AI framework expand or differ from traditional models of personal responsibility in public health?

Question 8.2. In what ways can AI enhance an individual's motivation, capability, and opportunity to make healthier choices?

Question 8.3. What are the limitations of relying on AI for personal risk prediction and health education, especially in low-resource settings?

Question 8.4. What ethical concerns arise when AI tools are used for behavioral nudging and coaching in public health?

Question 8.5. What role should equity considerations play when assigning personal responsibility through AI-driven frameworks?

Question 8.6. How does the PAPO model translate broad public policies into personalized opportunities for individuals?

References

Alaa, A. M., Bolton, T., Angelantonio, E. D., Rudd, J. H. F., & Schaar, M. D. (2019). Cardiovascular Disease Risk Prediction Using Automated Machine Learning: A Prospective Study of 423,604 UK Biobank Participants. *Plos One, 14*(5), e0213653. https://doi.org/10.1371/journal.pone.0213653

Arno, A., & Thomas, S. (2016). The Efficacy of Nudge Theory Strategies in Influencing Adult Dietary Behaviour: A Systematic Review and Meta-Analysis. *BMC Public Health, 16*(1). https://doi.org/10.1186/s12889-016-3272-x

Barello, S., Triberti, S., Graffigna, G., Libreri, C., Serino, S., Hibbard, J., & Riva, G. (2016). eHealth for Patient Engagement: A Systematic Review. *Frontiers in Psychology, 6*. https://doi.org/10.3389/fpsyg.2015.02013

Centers for Disease Control and Prevention, Agency for Toxic Substances and Disease Registry. (2024). *CDC/ATSDR Social Vulnerability Index*. https://www.atsdr.cdc.gov/place-health/php/svi/index.html

Chen, T., & Guestrin, C. (2016). *XGBoost*. Paper presented at the Proceedings of the 22nd ACM SIGKDD International Conference on Knowledge Discovery and Data Mining, 785–794. https://doi.org/10.1145/2939672.2939785

Choudri, B. S., Nasiri, N. A., Charabi, Y., & Al-Awadhi, T. (2020). Ecological and Human Health Risk Assessment. *Water Environment Research, 92*(10), 1440–1446. https://doi.org/10.1002/wer.1382

Cochrane. (2024). *Cochrane*. https://www.cochrane.org

Conn, V. S., & Ruppar, T. M. (2017). Medication Adherence Outcomes of 771 Intervention trials: Systematic Review and Meta-Analysis. *Preventive Medicine, 99*, 269–276. https://doi.org/10.1016/j.ypmed.2017.03.008

Corbett, A. T., & Anderson, J. R. (1995). Knowledge Tracing: Modeling the Acquisition of Procedural Knowledge. *User Modelling and User-Adapted Interaction, 4*(4), 253–278. https://doi.org/10.1007/bf01099821

Natekin, A., & Knoll, A. (2013). Gradient boosting machines, a tutorial. *Frontiers in Neurorobotics, 7*. https://doi.org/10.3389/fnbot.2013.00021

Desye, B. (2024). *Perspective Chapter: Application of Environmental Epidemiology for Exposure and Health Risk Assessment*. https://doi.org/10.5772/intechopen.105684

Ester, M., Kriegel, H. P., Sander, J., & Xu, X. (1996). A *Density-Based Algorithm for Discovering Clusters in Large Spatial Databases with Noise*. Proceedings of the 2nd International Conference on Knowledge Discovery and Data Mining (KDD-96), 226–231. https://www.aaai.org/Papers/KDD/1996/KDD96-037.pdf

Friedman, J. H. (2001). Greedy function approximation: A gradient boosting machine. *The Annals of Statistics, 29*(5). https://doi.org/10.1214/aos/1013203451

Gao, Y., Xiong, Y., Gao, X., Jia, K., Pan, J., Bi, Y., Dai, Y., Sun, J., Wang, M., & Wang, H. (2023). *Retrieval-Augmented Generation for Large Language Models: A Survey*. https://arxiv.org/abs/2312.10997

Gilpin, L. H., Bau, D., Yuan, B. Z., Bajwa, A., Specter, M., & Kagal, L. (2018). *Explaining Explanations: An Overview of Interpretability of Machine Learning*. Paper presented at the 2018 IEEE 5th International Conference on Data Science and Advanced Analytics (DSAA), 80–89. https://doi.org/10.1109/dsaa.2018.00018

Guidotti, R., Monreale, A., Ruggieri, S., Turini, F., Giannotti, F., & Pedreschi, D. (2018). A Survey of Methods for Explaining Black Box Models. *ACM Computing Surveys, 51*(5), 1–42. https://doi.org/10.1145/3236009

Hibbard, J. H., Stockard, J., Mahoney, E. R., & Tusler, M. (2004). Development of the Patient Activation Measure (PAM): Conceptualizing and Measuring Activation in Patients and Consumers. *Health Services Research, 39*(4p1), 1005–1026. https://doi.org/10.1111/j.1475-6773.2004.00269.x

Hochreiter, S., & Schmidhuber, J. (1997). Long Short-Term Memory. *Neural Computation, 9*(8), 1735–1780. https://doi.org/10.1162/neco.1997.9.8.1735

Hosmer, D. W., & Lemeshow, S. (2000). *Applied Logistic Regression*: Wiley. https://doi.org/10.1002/0471722146

Izacard, G., Lewis, P., Lomeli, M., Hosseini, L., Petroni, F., Schick, T., Dwivedi-Yu, J., Joulin, A., Riedel, S., & Grave, E. (2022). *Few-shot Learning with Retrieval Augmented Language Models*. https://arxiv.org/abs/2208.03299

Jain, A. K., Murty, M. N., & Flynn, P. J. (1999). Data Clustering: A Review. *ACM Computing Surveys, 31*(3), 264–323. https://dl.acm.org/doi/https://doi.org/10.1145/331499.331504

Laguarta, J., Hueto, F., & Subirana, B. (2020). COVID-19 Artificial Intelligence Diagnosis Using Only Cough Recordings. *IEEE Open Journal of Engineering in Medicine and Biology, 1*, 275–281. https://doi.org/10.1109/ojemb.2020.3026928

Lea, C., Flynn, M. D., Vidal, R., Reiter, A., & Hager, G. D. (2017). *Temporal Convolutional Networks for Action Segmentation and Detection*. https://doi.org/10.1109/cvpr.2017.113

McLachlan, S., Dube, K., Hitman, G. A., Fenton, N. E., & Kyrimi, E. (2020). Bayesian Networks in Healthcare: Distribution by Medical Condition. *Artificial Intelligence in Medicine, 107*, Article 101912. https://doi.org/10.1016/j.artmed.2020.101912

Melvin, S., Jamal, A., Hill, K., Wang, W., & Young, S. D. (2019). Identifying Sleep-Deprived Authors of Tweets: Prospective Study. *JMIR Mental Health, 6*(12), Article e13076. https://doi.org/10.2196/13076

Michie, S., van Stralen, M. M., & West, R. (2011). The Behaviour Change Wheel: A New Method for Characterising and Designing Behaviour Change Interventions. *Implementation Science, 6*, 42. https://doi.org/10.1186/1748-5908-6-42

Munro, S., Lewin, S., Swart, T., & Volmink, J. (2007). A Review of Health Behaviour Theories: How Useful are These for Developing Interventions to Promote Long-Term Medication Adherence for TB and HIV/AIDS? *BMC Public Health, 7*(1). https://doi.org/10.1186/1471-2458-7-104

Patel, M. S., Asch, D. A., & Volpp, K. G. (2015). Wearable Devices as Facilitators, Not Drivers, of Health Behavior Change. *JAMA, 313*(5), 459. https://doi.org/10.1001/jama.2014.14781

Rabiner, L. R. (1989). A Tutorial on Hidden Markov Models and Selected Applications in Speech Recognition. *Proceedings of the IEEE, 77*(2), 257–286. https://doi.org/10.1109/5.18626

Ryan, R. M., & Deci, E. L. (2000). Self-Determination Theory and the Facilitation of Intrinsic Motivation, Social Development, and Well-Being. *American Psychologist, 55*(1), 68–78. https://doi.org/10.1037/0003-066x.55.1.68

van der Maaten, L., & Hinton, G. (2008). Visualizing Data Using t-SNE. *Journal of Machine Learning Research, 9*(86), 2579–2605. http://jmlr.org/papers/v9/vandermaaten08a.html

University of Wisconsin-Madison. (2023). *Neighborhood Atlas—Area Deprivation Index.* https://www.neighborhoodatlas.medicine.wisc.edu/

Wolters, K. (2024). *UpToDate.* https://www.wolterskluwer.com/en/solutions/uptodate

Yeung, C.-K., & Yeung, D.-Y. (2018). *Addressing Two Problems in Deep Knowledge Tracing via Prediction-Consistent Regularization.* Paper presented at the Proceedings of the Fifth Annual ACM Conference on Learning at Scale, 1–10. https://doi.org/10.1145/3231644.3231647

Zhang, H.-Y., & Pan, T. (2022). Public Health Risk Assessment and Prevention Based on Big Data. *Journal of Environmental and Public Health, 1.* https://doi.org/10.1155/2022/7965917

Part V
Living with AI

Chapter 9
From Acceptance to Thinking Partner

9.1 Introduction

Traditional "User Acceptance"

"User acceptance" originated from the old technology era (e.g., software, the internet, and smartphones), and acceptance refers to the willingness to use a tool to complete a task. With the internet, you searched. With smartphones, you choose what to click. For that old technology, several technology acceptance models exist, including TAM (Technology Acceptance Model) and UTAUT (Unified Theory of Acceptance and Use of Technology).

Technology Acceptance Model (TAM)

TAM (proposed in 1986) explains how users come to accept and use a technology (Venkatesh & Davis, 2000). It's centered around perceived usefulness and perceived ease of use, which influence attitude toward use and eventually actual usage (see Table 9.1).

Unified Theory of Acceptance and Use of Technology (UTAUT)

UTAUT (proposed in 2003) integrates eight models, including TAM, TPB (Theory of Planned Behavior), and DOI (Diffusion of Innovations Theory), into a unified theory (Venkatesh et al., 2016). UTAUT identifies four core determinants of user acceptance and usage behavior, moderated by individual factors such as age, gender, experience, and voluntariness (see Table 9.2).

Why "Acceptance" Feels Incomplete for AI?

The short answer is that ***AI is not just a tool***. AI doesn't just perform a task; it also learns from its experiences. It collaborates, learns, and sometimes leads. ***AI is a new "intelligence"***, which can make suggestions that may reshape your goals, values, or worldview. The relationship between human and AI is dynamic, co-evolving, and often ambiguous. It challenges how we think, decide, and feel. The old user

M. Wu, *Artificial Intelligence in Public Health*,
https://doi.org/10.1007/978-3-032-15872-7_9

Table 9.1 Technology acceptance model (TAM)

Key constructs	Descriptions
Perceived Usefulness (PU)	Using this system will enhance my job performance
Perceived Ease of Use (PEOU)	Using the system will be free of effort
Attitude Toward Using (A)	I have a favorable/unfavorable view of using it
Behavioral Intention (BI)	I intend to use it regularly
Actual System Use	Objective or self-reported use

Table 9.2 Unified theory of acceptance and use of technology (UTAUT)

Key constructs	Descriptions
Performance Expectancy (PE)	I believe this will help me do better
Effort Expectancy (EE)	It is easy to use
Social Influence (SI)	People who are important to me think I should use it
Facilitating Conditions (FC)	I have the resources and support to use it
Behavioral Intention (BI) and Use Behavior	I intend to use this technology in the future

acceptance models assume the user evaluates a tool. AI isn't just a tool. It is interactive (learns from users), generative (creates outputs you didn't explicitly request), adaptive (changes with feedback and context), persuasive (influences your thoughts, beliefs, and emotions), and unpredictable (may surprise, confuse, or even shape your goals).

AI is fundamentally different from previous waves of technology (like the Internet or smartphones) when it comes to user acceptance. You adapt to your new smartphone and accept the Internet. You adapt to AI, and AI can also adapt to you. Because AI can adapt to people, rather than just waiting for people's changes, the AI adoption rate will be much faster, and there will be a shorter time for widespread adoption than the Internet or other old technologies. AI will be a transformative force, and you should be aware that it is already here.

9.2 New Constructs for AI Adoption Models

"User acceptance" models for AI must include new components (constructs or indicators), such as cognitive alignment (do I understand how it thinks?), emotional comfort (do I feel respected, safe, supported?), ethical trust (does it align with my values and autonomy?), and relational engagement (do I want to continue using it over time?).

Table 9.3 Some constructs for AI-related acceptance models

Possible constructs	Definition	Core questions
Perceived anthropomorphism (Alabed et al., 2022; Ma et al., 2025)	Extent to which users perceive human-like qualities in the AI (e.g., voice, emotions, social presence)	"Does this AI seem human-like in the way it interacts?" "Do I feel like I'm talking to a human?"
Perceived intelligence (Ling et al., 2023)	How smart, responsive, or capable the AI appears	"Does this AI provide intelligent responses?" "Can this AI understand complex situations or requests?"
Trust in AI (Zhao et al., 2025)	User's willingness to rely on the AI's recommendations and behavior	"Can I trust this AI to act in my best interest?" "Does this AI behave in a reliable and predictable way?"

Adaptability

One of AI-specific constructs added into AI-augmented models is "perceived adaptability" (Park et al., 2024). It is about how well the AI adjusts to user needs, preferences, and context over time. The core question is "The AI system adapts to my behavior and preferences effectively." AI applications can adapt to human needs through reinforcement learning, personalizing behavior, and recommendations. AI can learn from feedback loops and reflective use. In short, AI can grow with the user and changing environments.

More Constructs for AI-Related Acceptance Models

AI-related user acceptance model will be designed explicitly for AI systems, particularly those that exhibit human-like, intelligent, or autonomous behaviors. It should include some new factors (e.g., trust in AI), shown in Table 9.3.

9.3 Rethinking Trust in AI

Suppose that AI is like a teammate. You won't pass the ball unless you trust they'll play fair and help you win. When you go to a new park to join a pickup soccer game on the weekend, how do you earn the trust of strangers? There are several stages for establishing trust, such as playing defense first and passing the ball to key players (instead of carrying it by yourself). Finally, someone trusts you and starts passing the ball to you.

Trust in AI was the number one factor that predicted whether people would use the AI or not, even more than how smart or functional it seemed. People don't use things they don't trust, especially when it comes to health, safety, or decisions that matter. In this session, let's construct a layered view of trust evolution in AI, such as initial trust, deep trust, and sustained trust.

Stage 1. Transparency and Explainability (Initial Trust)

Transparency (Fine & Marsh, 2024; Yu et al., 2023)

It is about how much the AI system reveals itself. It is like looking under the hood of a car. You don't need to be a mechanic to feel better seeing under the hood. The same goes for AI. Early trust comes from seeing that it's not magic, but built on logic, data, and explainable decisions. We should remember that "***trust doesn't mean perfect understanding and just be transparent for the user.***" Some AI models are easier to understand (and explain), while others are more like "black boxes" (see Table 9.4).

Explainability (Cheung & Ho, 2024; Duarte et al., 2023)

It is about how well it can communicate its decisions to others. It is like asking why the GPS told you to take a detour. It's okay that some AI models are too complex to fully understand, if they demonstrate their reasoning, acknowledge their limits, and are guided by human ethics and oversight. Let's look at some examples for AI explanations in Table 9.5.

AI applications should help users establish their initial trust through better transparency and explainability. This doesn't mean users must fully understand how the

Table 9.4 Transparency level for some common AI models

Transparency level	AI model type	Notes
High	Rule-based systems	Fully transparent; every step traceable
	Linear models	Easily show how input variables contribute
Medium–high	Decision trees	You can trace decision paths, but may be large
Medium–low	Random forest	Each tree is explainable, but the ensemble is complex
	Gradient boosting machines	Performance is high, but harder to interpret
Low	Support vector machines (SVM)	Mathematical boundaries, not intuitive
	Neural networks (NN)	Many layers; billions of weights, not human-readable
Very low	Transformers/LLMs (Long Short-Term Memory) (e.g., ChatGPT)	Internals unclear, but can "talk through" answers
	Reinforcement learning agents	Behavior evolves from trial-and-error

Table 9.5 Some examples of AI explanations

No.	Examples of AI explanations
1	"This AI uses a complex model like doctors do. It's trained on thousands of examples and looks for patterns"
2	"We use explainability tools to show what factors influenced the decision, like age, activity, or symptoms"
3	"Here's why the AI gave this suggestion: (1) High blood pressure, (2) Family history, (3) Low exercise. Let's explore together"
4	"The system looked at your age, BMI, and recent labs. Most similar patients had higher risk. That's why it flagged you"
5	"You asked: Should I be concerned about high cholesterol? Based on your age (52), total cholesterol of 250 mg/dL, and low physical activity, you may be at increased risk for heart disease"

AI works. It means they should feel confident that the system is accountable, fair, and designed to be understood at the right level.

Stage 2. Co-thinking and Alignment (Deep Trust)

Trust starts small and grows over time through interaction. To trust AI, you must use it. Use it only long enough to see how it behaves over time. If you stop using AI too soon, you don't build the "mental model" of how it thinks. You may never learn how to correct or guide it. You don't have deep trust and may become skeptical or dismissive. Deep trust doesn't come from believing the AI is perfect, but rather from seeing that the AI learns alongside you, listens, adapts, and improves.

Socratic AI (Sak et al., 2025)

It is a type of AI that builds trust by engaging you in thoughtful dialogue. It is like a teacher using the Socratic method: "Instead of giving you the answer, it asks the right questions to help you think."

Adaptive Reasoning Agents (Joseph et al., 2025; Marah & Challenger, 2024)

They are a type of AI that reason step by step (not just make a prediction), and adapt their logic based on the user, the problem, or new feedback. The adaptive reasoning agents can explain and revise their thinking in response to what *you* say or do. They are not rigid calculators, but behave more like thoughtful, flexible problem-solvers ("new intelligence"). For example, an AI decision support tool to help a clinician decide on a treatment plan for a patient. The AI offers an initial recommendation. The clinician disagrees or tweaks it. The AI adjusts and offers a new suggestion based on feedback.

AI applications should help users establish their deep trust with co-thinking techniques (e.g., Socratic AI or adaptive reasoning agents). Trust grows over time through trial, correction, and learning together.

Stage 3. Fairness, Ethics, and Inclusion (Sustained Trust)

In public health, trust is not just personal, but it's collective. Trust becomes a social contract. Sustained trust is not losing confidence in AI applications in public health over time. People will lose trust if they feel AI is biased, mistreats some groups, ignores cultural or social realities, or violates shared ethical norms.

Fairness

AI applications should perform equally well across demographic groups. In public health, we work with diverse populations. In the real world, vulnerable communities already face systemic inequalities. If AI amplifies those inequalities, it breaks trust. Fair AI would be trained in diverse data and continuously checked across groups. At the very least, AI should be transparent about its limitations (e.g., having more historical data on one group than others). Fairness-aware machine learning is an algorithm that adjusts for imbalances or bias in data. Equity-aware risk stratification applications in public health can leverage the powerful adaptive AI capabilities to address complex social determinants situations (see Chap. 7).

Ethics

AI should respect privacy, autonomy, and informed choice (Alanzi et al., 2023; Benzinger et al., 2023). Users lose trust if they think data is being used without consent or sold/shared unethically. For privacy, AI applications should comply with ethical practice in regulations (e.g., GDPR (General Data Protection Regulation), EU AI ACT, HIPAA (Health Insurance Portability and Accountability Act)), such as data minimization (only collect what's needed), differential privacy (mask personal identity in model training), and federated learning (AI learns across devices without pulling user data to central servers). For autonomy, AI applications should employ ethical practices, such as human-in-the-loop models (where AI provides options and the user chooses), nudging transparency (explaining when AI suggests a change or behavior), and reversible suggestions (allowing users to override or question AI outputs). For informed choice, AI applications should employ ethical practices, such as explainability (XAI) (providing a plain-language explanation behind AI decisions), confidence scores (informing users of the certainty of AI predictions), and clear, readable disclosures of terms and data use.

Inclusion (Shams et al., 2023)

AI supports different cultures, values, and voices. AI applications should adapt language, tone, examples, and advice to users. Various users' identities are supported by AI Chatbots that use multilingual NLP (Natural Language Processing) to understand and respond in multiple native languages or dialects.

AI applications should help users build sustained trust by showing that they are fair, ethical, and inclusive. Users should feel confident that the AI treats everyone fairly, respects their rights and values, and includes diverse voices, without leaving out marginalized groups.

9.4 A New Model for Human-AI Thinking Partnership

When the author develops "meta-AI homework," we ask students not to treat AI as a shortcut but to treat AI as a "thinking partner." AI (e.g., ChatGPT) can earn students' trust when students think with AI, and AI can align with students' reasoning. Why not develop a new model when we treat AI as a "thinking partner?" This textbook proposes a new model for human-AI thinking partnership: *"AI thinking partnership model" (ATPM).* Let me define the ATPM as follows.

AI thinking partnership model (ATPM): ATPM is a new framework developed to guide the personalized, evolving relationship between humans and increasingly intelligent AI systems. This model will be used to improve or evaluate current AI applications. ATPM includes six dimensions, which are "trust," "value alignment," "cognitive load fit," "control and autonomy," "adaptability over time," and "emotional resonance."

What is ATPM?

The AI thinking partnership model (ATPM) has six clear, user-centered indicators. Table 9.6 shows "dimension names" (indicators), "core questions", "what it measures", and "examples of AI evidence" of ATPM.

Target the Future AI Applications

It is highly likely that "personalized, evolving, emotionally and cognitively integrated AI systems" will dominate the future. To meet this need, ATPM has been developed as the foundation for next-generation human–AI interaction.

How do We Use ATPM?

To evaluate an AI application, each dimension can be scored on a 1–5 scale (via user self-report, system analytics, or adaptive survey). Together, they form a personalized "*Partnership Index*" that evolves over time.

Future Work for ATPM

Researchers and developers of AI applications are welcome to explore ATPM for improving or evaluating their applications. Specific diagnostic tools are needed to quickly score each dimension (e.g., trust or cognitive load fit). For example, suppose the "cognitive load fit score" for an AI application drops. In that case, ATPM tools can provide simplified answers for users or developers. Future research on personalization factors can be integrated into ATPM. For example, users can select which dimensions matter most to them. For trust or control, users can set "selective forgetting" ranges for data-driven AI models.

Table 9.6 AI thinking partnership model (ATPM)

Dimension	Core question	What it measures	Examples of AI evidence
Trust	"Do I feel safe and confident using this AI?"	Reliability, transparency, and dependability	Override rate, re-use frequency, response explanation use
Value alignment	"Does this AI help with what really matters to me?"	Goal support, values match, relevance	Task success, goal achievement logs, user-customized goals
Cognitive load fit	"Is this AI helpful without overwhelming me?"	Clarity, simplicity, and thinking support	Info density, question simplification, user feedback on overload
Control and autonomy	"Am I in control of how this AI behaves?"	Agency, reversibility, customization	Frequency of manual edits, settings changes, override ability
Adaptability over time	"Is this AI improving in how it works with me?"	Learning, personalization, responsiveness to feedback	Memory use, personalization patterns, version improvement logs
Emotional resonance	"Does this AI emotionally support or suit me?"	Empathy, emotional tone fit, motivational support, feeling "understood"	Sentiment-matching responses, adaptive tone based on user emotion, comfort or encouragement prompts, avoidance of emotionally jarring responses, positive emotion in user feedback, stress-reduction, or regulation support

9.5 Discussion Questions

Question 9.1. What does it mean to "live with AI," and how might this reshape our expectations for long-term user acceptance?

Question 9.2. How do traditional user acceptance models (e.g., TAM, UTAUT) fall short when applied to AI applications in public health?

Question 9.3. What role does adaptability play in ensuring AI tools remain relevant as user needs and public health challenges evolve?

Question 9.4. How is trust in AI different from trust in traditional technologies, and why is it important to distinguish between initial, deep, and sustained trust?

Question 9.5. In what ways can "cognitive load fit" influence whether users successfully adopt and continue to use AI applications?

Question 9.6. How might emotional resonance strengthen or weaken public trust in AI for health-related decision-making?

References

Alabed, A., Javornik, A., & Gregory-Smith, D. (2022). AI Anthropomorphism and Its Effect on Users' Self-congruence and Self–AI Integration: A Theoretical Framework and Research Agenda. *Technological Forecasting and Social Change*. https://doi.org/10.1016/j.techfore.2022.121786

Alanzi, T., Alhajri, A., Almulhim, S., Alharbi, S. M., Alfaifi, S., Almarhoun, E., Mulla, R., Alasafra, Z. O., Alalwan, Z., Alnasser, F., Almukhtar, F., Al-Ghadeer, F., Amro, S., Alodhayb, I., & Alanzi, N. (2023). Artificial Intelligence and Patient Autonomy in Obesity Treatment Decisions: An Empirical Study of the Challenges. *Cureus*. https://doi.org/10.7759/cureus.49725

Benzinger, L., Ursin, F., Balke, W. T., Kacprowski, T., & Salloch, S. (2023). Should Artificial Intelligence Be Used to Support Clinical Ethical Decision-Making? A Systematic Review of Reasons. *BMC Medical Ethics, 24*(1). https://doi.org/10.1186/s12910-023-00929-6

Cheung, J. C. T., & Ho, S. S. (2024). Explainable AI and Trust: How News Media Shapes Public Support for AI-Powered Autonomous Passenger Drones. *Public Understanding of Science, 34*(3), 344–362. https://doi.org/10.1177/09636625241291192

Duarte, R. B., Correia, F., Arriaga, P., & Paiva, A. (2023). AI Trust: Can Explainable AI Enhance Warranted Trust? *Human Behavior and Emerging Technologies*, 1–12. https://doi.org/10.1155/2023/4637678

Fine, A., & Marsh, S. C. (2024). Judicial Leadership Matters (Yet Again): The Association Between Judge and Public Trust for Artificial Intelligence in Courts. *Discover Artificial Intelligence, 4*(1). https://doi.org/10.1007/s44163-024-00142-3

Joseph, T., Gowrie, S., Montalbano, M. J., Bandelow, S., Clunes, M. T., Dumont, A. S., Iwanaga, J., Tubbs, R. S., & Loukas, M. (2025). The Roles of Artificial Intelligence in Teaching Anatomy: A Systematic Review. *Clinical Anatomy, 38*(5), 552–567. https://doi.org/10.1002/ca.24272

Ling, E. C., Tussyadiah, I., Liu, A., & Stienmetz, J. L. (2023). Perceived Intelligence of Artificially Intelligent Assistants for Travel: Scale Development and Validation. *Journal of Travel Research, 64*(2), 299–321. https://doi.org/10.1177/00472875231217899

Ma, N., Khynevych, R., Hao, Y., & Wang, Y. (2025). Effect of Anthropomorphism and Perceived Intelligence in Chatbot Avatars of Visual Design on User Experience. *Frontiers in Computer Science, 7*. https://doi.org/10.3389/fcomp.2025.1531976

Marah, H., & Challenger, M. (2024). Adaptive Hybrid Reasoning for Agent-Based Digital Twins of Distributed Multi-robot Systems. *SIMULATION, 100*(9), 931–957. https://doi.org/10.1177/00375497231226436

Park, J., Woo, S. E., & Kim, J. (2024). *Attitudes Towards Artificial Intelligence at Work: Scale Development and Validation*. https://doi.org/10.31234/osf.io/sxdp9

Sak, M. E., Sonlu, S., & Güdükbay, U. (2025). Talk With Socrates: Relation Between Perceived Agent Personality and User Personality in LLM-Based Natural Language Dialogue Using Virtual Reality. *Computer Animation and Virtual Worlds, 36*(3). https://doi.org/10.1002/cav.70033

Shams, R. A., Zowghi, D., & Bano, M. (2023). AI and the Quest for Diversity and Inclusion: A Systematic Literature Review. *AI and Ethics, 5*(1), 411–438. https://doi.org/10.1007/s43681-023-00362-w

Venkatesh, V., & Davis, F. D. (2000). A Theoretical Extension of the Technology Acceptance Model: Four Longitudinal Field Studies. *Management Science, 46*(2), 186–204. https://doi.org/10.1287/mnsc.46.2.186.11926

Venkatesh, V., Thong, J. Y. L., & Xin, X. (2016). Unified Theory of Acceptance and Use of Technology: A Synthesis and the Road Ahead. *Journal of the Association for Information Systems, 17*(5), 328–376. https://doi.org/10.17705/1jais.00428

Yu, L., Li, Y., & Fan, F. (2023). Employees' Appraisals and Trust of Artificial Intelligences' Transparency and Opacity. *Behavioral Sciences, 13*(4), 344. https://doi.org/10.3390/bs13040344

Zhao, X., You, W., Zheng, Z., Shi, S., Lu, Y., & Sun, L. (2025). How Do Consumers Trust and Accept AI Agents? An Extended Theoretical Framework and Empirical Evidence. *Behavioral Sciences, 15*(3), 337. https://doi.org/10.3390/bs15030337

Chapter 10
AI and Workforce for Public Health

10.1 AI for Current Workforce's Continuous Education

Risks for AI Replacement

Are there risks for job displacement in the artificial intelligence (AI) era for the current public health workforce? There are some repetitive clerical works in public health, such as data entry and patient appointment scheduling. Let's explore this question using various approaches.

Data Entry

Does it have a high risk for AI replacement? Let's explore data entry in Table 10.1. In short, data entry is easy for AI to replace based on the conceptual analysis of this job type.

Appointment Scheduling

Let's further explore the "appointment scheduling" job type with the technology-based approach in Table 10.2. In short, AI non-human functions provide more benefits than a person. The conclusion is that the appointment scheduling will be replaced with AI.

When this book is written in 2025, it's early adoption of AI. Based on the discussion of user acceptance of AI in Chap. 9, AI is different from other technologies, and AI may have a fast adoption (Ding et al., 2024). The workforce issue is a big question for everyone in the AI era. In the future, there will be an abundance of jobs for us or a widening inequality (polarization). One thing is essential for changing the results of the workforce, and that is education. One reason for writing this textbook is to improve AI literacy for public health students, practitioners, or officials. Only through education can someone adapt to the AI era and become an AI-augmented worker.

M. Wu, *Artificial Intelligence in Public Health*,
https://doi.org/10.1007/978-3-032-15872-7_10

Table 10.1 Data entry and management

Human cognitive functions for data entry	Descriptions	Examples of AI mimic functions (difficulty level)
Perceptual speed	Quickly recognizing and processing numbers, codes, or text	AI excels at rapid text/number recognition. OCR (optical character recognition) converts images or scanned documents into text. NLP can extract entities, classify content, etc. (Easy)
Error monitoring	Detecting and correcting inconsistencies (e.g., mismatched lab results)	AI detects inconsistencies using rule-based checks. (Easy)
Working memory	Temporarily holding information (e.g., a patient ID) while transferring it between systems	Computers are good at memory and temporary data holding is trivial for AI. (Easy)
Attention (sustained and selective)	Maintaining focus over long periods while entering data; filtering out irrelevant information	AI doesn't fatigue; sustains focus indefinitely. (Easy)

Table 10.2 Patient appointment scheduling from technology-based analysis

AI strength	How it helps scheduling	Human bottleneck it removes
Massive parallel processing	Check many clinicians, rooms, and insurance constraints simultaneously	Staff must juggle calendars one call at a time
High-speed data ingestion	Instantly read insurer rules, provider availability, patient preferences	Humans sift through screens or desk calendars
Memory at scale	Recall every patient's past visits, authorizations, prep instructions	Staff rely on EHR look-ups and sticky notes
24/7 operation	Offer after-hours booking and same-day rescheduling	Offices close; call-backs create delays
Unbounded multimodal fusion	Accept voice (IVR (Interactive Voice Response)), text, portal, smartphone, or kiosk inputs	Traditional phone lines only
Exploration in non-intuitive spaces	Suggest split appointments, telehealth slots, or neighboring clinics the caller never considered	Humans default to familiar slots

"Upskilling" or "Reskilling"

AI data availability for public health in the US has benefited from the meaningful uses (MU) of EMR (Electronic Medical Record) since 2011. As a result of a decade of MU and subsequent health IT initiatives, thousands of hospitals, labs, and clinics now send data regularly to public health agencies, including immunizations, lab reports, syndromic surveillance data, and case reports. This data flows to federal (CDC (Centers for Disease Control and Prevention)), state, and local agencies, often *daily or in real-time.* Public health agencies now operate as de facto data centers, collecting, storing, integrating, and analyzing large volumes of health data, supporting decision-making, outbreak response, forecasting, policy development, and maintaining infrastructure, interoperability standards, and data governance practices. Data science and AI are essential, not optional, for public health. We urgently need a skilled workforce using AI tools to meet growing demands. It depends on the progress of continuous education of current workforces (e.g., AI literacy).

1. ***AI literacy***

After you go through this textbook, you will have clear concepts of AI and a big picture of AI applications in public health (such as key AI components, design models, evaluation, data issues, public health domain data, case studies of AI applications in public health, user acceptance, challenges, and opportunities).

There is a cognitive load shift in the AI era from searching to judging. The past information overload is "drinking from a firehose". AI solves this by providing a single, streaming output. The new problem is cognitive overload of verification. Your role shifts from being a finder of information to being an analyst, judge, and validator of AI-generated intelligence. As a key part of AI literacy, each AI output must be met with critical questions with constant and vigilant skepticism. You should have good prompt skills and know how to question AI systems to test their limits and reveal uncertainty.

2. ***Using chatbots (e.g., ChatGPT) for just-in-time learning***

"Meta-AI homework" in this textbook will train you to become an advanced AI user, treating AI as a thinking partner. With enough practice, you can understand what you want and what AI can help you. For example, you can critically evaluate AI outputs (e.g., spotting hallucinations in ChatGPT summaries). Generative AI (e.g., ChatGPT) provides a just-in-time learning option for public health practitioners, and you should be "upskilled" to be comfortable using it. For example, many practicing epidemiologists were trained before genomics and AMR became central topics. During real work, epidemiologists can ask AI questions on demand, such as, "What is OXA-48 resistance?" or "How do we interpret SNP distances in WGS clustering?"

3. ***AI for data management***

Chapter 5 helps you establish a clear concept map of AI data issues. After seeing many public health domain data from AI pipeline perspectives in Chap. 6, you could manage your data for initial training or continue retraining AI models for your tasks. With clear concepts about AI data issues, you can quickly choose AI tools to facilitate your data management. Those AI tools will automate data entry, cleaning, or fusion. AI is growing so fast. When you read this textbook, more powerful AI tools for data management may be available and directly prepare synthetic training data (static, streaming, and self-report data) for you.

4. ***AI for reporting***

AI tools for reporting will be helpful for your daily work. You can follow up on the progress of AI reporting tools' new functions, such as generating templated reports from structured data, exporting AI outputs as specific formats (e.g., PDFs), generating text summaries of data, creating visualizations, assisting in prompt-based data querying, and translating or rephrasing reports. At this time, you should be cautious about the quality of the AI reporting tools, such as AI hallucinating statistics or sources. Validation and human review are needed for AI reporting.

5. ***Other jobs for AI development teams***

Suppose some of you are interested in switching careers from public health workforce to data annotator or human feedback specialist in an AI development team. In that case, there are some tasks to do in the new jobs, such as labeling datasets for training AI models (e.g., tagging EHR notes for disease classification) and fine-tuning models with human feedback.

6. ***AI application design***

Chapter 3 prepares you with related knowledge of the design of AI applications. For example, you need to identify unmet needs as a public health practitioner. Chapter 3 provides many methods to systematically identify realized and unrealized needs. Our design models will help you to collaborate with developers to translate public health requirements (tasks or human cognitive functions) into technical specs (AI model selections).

7. ***AI evaluation and ethics***

Chapter 4 prepares you with basic evaluation knowledge for AI evaluation and ethics. There are some AI audit models for bias. Guidelines for AI use in public health policy (e.g., privacy safeguards for digital surveillance) will be developed in the future. There will be a bright future for you to "upskill" and become an expert in AI alignment and AI safety (Festor et al., 2022; Nissenbaum, 2024).

8. ***AI-driven scientific research work***

It's exciting to anticipate the AI-driven breakthroughs that lie ahead for public health. Suppose you have a solid public health education foundation (e.g., MPH (Master of Public Health) or PhD). In this case, you can "upskill" to gain the skills to conduct AI-powered research in public health. *What are the most significant research questions in a specific public health domain?* AI can help you with this as a thinking partner! Your domain expertise in public health will enable the structured conceptual thinking required to effectively use AI's potential in research.

10.2 AI for Public Health Education

Messy World

Daily, you will hear bad news about natural disasters like floods, hurricanes/typhoons, earthquakes, wildfires, heat waves/cold waves, droughts, tsunamis, landslides, and volcanic eruptions. In addition, there is more news about biological disasters, such as pandemics and vector-borne outbreaks. On top of that, unfortunately, there are more man-made disasters, such as chemical spills/exposures, radiological/nuclear incidents, infrastructure failures, mass casualty events, wars, refugee crises, food insecurity, etc. We live in a messy world, and our public health professionals must handle public health issues to respond to those disasters. The public demands that public health professionals have high critical thinking skills and be capable of handling new case scenarios. Fortunately, AI is coming. Hopefully, our next-generation public health professionals can critically evaluate AI outputs. With AI helping to respond to disasters well, we expect to reach public health goals, and more people will live longer and better.

Meta-AI Homework (Treating AI as a Thinking Partner)

"Metacognition" was coined as thinking about thinking in 1979, emphasizing self-monitoring in learning (Flavell, 1979). The metacognitive awareness inventory (MAI) was developed to operationalize metacognition for assessments in 1994 (Schraw & Dennison, 1994). With ChatGPT's rise (launched in 2022), educators explored AI for metacognitive prompts (e.g., refining queries, bias-checking) (Di Martino et al., 2024; Zhu, 2025). In education, there is a long way to go for students to treat AI as a thinking partner rather than a shortcut. Educators should provide solutions for the problem, such as scaffolding strategies based on guided metacognition support. "Meta-AI homework" (see definition in Chap. 3) aims to guide students in reflecting on how they use AI, why they use it, and what they learn from it. AI literacy education has become significantly important (Long & Magerko, 2020), so meta-AI homework could be an advanced homework assignment format for AI education in the future.

Why Should Public Health Education Adopt "Meta-AI Homework"?

We hope our next-generation public health students can have system thinking skills (how parts interact in complex systems) and work well with AI tools (data management, reporting, or simulation) to solve problems (even with incomplete information). Public health officials face high stakes in public health decisions and need AI help with structured reasoning. Public health workers need to quickly figure out why and how. They also need to handle ethical and practical trade-offs. "Meta-AI homework" focuses on the thinking processes and trains our students in adaptive and critical thinking. For example, students can ask AI, "How would you prioritize vaccines in a shortage?" then, you can evaluate AI output and debate AI-generated public health strategies. We can design a case scenario as a stress test for students. With enough practice, they will not freeze when they face real-world messiness (e.g., infectious disease breakouts or flooding).

Future public health professionals need to adopt Just-in-Time (JIT) learning. This learning approach involves acquiring knowledge and skills when required to respond to dynamic real-world challenges. However, traditional public health education remains outcome-based, relying on fixed content delivery and assessment. With "meta-AI homework" practices, our students can treat AI as a thinking partner, seeking, evaluating, and applying information in real-time scenarios. Students' domain knowledge learned from other public health courses helps them have structured conceptual thinking, which is vital for effectively using generative AI tools.

Tools for Educators to Create Meta-AI Homework

This textbook provides a framework as a lens to guide the creation of meta-AI homework assignments for AI in public health (see Appendix B). The design process draws on principles from metacognitive-guided questioning and educational scaffolding. The framework outputs are meta-AI homework templates. It shifts homework from outcome-based to process-oriented. The textbook uses case scenarios in public health to help educators understand and follow the metacognitive learning process. A rubric criterion is also attached as Appendix C for educators to grade students' meta-AI homework.

A meta-AI homework assignment sample is developed in this textbook (see Appendix A). Each homework assignment will include three metacognitive phases: a pre-task self-assessment, in-task guided questioning, and a post-task reflection, aligned to the cognitive stages of planning, monitoring, and evaluating.

In the future, an AI faculty co-pilot tool could be designed and developed to help instructors design course syllabi and create meta-AI homework related to each learning objective, which may integrate the homework development framework in Appendix B and grading criteria in Appendix C.

Evaluations of Meta-AI Homework

Students' experiences on the new meta-AI homework could be collected using subjective evaluation studies (e.g., surveys, interviews, observations). Based on the feedback from students, the meta-AI homework templates should be revised dynamically by public health educators during their practices. After more public health educators adopt meta-AI homework, evaluation studies, such as longitudinal studies, could be conducted to measure student metacognitive development and AI competency improvement over time. You can find more information about evaluation study design in Chap. 4.

10.3 AI for Public Health Informatics Education

Today, there are many jobs for public health informatics students in AI development for public health, such as AI trainer, data annotation lead, fine-tuning specialist, prompt engineer, AI safety researcher, and human-AI collaboration manager. Our informatics students can help with AI alignment. It ensures that the AI application's goals, actions, and behaviors align with human values, intentions, and safety requirements. Chapter 4 helps our public health informatics students with AI evaluation (e.g., BLEU (Bilingual Evaluation Understudy), ROUGE (Recall-Oriented Understudy for Gisting Evaluation) metrics).

Why is Public Health Informatics Education Important in the AI Area?

An integrated development environment (IDE) is specific software for developing other applications. AI IDEs now take over much of the coding work. When you read this textbook, AI IDEs may become multi-agent systems (design, code, test, debug, deploy), and no-code software development is widely viable for non-developers with domain knowledge and precise requirements (Ali, 2023). At that time, public health informatics became even more critical, especially in designing and evaluating public health software.

Why is public health informatics education important in the AI era? Firstly, AI can write code but not goals or ethics. AI doesn't know why a surveillance system is needed, what outcomes matter, or what risks to avoid (e.g., bias, equity, data privacy). That's where public health experts lead. Secondly, public health informatics bridges the gap. Professionals trained in informatics translate public health needs into system designs (see Chaps. 3, 7, and 8). Public health informatics students will define *what* data is required, guide *how* it should be collected, integrated, and used (see Chaps. 5 and 6), and evaluate *whether* the system helps improve health outcomes or adds noise (see Chap. 4. Thirdly, AI IDEs are tools, not thinkers. Even if you can describe a system in natural language and the AI codes it, you must still define workflows and validation rules (see case scenarios in Chaps. 7 and 8). You must evaluate system accuracy, bias, or unintended consequences (see case scenarios in Chap. 4).

In the AI era, public health informatics' new roles are to design workflows and goals for AI to implement, directly prompt AI IDEs, validate outputs, and evaluate fairness, real-world impact, bias, and trust. In short, public health informatics bridges human and AI collaboration in public health.

Projects for Public Health Informatics Education

The goals of public health informatics are to teach students critical data reasoning, to simulate real-world complexity (public health decisions involve medicine, policy, ethics, and technology), and to train adaptive problem-solving (no single correct answer). For example, the teacher can choose case scenarios like disease monitoring. One objective is to select AI models in the different stages of disease monitoring, paired with metacognitive questions targeting hypothesis generation and uncertainty evaluation. Before acting on any data, we need an AI system to clean it. A project will focus on the first stage of disease monitoring, such as signal refinement and noise filtering. This project can help students understand input data (e.g., chief complaints in clinic visits, self-reported symptoms, syndromic data, reports from sentinel healthcare providers, search engine trends, and social media signals). The project helps students select AI models (e.g., feature selection) to filter out false signals, misreported cases, and background noise (e.g., weekend effects).

10.4 Directions of Higher Education Reform

Why Do We Need Higher Education Reform in the Age of AI?

There are many reasons for this. First, the world is changing faster than curricula. AI, climate change, globalization, and shifting job markets are reshaping what students need to know and how they learn. Secondly, AI disrupts traditional academic roles. AI can write essays, generate code, and summarize research, which challenges the conventional understanding of what constitutes "do" scholarly work. Finally, universities risk losing relevance. Suppose higher education becomes a credentialing factory instead of a space for deep thinking and societal leadership. In that case, it will be bypassed by faster, cheaper alternatives.

Reform Directions

We urgently need better, wiser, and more human-centered education, as AI reshapes every domain of life. The first important task is to identify the direction for higher education reform in the era of AI. Let me propose the concepts of "AI-informed liberal education" and "AI-integrated scientific education" below.

> **AI-informed liberal education**: Combines the values of critical thinking, creativity, and civic responsibility with an understanding of AI. It helps students ask better questions and think with and about AI.
>
> **AI-integrated scientific education:** Combines science and technology training with hands-on use of AI. It helps students solve problems, analyze data, and design intelligent systems using AI tools—while cultivating data-informed judgment, experimental curiosity, and systems understanding.

The core values of traditional liberal education are critical thinking, creativity, and civic engagement. Table 10.3 provides new meanings of core values in the AI era.

Let's summarize the core processes and purposes of scientific education as follows. First, students need to identify scientific questions. Our education will prepare students to develop curiosity, critical thinking, and the ability to frame meaningful, relevant scientific problems. Secondly, professors in a university teach students to experiment or prototype. Students can learn methods and tools. They can

Table 10.3 The core values of "AI-informed liberal education"

Core values of liberal education	New meanings in the age of AI
Critical thinking	AI automates answers, but not judgment Students must learn to evaluate evidence, challenge assumptions, and discern truth in an AI-saturated information environment Critical thinking helps prevent misuse or blind trust in AI outputs
Creativity	AI is good at recombination, but not original insight or human imagination Creativity drives new ideas, innovative solutions, and human-centered design In fields from art to science to health, creativity will define what humans bring uniquely in partnership with AI
Civic engagement	AI affects policy, justice, media, education, and health We need educated citizens who understand the social implications of AI and advocate for equity, accountability, and democracy Without civic-minded graduates, AI could widen societal gaps and erode public trust

build models or create prototypes to test hypotheses. Finally, the goal of education is to help graduates discover or innovate. Students will analyze results, synthesize knowledge, and generate new insights or technologies that advance understanding or solve real-world problems. AI can empower all processes beyond those listed above (see Table 10.4).

In the future, our society will need some builders of AI, graduates from "AI-integrated scientific education." They are core developers, AI engineers, and data scientists. They design and implement algorithms and infrastructure. Our society will need more bridges to AI, graduates from "AI-informed liberal education." They

Table 10.4 The key processes of "AI-integrated scientific education"

Processes of scientific education	Data-informed judgment	Experimental curiosity	Systems understanding
Identify questions	Refine questions with AI insights and critical evaluation	Explore AI-suggested hypotheses and gaps	Frame questions in complex, AI-mapped systems
Experiment/prototype	Design and evaluate AI-aided experiments	Rapidly test and iterate with AI automation	Simulate and predict system behaviors with AI
Discover/innovate	Decide which AI-generated discoveries to trust and develop	Co-create new knowledge and solutions with AI collaborators	Innovate models that capture dynamic, interconnected realities

are professionals across domains (health, law, education, government, business, etc.) who use, question, interpret, and apply AI responsibly in real-world settings.

10.5 Discussion Questions

Question 10.1. What are the most critical AI competencies that current public health professionals should prioritize learning? How can organizations support continuous AI education without overwhelming their workforce?

Question 10.2. What barriers might institutions face when integrating AI into public health curricula, and how can they overcome them?

Question 10.3. How can Meta-AI homework (see Appendix A) improve critical thinking and self-regulated learning compared to traditional homework approaches?

Question 10.4. As AI-integrated development environments (IDEs) (automated coding) become more powerful, how might this shift create new opportunities for public health informatics students who excel in design thinking but lack traditional programming skills? At the same time, what unique risks could arise if design-focused professionals heavily rely on AI-generated code with AI IDEs without proper technical oversight?

Question 10.5. How can universities redesign curricula in the AI era? What specific pedagogical strategies or interdisciplinary collaborations could make this successful?

References

Ali, J. M. (2023). AI-driven Software Engineering. *Advances in Engineering Innovation, 3*(1), None-None. https://doi.org/10.54254/2977-3903/3/2023030

Di Martino, V., Falzone, Y., Gulbay, E., La Marca, A., Leone, A., Longo, L., & Di Carlo, D. (2024). Empowering Higher Education with ChatGPT: Innovating University Instructional Design. In *Communications in Computer and Information Science* (pp. 398–409): Springer Nature Switzerland. https://doi.org/10.1007/978-3-031-67351-1_27

Festor, P., Jia, Y., Gordon, A., Faisal, A. A., Habli, I., & Komorowski, M. (2022). Assuring the Safety of AI-based Clinical Decision Support Systems: A Case Study of the AI Clinician for Sepsis Treatment. *BMJ Health & Care Informatics, 29*(1), Article e100549. https://doi.org/10.1136/bmjhci-2022-100549

Flavell, J. H. (1979). Metacognition and Cognitive Monitoring: A New Area of Cognitive-Developmental Inquiry. *American Psychologist, 34*(10), 906–911. https://doi.org/10.1037/0003-066x.34.10.906

Long, D., & Magerko, B. (2020). *What Is AI Literacy? Competencies and Design Considerations.* Proceedings of the ACM CHI Conference on Human Factors in Computing Systems, 1-16. https://doi.org/10.1145/3313831.3376727

Nissenbaum, H. (2024). AI Safety: A Poisoned Chalice? *IEEE Security & Privacy, 22*(2), 94–96. https://doi.org/10.1109/msec.2024.3356848

Schraw, G., & Dennison, R. S. (1994). Assessing Metacognitive Awareness. *Contemporary Educational Psychology, 19*(4), 460–475. https://doi.org/10.1006/ceps.1994.1033

Zhu, M. (2025). Leveraging ChatGPT to Support Self-Regulated Learning in Online Courses. *TechTrends*. https://doi.org/10.1007/s11528-025-01075-z

Part VI
Futures

Chapter 11
Challenges and Opportunities in the Future

11.1 Challenges for AI in Public Health

Artificial intelligence (AI) has many challenges in public health, and it's hard to list them all. A picture is worth a thousand words. Two figures are created to group them based on the domain and urgency.

Urgent Challenges

Some urgent challenges are summarized in Fig. 11.1, and more researchers can participate in solving those urgent unmet needs in AI for public health.

Natural sciences will dominate urgent challenges to fix AI technical issues (e.g., pandemic forecasting, contact tracing, diagnostic bias, and antibiotic resistance), so I put natural science at the top of Fig. 11.1. There are many challenges on the social sciences side. Vaccine equity is about AI allocating doses fairly. AI workforce displacement is about worries about replacing community health workers. Health misinformation can be AI-generated anti-vaccine content on social media. Algorithmic triage is about allocating beds during crises (It involves ethics).

When the mass adoption of the Internet happened, I started feeling the impact of the technological breakthrough. My favorite movie video rental stores disappeared. My favorite bookstores are closed. I stopped reading paper-based newspapers or magazines. I stopped watching TV. I started struggling with "fake news" in social media and do fact-checking on online information. As a professor at college, I started worrying about teacher jobs that would be replaced by online education. Now, AI (another technology breakout) is coming. Our cars may become intelligent robots, and we are in the robot's hug when we travel. Imagine that you can chat with your car to change the car's temperature, and your vehicle will recommend a delicious restaurant in the next town. Maybe it's the early adoption of AI in 2025, but the mass adoption of AI is coming to the corner. One thing for sure is that AI will change our life again.

M. Wu, *Artificial Intelligence in Public Health*,
https://doi.org/10.1007/978-3-032-15872-7_11

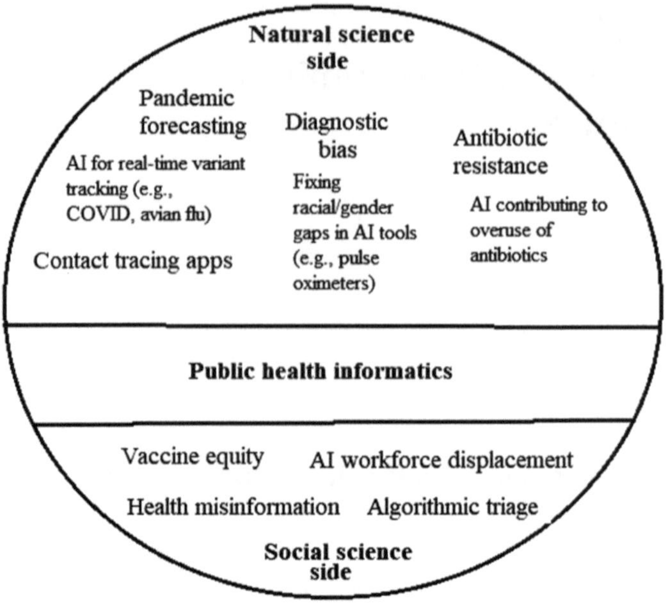

Fig. 11.1 Urgent challenges of AI in public health

Long-Term Challenges

Some long-term challenges are summarized in Fig. 11.2, and more researchers can participate in solving those long-term challenges in AI for public health. Social sciences (e.g., AI clinical adoption) will shape long-term systems, so I put social science at the top of the figure.

Global AI governance is about who controls pandemic-response algorithms. Mental health bots are about how to regulate AI therapists. One health integration is AI linking animal, human, and environmental data. Post-labor healthcare is about universal-based income and retraining if AI automates half of the jobs. AI-augmented human is about neural implants for chronic disease management. Climate-disease models are about predicting malaria or dengue shifts from warming. Precision medicine leverages genomic data to enable AI-driven, personalized treatment strategies at scale. Synthetic biology is about AI-designed pathogens or therapies.

Public Health Informatics

Our public health informatics will bridge natural sciences (e.g., AI models) and social sciences (e.g., user trust). Chapters 3, 5, 6, 7, and 8 prepare our public health informatics students about the design and development of AI applications in public health, and Chaps. 4, 9, 10, and 11 will prepare you for evaluation, use acceptance (e.g., trust), workforce, and challenges of AI applications. Therefore, I put our public health informatics in the center and between natural sciences and social sciences in

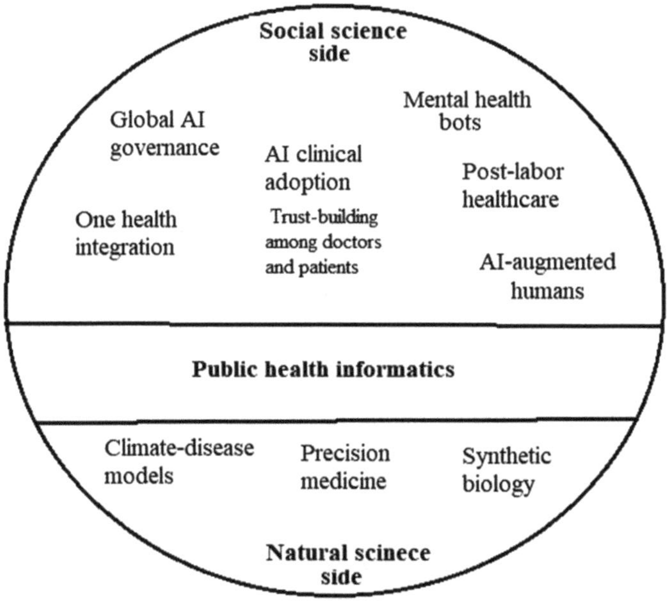

Fig. 11.2 Long-time challenges of AI in public health

both Figs. 11.1 and 11.2. You are in a unique position and have the potential to innovatively contribute to AI applications in public health.

11.2 Opportunities for AI in Public Health

"Matthew Effect (The Rich Get Richer)" (Merton, 1968)

Public health is a "data-rich" field, particularly for studying systemic factors that shape health outcomes. The 'Matthew effect' discusses how advantages accumulate for those already well-resourced.

Step 1. More Data Leads to Better AI

This is an opportunity for AI in public health to get started early, because public health is a "data-rich" field. Chapters 1, 5 and 6 explain big data in public health. Public health does have high-quality datasets (e.g., meaningful use of EHRs (Electronic Health Records), WHO (World Health Organization), and CDC (Centers for Disease Control and Prevention)), peer-reviewed studies, and real-time surveillance. For example, sepsis is a life-threatening medical condition that happens when the body's response to an infection spirals out of control. AI can detect sepsis early using EHR data. An AI tool, *Sepsis Watch*, was developed at Duke University Health System

(Sendak et al., 2020). Data sources are historical EHR data (e.g., vital signs, lab results, nurse notes). The AI models are deep learning-based early warning systems. The AI tool detected sepsis risk hours before clinical diagnosis, allowing earlier intervention, which is crucial for saving lives.

Step 2. Better AI Leads to More Usage of AI

Users trust AI outputs in public health will generate even more real-world usage of AI applications in public health. For example, TB (tuberculosis) is a severe infectious disease. AI models like "Computer-Aided Detection for TB" (CAD4TB) are used to interpret chest X-rays. Studies showed that CAD4TB could detect TB with sensitivity comparable to that of human radiologists (Qin et al., 2021). Because the AI system performs reliably, clinicians trust it. This trust has led to scaling up deployment in national screening programs and integration with mobile health units (Codlin et al., 2021).

Step 3. More Usage of AI Leads to More Data

Every interaction feeds back in improving the system. For example, AI chatbots can screen for COVID-19 symptoms. CDC and Microsoft's COVID-19 Self-Checker were developed to help people decide whether they needed COVID testing or emergency care (Shah et al., 2023). Data from each user interaction (symptoms entered, questions asked, recommendations followed) was logged (with privacy safeguards). Over time, AI developers used this real-world usage data to improve question phrasing, refine symptom-to-risk pathways, reduce false alarms, and tailor guidance for different demographics (e.g., older adults, pregnant women).

Step 4. More Data Leads to Even Better AI

The loop continues and may accelerate AI dominance in public health. In the end, AI applications in public health may become a successful story.

Health Literacy

For personal responsibilities in public health, AI is an opportunity for equal access to health knowledge. There is a knowledge gap between healthcare providers (e.g., medical doctors and nurses) and the public. An AI health agent (e.g., Robotics) or generative AI (e.g., ChatGPT) will be an AI doctor or an AI nurse who will help you access health knowledge anytime and anywhere. It's an opportunity for software companies to successfully launch personal health records or telehealth service systems, achieving a better adoption rate due to improved health literacy for all citizens.

11.3 AI Ethics

After you read this textbook and realize AI's power, fast growth is expected. The constraints of AI may shift from technical bottlenecks (e.g., computing or data) to challenges of control (human vs non-human), safety (unintended use, misuse, harm), alignment, and societal adoption. Chapter 3 discusses the ethical considerations and regulations. However, developing an ethical-based design model for AI applications in public health is more urgent. The design model can initially directly integrate AI ethics into the design processes. This is a challenge and an opportunity for more researchers to participate in developing this ethical-based design model, which should include some key components as below. First, AI control is the key, especially when AI (robotics) is becoming more powerful and complex. The role of responsibility and accountability among humans and AI should be clearly defined early. We cannot simply depend on AI. Many community society systems are fragile. AI failures might be catastrophic and complex to diagnose and fix. Second, AI safety should be embedded in the testing stages of this AI design model, including unintended uses, misuse, or harm. Third, AI should align with human values. We should avoid a powerful AI system pursuing a poorly specified goal. Finally, societal adoption of AI is a big issue. It includes the AI "black box problem," which makes it difficult for humans to understand how AI decides. AI hallucination and bias should be detected and debugged. Massive workforce displacement may exist before policy on places (e.g., AI taxes or universal basic income).

11.4 Rethinking Higher Education in the Age of AI

Challenges: The Higher Education Crisis[1]

Higher education's focus has shifted from intellectual inquiry to workforce preparation in the past two decades. Ironically, the very jobs targeted by this "job-readiness" model are among those most vulnerable to automation by AI. Some jobs that typically require a college degree are also vulnerable to AI automation, especially as generative and analytical AI tools improve. These include roles such as bookkeeper or claims processor. This will be a new crisis for most institutions, which remain unprepared for AI's profound impact on knowledge, learning, and work.

Opportunities: Reclaiming Higher Education's Purpose

The future will belong to those who can ask better questions, reason both with and against AI, and exercise judgment, ethics, and imagination in increasingly complex human–AI systems. This demands a bold rethinking of higher education's

[1] With over two decades of teaching at a public university in the United States, I have witnessed a significant increase in college tuition costs and a shift toward higher education models focused on career preparation and job readiness.

core mission. Universities must rediscover their original purpose: not to train task performers, but to cultivate thinkers, creators, and citizens. Higher education should help students thrive in ambiguity, not just follow instructions. AI challenges us to re-center education on what makes us most human: curiosity, reflection, imagination, and connection.

Higher education needs to find its new directions, such as "AI-informed liberal education" and "AI-integrated scientific education" (see Chap. 10). This presents an opportunity for reform in higher education. AI provides the urgency for this. Universities that embrace this moment will not only renew their educational mission but also cultivate the next generation of thinkers, builders, and bridge-makers who can lead human-centered AI applications across disciplines. Through this book, we've explored innovations such as PMCO-AI (Personalized Motivation, Capability, Opportunity-AI), PAPO (Policy-Aware Personalized Opportunity), ATPM (AI Thinking Partner Model), and meta-AI homework projects as examples of how AI can support personalized, reflective, and adaptive learning. AI can become a collaborator that amplifies human insight to prevent diseases, live longer, and live better.

11.5 Predictions About AI Cultures in Public Health

AI is evolving too quickly to be certain. It's highly risky to predict the future of AI cultures in public health. I offer a way to think about the future as follows.

- **Open-source AI health commons**: Major public health organizations (e.g., WHO, CDC, NGOs (Non-Governmental Organizations)) will host open AI models trained on global but anonymized health data.
- **Prompt literacy for public health workers**: Public health workers and students will learn *prompt literacy (dialogue and play)* alongside epidemiology.
- **Equity and governance frameworks**: Every health AI project will come with equity audits, bias reports, and community oversight boards, just like IRB (Institutional Review Board) for human studies.
- **Global–local AI health mosaic**: AI health tools will blend knowledge from multiple cultural contexts. Acceptance will rise when people see their cultural identity reflected in AI health tools.
- **Grassroots AI communities**: Small AI communities will form around specific health issues, such as diabetes patient groups, climate-health activists, and local NGOs.

Public health professionals, policymakers, and communities all have a role in shaping the culture of AI in public health. These futures are your choices today. Ethical access to AI in public health (e.g., sharing satellite data or disease prediction AI models) is an opportunity for humans to review our lives on earth again and reform our workflow in public health (not repeat previous situations). At the end of this textbook, let's revisit our definition of public health: "*prevent disease, live longer, and live better* ***through organized efforts of societies***."

11.6 Discussion Questions

Question 11.1. What are the most urgent challenges facing AI in public health today, and how do they differ from long-term challenges?

Question 11.2. How can public health informatics, as a data-rich field, be leveraged responsibly to maximize the benefits of AI?

Question 11.3. What is the "Matthew Effect" in the context of AI, and how might it worsen or improve health equity?

Question 11.4. In what ways can AI support health literacy and ensure equal access to health knowledge for diverse populations?

Question 11.5. What principles should guide ethical access to AI in public health, primarily when resources are unevenly distributed?

Question 11.6. How might higher education reform prepare future public health professionals to address both the anxieties and opportunities of AI adoption?

References

Codlin, A. J., Dao, T. P., Vo, L. N. Q., Forse, R. J., Vinh, T. V., Dang, H., Nguyen, L. H., Hoa, N. B., Nhung, N. V., Annerstedt, K. S., Squire, B., Lonnroth, K., & Caws, M. (2021). Independent Evaluation of 12 Artificial Intelligence Solutions for the Detection of Tuberculosis. *Scientific Reports, 11*(1). https://doi.org/10.1038/s41598-021-03265-0

Merton, R. K. (1968). The Matthew Effect in Science: The Reward and Communication Systems of Science are Considered. *Science, 159*(3810), 56–63. https://doi.org/10.1126/science.159.3810.56

Qin, Z. Z., Ahmed, S., Sarker, M. S., Paul, K. K., Adel, A. S. S., Naheyan, T., Barrett, R., Banu, S., & Creswell, J. (2021). Tuberculosis Detection From Chest X-Rays for Triaging in a High Tuberculosis-Burden Setting: An Evaluation of Five Artificial Intelligence Algorithms. *The Lancet Digital Health, 3*(9), e543–e554. https://doi.org/10.1016/s2589-7500(21)00116-3

Sendak, M. P., Ratliff, W., Sarro, D., Alderton, E., Futoma, J., Gao, M., Nichols, M., Revoir, M., Yashar, F., Miller, C., Kester, K., Sandhu, S., Corey, K., Brajer, N., Tan, C., Lin, A., Brown, T., Engelbosch, S., Anstrom, K., … O'Brien, C. (2020). Real-World Integration of a Sepsis Deep Learning Technology Into Routine Clinical Care: Implementation Study. *JMIR Medical Informatics, 8*(7), e15182. https://doi.org/10.2196/15182

Shah, A. B., Oyegun, E., Hampton, W. B., Neri, A., Maddox, N., Raso, D., Sandhu, P., Patel, A., Koonin, L. M., Lee, L., Roper, L., Whitfield, G., Siegel, D. A., & Koumans, E. H. (2023). Engagement with the Centers for Disease Control and Prevention Coronavirus Self-Checker and Guidance Provided to Users in the United States from March 23, 2020, to April 19, 2021: Thematic and Trend Analysis. *Journal of Medical Internet Research, 25*, Article e39054. https://doi.org/10.2196/39054

Appendix A
A Meta-AI Homework Sample

Meta-AI Homework: Air Pollution

> **Case scenario**: *Most students in a class think that air pollution is their city's most significant public health issue. Please use generative AI (e.g., ChatGPT) as* ***a thinking partner****to explore the issue.*

Possible Learning Objectives (Treating AI as a Thinking Partner):

- What is AQI?
- Identify major sources of air pollution in your town.
- Explain health effect of air pollution in your town.
- Describe regulatory rules on air pollution.
- Interpret AQI data.
- Analyze intervention.
- Define how generative AI (e.g., ChatGPT) works and its limitations on air pollution issues.
- Identify common AI biases/hallucinations in environmental health data (e.g., outdated statistics, fabricated sources).

Tasks

1. Read "Case scenario" and "learning objectives" above.
2. Answer guided questions below (see Table A.1) and plan AI prompts.
3. Use AI chatbots (e.g., ChatGPT): Run queries, refine prompts, and verify AI responses (e.g., cross-check facts with trusted sources).
4. Submit original and refined AI prompts, which show iterative improvement.
5. Submit a 200-word (or audio/video) reflection on your learning process.
6. Sumit AI-generated answers (screen copies or text output) (optional).

M. Wu, *Artificial Intelligence in Public Health*,
https://doi.org/10.1007/978-3-032-15872-7

Table A.1 Guided questions for metacognitive learning

Stages	Guided questions
Pre-task self-assessment (planning stage)	What do I already know about air pollution in my city? What specific aspects of air pollution do I want to investigate? (Defining focus areas, e.g., sources, health effects, policies) How can I use AI to identify reliable databases (e.g., EPA AirData, WHO repositories) or detect biased sources?
In-task guided questioning (monitoring stage)	Am I staying focused on my research questions, or am I getting off track? Can AI suggest alternative keywords or research gaps? Should I adjust my approach if I'm not finding enough information? Am I finding reliable sources? How do I verify their credibility? Is this AI output credible? How do I verify them? How does this compare to WHO/CDC data? How can I use AI tools to cross-check claims or detect misinformation? Could AI summarizers help filter irrelevant information? Do I understand the data I've collected, or do I need to clarify certain terms/concepts?
Post-task reflection (evaluating stage)	When should I not use AI? Was AI more useful for data collection, analysis, or communication? Did AI tools help or hinder my understanding? How? Did AI expose any biases in my initial assumptions? What were the most important findings about air pollution in my city? How has my understanding of air pollution changed after this exploration? What strategies worked well, and what would I do differently next time?

Appendix B
A Meta-AI Homework Development Framework

Educators design meta-AI homework for students interacting with AI (e.g., ChatGPT). In short, Step 1 in the framework (see Table B.1) is to broadly list what educators want (public health and AI literacy learning objectives). Students need to figure out "*what to do*" while AI is working on "*how to do it.*" AI prefers students to be specific. Following Step 2 in the framework, educators design meta-AI homework assignments, which help students tell AI "*what to do specifically.*" The instructors can follow the framework below to develop a meta-AI homework.

Case Scenario:*In a public health class, a teacher asks students, "What is the most significant public health issue in our city?" Students may identify some issues about which they care most. These could be cardiovascular diseases (CVD), mental health disorders, or air pollution. The teacher chose the air pollution issue and plans to design a meta-AI homework assignment for students to explore air pollution issues in their city.*

M. Wu, *Artificial Intelligence in Public Health*,
https://doi.org/10.1007/978-3-032-15872-7

Table B.1 Meta-AI homework development framework

Metacognition theory	Descriptions (Principle, actions, and examples)
Step 1: Align with learning objectives (Flavell, 1979)	**Principle**: Require clear goals
	Action: Define a specific skill/knowledge goal for the homework (public health and AI literacy objectives)
	Examples: Choose public health objectives: Foundational knowledge (e.g., define key terms, identify major sources, explain health effect, describe regulatory roles) Analytical and applied skills (e.g., interpret AQI data, analyze interventions) Critical thinking (e.g., evaluate equity implications, critique policies) Civic engagement (e.g., engage stakeholders, advocate for solutions)
	Examples: Choose AI literacy objectives: Define how generative AI (e.g., ChatGPT) works and its limitations in public health contexts Identify common AI biases/hallucinations in environmental health data (e.g., outdated statistics, fabricated sources) Describe ethical guidelines for using AI in academic work (e.g., avoiding plagiarism, disclosing AI use) Construct effective prompts to retrieve localized air pollution data (e.g., "Compare AQI trends in [City] vs. national averages 2015–2024") Evaluate AI-generated summaries of air pollution studies using criteria like source citations and recency Analyze discrepancies between AI outputs and peer-reviewed literature (e.g., conflicting health risk estimates) Etc.
Step 2: Design guided questions (Schraw et al., 1994)	**Principle**: Enhances reflection using scaffolded self-questioning
	Action: Create tiered questions that prompt awareness of prior knowledge, monitoring understanding, and evaluating strategies

(continued)

Table B.1 (continued)

Metacognition theory	Descriptions (Principle, actions, and examples)
	Examples: Public health oriented guided questions: **Awareness of prior knowledge** What do I already know about air pollution in my city? What specific aspects of air pollution do I want to investigate? (Defining focus areas, e.g., sources, health effects, policies) What resources (websites, experts, data sources) will I need? (Planning research strategies) How will I organize my findings? (Deciding on notetaking or data-collection methods) **Monitoring understanding** Am I finding reliable sources? How do I verify their credibility? (Monitoring source quality) Am I staying focused on my research questions, or am I getting off track? (Self-regulating focus) Do I understand the data I've collected, or do I need to clarify certain terms/ concepts? (Checking comprehension) Should I adjust my approach if I'm not finding enough information? (Adapting strategies) **Evaluating strategies** What were the most important findings about air pollution in my city? (Summarizing key takeaways) What strategies worked well, and what would I do differently next time? (Assessing research methods) How has my understanding of air pollution changed after this exploration? (Evaluating knowledge growth) What further questions or actions could I take based on what I learned? (Extending learning beyond the task)

(continued)

Table B.1 (continued)

Metacognition theory	Descriptions (Principle, actions, and examples)
	Examples: AI literacy oriented guided questions **Awareness of prior knowledge** How can AI streamline my workflow? Could AI tools help summarize baseline knowledge? How can I use AI to identify reliable databases (e.g., EPA AirData, WHO repositories) or detect biased sources? Could AI tools assist with notetaking?" **Monitoring understanding** Is this AI output credible? How can I use AI tools to cross-check claims or detect misinformation? Could AI summarizers help filter irrelevant information? Should I use AI visualization tools to interpret complex air quality datasets? Can AI suggest alternative keywords or research gaps? **Evaluating strategies** When should I not use AI? Did AI tools help or hinder my understanding? How? Was AI more useful for data collection, analysis, or communication? Did AI expose any biases in my initial assumptions?
Step 3: Embed reflective prompts (Tanner, 2012)	**Principle**: Improves on explicit reflection
	Action: Add a "Process Summary" section (request students to submit short written responses or audio/video reflections)
	Examples: Describe one way your thinking changed during this assignment What step was most challenging? Why?
Step 4: Provide structured feedback (Cox, 2005)	**Principle**: Feedback should target thinking processes
	Action: Grade prompts and reflections using a rubric with criteria
	Examples: (See a sample of rubric criteria in Appendix C)
Step 5: Connect to real-world application (Schraw et al., 1994; Tanner, 2012)	**Principle**: Reinforced through relevance
	Action: End with an applied task

(continued)

Table B.1 (continued)

Metacognition theory	Descriptions (Principle, actions, and examples)
	Exams: Draft a commentary to local newspapers about air pollution in your city and apply your new knowledge to comment on current situations How might AI support advocacy on air pollution in your city (e.g., drafting policy briefs)?

References

Cox, M. T. (2005). Metacognition in Computation: A Selected Research Review. *Artificial Intelligence, 169*(2), 104–141. http://dx.doi.org/10.1016/j.artint.2005.10.009

Flavell, J. H. (1979). Metacognition and Cognitive Monitoring: A New Area of Cognitive-Developmental Inquiry. *American Psychologist, 34*(10), 906–911. http://dx.doi.org/10.1037//0003-066x.34.10.906

Schraw, G., & Dennison, R. S. (1994). Assessing Metacognitive Awareness. *Contemporary Educational Psychology, 19*(4), 460–475. https://doi.org/10.1006/ceps.1994.1033

Tanner, K. D. (2012). Promoting Student Metacognition. *CBE—Life Sciences Education, 11*(2), 113–120. https://www.lifescied.org/doi/10.1187/cbe.12-03-0033

Appendix C
A Grading Rubric for Meta-AI Homework[1]

Educators can use a sample rubric (see Table C.1) for grading meta-AI homework.

Table C.1 A sample of rubric for grading meta-AI homework for beginners

Criteria	5 (Excellent)	3 (Developing)	1 (Needs Work)
Clarity (40%) (Tanner, 2012)	Prompts are specific, unambiguous, and structured; Well-structured, error-free in reflection	Prompts are clear but occasionally vague or overly broad; Some organization issues in reflection	Prompts are unclear; Disjointed or incomplete in reflection
Critical Thinking (25%) (Cox, 2005; Flavell, 1979)	Identifies AI biases/ gaps, flags omissions; suggests fixes	Lists limitations without analysis	Accepts AI answers uncritically
Reflection Depth (20%) (Schraw et al., 1994; Tanner, 2012)	Detailed, connects to prior learning, link AI use to broader public health ethics	Basic ("AI helped"), surface-level analysis	Minimal or off-topic
Verification (15%)	Uses two or more authoritative sources to validate	Uses one source superficially	No fact-checking

[1] Public health educators can design, and revise evaluation metrics based on students' proficiency level (e.g., beginner vs. advanced) and the learning stage (e.g., initial exposure vs. mastery). The sample of the grading rubric (see Table C.1) is designed for beginners doing meta-AI homework. Clarity should have a higher weight early on for beginners to build foundational skills (e.g., prompt precision). It is a high priority to prevent garbage-in-garbage-out. For advanced users, critical thinking will have more weight.

M. Wu, *Artificial Intelligence in Public Health*,
https://doi.org/10.1007/978-3-032-15872-7

References

Cox, M. T. (2005). Metacognition in Computation: A Selected Research Review. *Artificial Intelligence, 169*(2), 104–141. http://dx.doi.org/10.1016/j.artint.2005.10.009

Flavell, J. H. (1979). Metacognition and Cognitive Monitoring: A New Area of Cognitive-Developmental Inquiry. *American Psychologist, 34*(10), 906–911. http://dx.doi.org/10.1037//0003-066x.34.10.906

Schraw, G., & Dennison, R. S. (1994). Assessing Metacognitive Awareness. *Contemporary Educational Psychology, 19*(4), 460–475. https://doi.org/10.1006/ceps.1994.1033

Tanner, K. D. (2012). Promoting Student Metacognition. *CBE—Life Sciences Education, 11*(2), 113–120. https://www.lifescied.org/doi/10.1187/cbe.12-03-0033

Appendix D
A List of Case Scenarios for the Evaluation Study Design

AI promises significant gains in public health, but without proper evaluation, we risk bias, harm, wasted resources, or loss of trust. Public health agencies, funders, and journals now demand impact, equity, and real-world effectiveness evidence. You can design your evaluation projects for grant proposals or journal papers based on evaluation methods in Case scenarios 4A, 4B, 4C, and 4D in Chap. 4.

- Case scenarios 4A: Evaluation study design about the accuracy of AI chatbots for health information about cataract surgery
- Case scenarios 4B: Evaluation study design about the accuracy of AI doctors by comparing with medical students
- Case scenarios 4C: Evaluation study design about the accountability of self-driving cars
- Case scenarios 4D: Evaluation study design about the user experience of AI mental health support

M. Wu, *Artificial Intelligence in Public Health*,
https://doi.org/10.1007/978-3-032-15872-7

Appendix E
A List of Case Scenarios for AI Application Design

AI in public health is a wide-open field, with plenty of space for newcomers, whether you're a student, researcher, or a startup. It's an excellent time to join, participate, or prototype AI applications for public health. Before you can run, you need to walk through case scenarios in Chaps. 7 and 8 and learn how to select AI techniques for various public health tasks. Each design includes AI model selections with input and output information for each step.

- Case scenarios 7a: Design for respiratory diseases monitoring
- Case scenarios 7b: AMR-related epidemiological investigations
- Case scenarios 7c: AMR-related infection forecasting
- Case scenarios 7d: EquiRisk on diabetes within food deserts
- Case scenarios 8a: Personalized health risk management
- Case scenarios 8b: Personalized health education
- Case scenarios 8c: Medication adherence support
- Case scenarios 8d: PAPO-heatwave AI

M. Wu, *Artificial Intelligence in Public Health*,
https://doi.org/10.1007/978-3-032-15872-7

Index

M. Wu, *Artificial Intelligence in Public Health*,
https://doi.org/10.1007/978-3-032-15872-7

S

T

U

MIX
Papier aus verantwortungsvollen Quellen
Paper from responsible sources
FSC® C105338

If you have any concerns about our products,
you can contact us on
ProductSafety@springernature.com

In case Publisher is established outside the EU,
the EU authorized representative is:
Springer Nature Customer Service Center GmbH
Europaplatz 3, 69115 Heidelberg, Germany

Printed by Libri Plureos GmbH
in Hamburg, Germany